Use R!

This series of inexpensive and focused books on R is aimed at practitioners. Books can discuss the use of R in a particular subject area (e.g., epidemiology, econometrics, psychometrics) or as it relates to statistical topics (e.g., missing data, longitudinal data). In most cases, books combine LaTeX and R so that the code for figures and tables can be put on a website. Authors should assume a background as supplied by Dalgaard's Introductory Statistics with R or other introductory books so that each book does not repeat basic material.

How to Submit Your Proposal

Book proposals and manuscripts should be submitted to one of the publishing editors in your region per email - for the list of statistics editors by their location please see https://www.springer.com/gp/statistics/contact-us. All submissions should include a completed Book Proposal Form.

For general and technical questions regarding the series and the submission process please contact Faith Su (faith.su@springer.com) or Veronika Rosteck (veronika.rosteck@springer.com).

Ottar N. Bjørnstad

Epidemics

Models and Data Using R

Second Edition

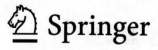

Ottar N. Bjørnstad
Center for Infectious Disease Dynamics
Pennsylvania State University
University Park, PA, USA

ISSN 2197-5736   ISSN 2197-5744   (electronic)
Use R!
ISBN 978-3-031-12055-8   ISBN 978-3-031-12056-5   (eBook)
https://doi.org/10.1007/978-3-031-12056-5

This Springer imprint is published by the registered company Springer Nature Switzerland AG
The registered company address is: Gewerbestrasse 11, 6330 Cham, Switzerland

For Katriona, Esme, and Michael

Preface

Preface to Second Edition

As with the first edition, the second edition has further benefitted heavily from input from numerous people, particularly my various students, postdocs, and collaborators. The book club at the London School of Tropical Medicine and Hygiene provided valuable feedback on the first edition clarifying how the text should be better fleshed out and organized. Reorganizing, restructuring, and recoding meant that the current material is not fully back-compatible, so the epimdr2 R package should be used with the new edition. Typesetting of equations has been changed for clarity and shinyApps has largely been reparameterized with reproduction number, R_0, rather than transmission rate (β) since that is more intuitive. The SARS-CoV-2 pandemic spurred significant new analyses of infectious disease dynamics. Much of the new age-structured modeling in Chap. 4 were developed with Jessica Metcalf, Ruiyun Li, and Dami Pak. The catalytic model is now discussed in a separate chapter (Chap. 5). New competing strain models have been added (Sect. 3.12). The chapter on networks has been greatly expanded. Functions for automation of Jacobian matrices and next generation calculation are presented. A new chapter on invasion and persistence (Chap. 15) has new treatment of zoonoses including visits on branching processes, spatial diffusion, synchrony, and metapopulation persistence. New data sets were provided by Lance Waller and Laura Pomeroy as well as various publicly available sources. Rustom Antia has kindly helped me better understand the rudiments of adaptive immunity and immune memory.

To understand the philosophy behind this text, I encourage any reader to peruse the preface to the first edition.[1] While the R ecosystem is evolving rapidly, I have deliberately striven to use generic S3 code for all calculations (except for occasional straying for animations, etc., in accompanying shinyApps) for the reason that I didactically believe that the logic of programming with data laid out by Chambers (1998) is the simplest and most elegant way. With respect to mathematical sym-

---

[1] The preface to the first edition has been updated so chapter and section labels are consistent with the new text.

bols, I have tried as best as possible to be consistent in usage (thus some changes in notation from first edition) such that, for example, β is generally used for transmission, ϕ for force of infection, ω for loss of immunity, rates are lowercase Greek, and probabilities are uppercase Greek. The text covers a lot of material though, so keeping the Greek alphabet soup sorted has been challenging.

In addition to previous funding, this text has also benefitted from support from the Norwegian Research Council. The text and associated teaching materials have been my main passion for almost a decade.

University Park, PA, USA   Ottar N. Bjørnstad
May 2022

Preface to First Edition

Despite an undergraduate degree in Zoology and a MSc on the behavior of voles, I have long been fascinated by theoretical biology and the relationship between models and data, and the feedback between statistical analysis and conceptual developments in the area of infectious disease dynamics, in particular, and ecological dynamics in general. My perpetual frustration has been to read all the wonderfully clever books and journal articles exuding all sort of nifty maths and stats, but not quite being able to *do* any of it myself when it came to infectious diseases that I care about. This frustration led me to make myself some worked examples of all this cleverness. Over the years the stack of how-to's has grown, and the following chapters are an attempt at organizing these so they may be useful to others. I have tried to organize the chapters and sections in a reasonably logical way: Chaps. 2–11 is a mix and match of models, data and statistics pertaining to local disease dynamics; Chaps. 12–15 pertains to spatial and spatiotemporal dynamics; Chap. 16 highlights similarities between the dynamics of infectious disease and parasitoid–host dynamics; Finally, Chaps. 17–18 overviews additional statistical methodology I have found useful in the study of infectious disease dynamics. Some sections are marked as "advanced" for one of two reasons: (i) either the maths or stats is a bit more involved and/or (ii) the topic in focus is a bit more esoteric. Although not marked as such, most of Chap. 11 is advanced in this respect. While less run-of-the-mill, I have thought it important to include these sections, because they cover topics that may be less easy to find code for elsewhere.

I have had invaluable help from students, colleagues and collaborators in my quest. The pre-conference workshops of "Ecology and Evolution of Infectious Disease" that I co-taught between 2005 and 2008 enhanced my motivation to annotate many worked examples; Bare-bones of several of the following sections were written during frantic 24hrs stints prior to these workshops. Much of the other material arose from interactions with students and post-docs at Pennsylvania State University's Center for Infectious Disease Dynamics (CIDD). Parts of the epidemics on networks and the R_0 removal estimator is from Matt Ferrari's PhD research, the age-structured SIR simulator and the SIRWS model is from Jennie Lavine's PhD work. Working with distributed-delay models has been a collaboration with Bill Nelson and my students Lindsay Beck-Johnson and Megan Greischar. Angie Luis and I cooked up the code to do transfer functions in R as part of her PhD research. Much of the code on the catalytic model is from collaborations with Laura Pomeroy and then-CIDD postdoctoral fellows Grainne Long and Jess Metcalf. The in-host TSIR was also a collaboration with Jess. The Gillespie code arose from collaborations with postdoctoral fellow Shouli Li and my honor student Reilly Mummah. Reilly also taught me how to write my first shinyApp. Away from Penn State, Aaron King and Ben Bolker have at various times been unbelievably patient in teaching me bits of maths I didn't understand. Roger Nisbet painstakingly guided me through my first transfer functions during my postdoctoral fellowship at NCEAS. During the same period Jordi Bascompte introduced me to coupled-map lattice models. Finally,

Bryan Grenfell showed me wavelets and introduced me to the field of infectious disease dynamics some 20 years ago.

The data used has been kindly shared by Janis Antonovics, Jeremy Burdon, Rebecca Grais, Sylvije Huygen, Jenn Keslow, Sandy Leibhold, Grainne Long and Mary Poss. The first draft of the text was completed while I was on sabbatical at the University of Western Australia and University of Oslo/the Norwegian Veterinary Institute during 2017. My work leading up to this text has variously been funded by the National Science Foundation, the National Institute of Health, the US Department of Agriculture and the Bill and Melinda Gates Foundation.

Contents

Chapter 1
Introduction

1.1 Preamble

The use of mathematical models to understand infectious disease dynamics has a very rich history in epidemiology. Kermack and McKendrick (1927) is the seminal paper that introduced the equations for the general Susceptible–Infected–Removed model and showed how a set of restrictive assumptions lead to the standard SIR model of ordinary differential equations. During the 1950s and early 1960s, stochastic theories of disease dynamics were developed by Bailey (1957) and Bartlett (1960a). Bartlett (1956, 1960b) further pioneered the use of Monte Carlo simulations of epidemics with the aid of *electronic computers* (as opposed to regular human computers), while Muench (1959) proposed the catalytic framework for understanding age-incidence patterns.[1] The decades to follow saw broad expansions of theories as well as a surge in real-life application of mathematics to dynamics and control of infectious disease.

There are several excellent textbooks of mathematical epidemiology including Anderson and May (1991) and Keeling and Rohani (2008). The purpose of the current text is not to replicate these efforts but rather use these frameworks as a starting point to discuss practical implementation and analysis. The discussion will be centered around a somewhat haphazard collection of case studies selected to explore various conceptual, mathematical, and statistical issues. The text is designed to be more of a practicum in infectious disease dynamics.

The dynamics of infectious diseases shows a wide diversity of pattern. Some have locally persistent chains of transmission others persist spatially in consumer–resource metapopulations. Some infections are prevalent among the young, some among the old, and some are age-invariant. Temporally, some diseases have little variation in prevalence, some have predictable seasonal shifts, and others exhibit vi-

---

I recommend that readers peruse the preface to the first edition to get a sense of the intended purpose of this monograph.

[1] Though, as reviewed by Dietz and Heesterbeek (2002), the original calculations leading to the catalytic model were proposed by Daniel Bernoulli in the late eighteenth century.

O. N. Bjørnstad, *Epidemics*, Use R!, https://doi.org/10.1007/978-3-031-12056-5_1

olent epidemics that may be regular or irregular in their timing. Models and models with data have proved invaluable for understanding and predicting this diversity and thence help improve intervention and control. The following chapters are an attempt at providing some notes for a field guide for working with data, models, and models and data to understand epidemics and infectious disease dynamics in space and time.

1.2 In-Host Persistence

Infectious diseases can be classified according to their persistence within the host and attack rates with respect to age. Some infections result in life-long colonization of a host because the immune system does not clear them. Such in-host persistence may be because the immune system permits it—as for the many symbionts that are beneficial to the host (viz. commmensals and mutualists)—or because detrimental symbionts (viz. pathogens) are able to evade clearance. Examples of "in-host persistent" pathogens are retroviruses such as HIV, latent viruses such as herpes viruses, and a number of bacteria such as the causative agents of tuberculosis (*Mycobacterium tuberculosis*) and leprosy (*M. leprae*). There are also a large number of other chronic viruses (Virgin et al., 2009).

Acute infections, in contrast, result in transient colonization of the host—which in humans can last for days or months depending on the pathogen—followed by clearance. The clearance is usually immune-mediated, though some viruses like measles or canine distemper virus may run out of target cells to infect (Morris et al., 2018) and some pathogens may have a programmed life cycle within the host. Some coccidian pathogens within the genus *Eimeria*, for example, go through an exact number of replication cycles in the host (as merozoites) before all pathogen cells are expelled into the environment as oocysts (Smith et al., 2002b). The more common example of transience is due to immune-mediated clearance. Examples are plentiful and include acute viruses like measles and influenza, bacteria such as many that causes respiratory disease like bacterial meningitis (e.g., *Neisseria meningitidis*) or whooping cough (*Bordetella pertussis* and *B. parapertussis*), and protozoans such as those that cause malaria (*Plasmodium* spp.).

Among the acute infections, we distinguish between those that leave sterilizing immunity following clearance versus those that leave no or short-lived immunity. This can happen via a number of mechanisms including variable gene expression, rapid evolution, co-circulating strain clouds, or other immune evasive maneuvers. *Neisseria meningitidis* and its congener *N. gonorrhoeae* (which cause gonorrhea), for example, are thought to leave little effective immune memory because of the bacteria's ability to express a very variable arsenal of surface proteins (e.g., Stern et al., 1984; Tettelin et al., 2000). *Plasmodium falciparum* is comprised of a diverse set of strains with non-overlapping "antigenic repertoires" (as well as variable antigen expression) that allows repeat reinfection (e.g., Gupta et al., 1998). A number of common viral afflictions of children have a somewhat more limited strain diversity that may allow several reinfection cycles, but the immune system is ultimately able to cover their entire antigenic space. Examples include rotavirus (Pitzer et al., 2011) and the enterovirus complex that cause hand, foot, and mouth disease (Takahashi et al., 2016). Many influenza subtypes render effective immune memory short-lived because of rapid evolution; high mutation rates lead to antigenic drift and viral recombination during coinfection leads to antigenic shifts (Koelle et al., 2006). Moreover, many respiratory infections target the so-called permissive areas of the nasopharyngeal and upper respiratory tract. Endemic α- and β-coronavirus infections, for instance, result in production of protective antibodies and T-cell memory but reinfections are common because immune delivery is down-regulated in these areas (Lavine et al., 2021). Finally, many pathogens have various anti-immune devices. Respiratory syncytial virus, for example, uses molecular decoys against neutralizing antibodies (Bukreyev et al., 2008) and *Bordetella pertussis* employs the pertussis toxin to, at least transiently, inhibit recruitment of immune effector cells to sites of infection (Kirimanjeswara et al., 2005).

Many of the remaining acute, immunizing pathogens—the ones that result in a transient infection followed by life-long sterilizing immunity—are the poster children of mathematical epidemiology. Notable examples are among the classic vaccine-preventable viruses like measles, rubella, and smallpox. From a biological point of view, the complete failure of immune escape of these pathogens is somewhat mysterious (Kennedy & Read, 2017), but the resulting simple dynamical clockwork is a joy to anyone hoping to apply mathematics to understand the living world.

From an epidemiological point of view, it is important to make a functional, as opposed to taxonomical, classification of pathogens because it allows us to understand the differences in age-specific attack rates and contrasting disease dynamics. The acute, immunizing infections mainly circulate among the young and therefore comprise the many childhood infections because most or all older hosts are immune. From the point of view of the compartmental SIR-like formalism, it is natural to divide the host population in **S**usceptible, **I**nfected, and **R**emoved compartments and assume a unidirectional flow from susceptible children through immune ("removed") adults. In contrast, the prevalence of in-host persistent infections, such as the many chronic viruses (Virgin et al., 2009) and untreated life-long bacterial infections that cause tuberculosis and leprosy, will generally tend to accumulate with age. With respect to the SIR formalism, it is thus natural to consider a model with a unidirectional flow from the S compartment to a terminal I compartment. The acute but imperfectly immunizing infections may lead to relatively age-invariant attack rates with looped $S \to I \to S$ or $S \to I \to R \to S$ flows depending on the duration of immune protection (Fig. 1.1).

SIR-like frameworks predict the broad expectation for how age-prevalence curves will be modulated by factors such as age-specific pattern of mixing and differential mortality between infected and non-infected individuals (Chap. 4). Statistical epidemiology can subsequently be used to probe empirical patterns to discover subtleties in the dynamics of disease transmission that is hard to observe directly (Chap. 5).

1.3 Patterns of Endemicity

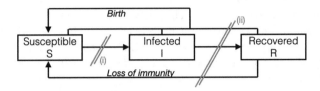

Fig. 1.1: The SIR(S) compartmental flow and the two bottlenecks for local persistence: (i) the transmission bottleneck for poorly transmitted infections and (ii) the susceptible bottleneck for highly transmissible, acute immunizing (or lethal) pathogens

We classify the dynamics of infectious disease according to broad patterns of endemicity. First, there is the distinction between locally persistent and locally non-persistence pathogens. Local persistence fails when a local chain of transmission breaks. This can happen for two very different reasons (Fig. 1.1): (i) the transmission bottleneck is when a pathogen is insufficiently transmissible to sustain a chain of transmission and (ii) at the opposite end of the spectrum is the susceptible bottleneck for acute pathogens that are so transmissible that they burn through susceptibles much faster than they are replenished. In measles, for example, prevaccination cities in the USA smaller than a critical community size (CCS) of 250k–500k did not produce enough susceptible children to sustain a local chain of transmission (Bartlett, 1960b) (Fig. 1.2). Recurrence of such pathogens typically involves spatial dynamics and persistence at the metapopulation scale through spread among asynchronous local host communities (Keeling et al., 2004) or core-satellite dynamics in which a few large cities above the CCS serve as persistent sources for spatial dissemination to communities below the CCS (Grenfell & Harwood, 1997; Grenfell et al., 2001). The 1988 and 2002 epidemics of a related morbillivirus, the phocine distemper virus (PDV) in European harbor seals, are other illustrations of locally non-persistent infections due to high transmission relative to susceptible recruitment rates (e.g., Swinton, 1998). Following introduction into each local population ("haul-out"), explosive local epidemics terminated after 1–4 months due to susceptible depletion. When such epidemics happens so fast that recruitment of susceptibles (through birth, immigration, or loss of immunity) is negligible during the course of the outbreak it is termed a closed epidemics. The closed epidemic is the focus of the standard Susceptible–Infected–Recovered model which is introduced in the first part of Chap. 2. We will discuss PDV spillover and invasion in more detail in Sect. 15.3. At the opposite end of the transmissibility spectrum, pathogens may bottleneck because transmission is too ineffective. In particular, if the reproduction number (R_0, the expected number of secondary cases from a primary case in a

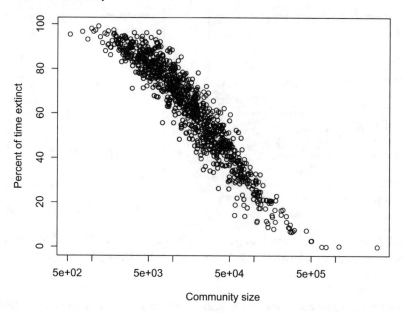

Fig. 1.2: Persistence of measles against population size for 954 cities and villages in prevaccination England and Wales (1944–1964). Communities below 500k exhibited occasional or frequent (depending on size) local extinction of the virus

completely susceptible population) is smaller than one, we see stuttering subcritical chains of transmission followed by pathogen fadeout. This is the case for many zoonoses such as monkey pox and Nipah (stage 3 zoonoses in the classification by Lloyd-Smith et al., 2009, Sect. 15.1). Persistent recurrence of these infections typically involves reservoir hosts and intermittent zoonotic reintroduction. For example, in their study of Lassa fever in Sierra Leone, Iacono et al. (2015) concluded that about 20% of the human cases were caused by human-to-human transmission (with an average reproduction number below one), while the remaining majority was caused by transmission from the multimammate rat (*Mastomys natalensis*) reservoir.

Locally persistent infections are commonly classified as (i) stable endemics that show little variation in incidence through time. Many STDs with SI- and SIS-like dynamics like gonorrhea (Fig. 1.3a) and HIV exhibit this pattern. (ii) Seasonal endemics that show low'ish-level predictable seasonal variation around some mean. Many endemic vector-borne and water-borne infections exhibit this pattern. A classic example is the seasonal two-peaked mortality rate from Cholera in the province of Dacca, East Bengal (King et al., 2008); the first peaks at the beginning of the monsoon season and the second toward the end (Fig. 1.3b) due to how water flow affects bacterial presence. Finally, (iii) recurrent epidemics that may be regular or irregular are characterized by violent epidemic fluctuations over time. Many acute,

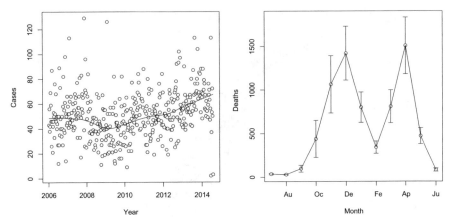

Fig. 1.3: **(a)** Weekly incidence of gonorrhea in Massachusetts (2006–2015) and **(b)** monthly average ($\pm$ SE) mortality from cholera in the Dacca district (1891–1940)

immunizing highly contagious pathogens—measles being the poster child—follow this pattern (Fig. 1.4), the determinants of which will be discussed in Chaps. 6 and 8.

1.4 R

To provide a cohesive framework for the practical calculations, all analyses are done in the open-source R language. All functions, data, and shinyApp's discussed in the text are contained in the epimdr2 package and all the code used is available in text format on the epimdr2 GitHub site https://github.com/objornstad/epimdr2. With the package and the code, everything contained herein should be fully reproducible. Figures 1.2 and 1.4 were for example generated using the following code:

```r
require(epimdr2)
#Fig 1.2
data(ccs)
plot(ccs$size, ccs$ext*100, log = "x", xlab =
    "Community size", ylab = "Percent
    of time extinct")

#Fig 1.3a
plot(magono$time, magono$number, ylab = "Cases",
    xlab = "Year")
lines(lowess(x = magono$time, y = magono$number, f = 0.4))

#Fig 1.3b
data(cholera)
ses = sesd = sesdv = rep(NA, 12)
ses[c(7:12, 1:6)] = sapply(split(cholera$Dacca,
```

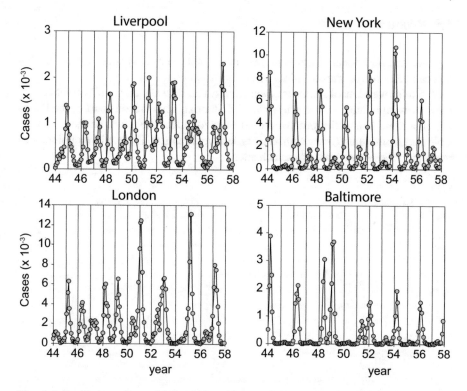

Fig. 1.4: Incidence of measles in various US and UK cities during the prevaccination era. The data represent fortnightly incidence (roughly corresponding to the virus' serial interval). The vertical bars mark annual intervals

```
    cholera$Month), mean, na.rm = TRUE)
sesd[c(7:12, 1:6)] = sapply(split(cholera$Dacca,
    cholera$Month), sd, na.rm = TRUE)
sesdv[c(7:12, 1:6)] = sesd/sqrt(length(split(cholera$Dacca,
    cholera$Month)))
require(plotrix)
plotCI(x = 1:12, y = ses, ui = ses + sesdv, li = ses -
    sesdv, xlab = "Month", ylab = "Deaths")
lines(x = 1:12, y = ses)
```

1.5 Resources

Updates and additional multimedia resources (including all R code) related to this text can be found on https://github.com/objornstad/epimdr2.

A 5 min overview of *Patterns of endemicity* can be watched from YouTube: https://www.youtube.com/watch?v=Mf_EZm5amxI. This video is part of the Pennsylvania State University produced epidemics MOOC. The entire course is accessible free from https://www.coursera.org/learn/epidemics. There will be pointers to relevant videos at the start of each chapter.

Part I
Time

Chapter 2
SIR

2.1 Introduction

The following 10 chapters are devoted to the study of patterns of infection over time and age. The current chapter introduces the basics of compartmental modeling of transmission dynamics. This is followed by a chapter with in-depth discussion of the reproduction number, R_0, which is the most important quantity for understanding epidemics of infectious agents. The subsequent chapters detail the importance of age structure and seasonality in shaping epidemics and pandemics as well as several important time series methods for characterizing and understanding temporal recurrence patterns of infection. The last two chapters explore how ideas from dynamical systems theory can help explain several very curious aspects of the waxing and waning of infection through time.

2.2 The SIR Model

In 1927, Kermack and McKendrick (1927) published a set of general equations (Breda et al., 2012) to better understand the dynamics of an infectious disease spreading through a susceptible population. Their motivation was

> One of the most striking features in the study of epidemics is the difficulty of finding a causal factor which appears to be adequate to account for the magnitude of the frequent epidemics of disease which visit almost every population [...] The problem may be summarized as follows: One (or more) infected person is introduced into a community of individuals, more

This chapter uses the following R packages: deSolve, phaseR, and shiny.
A conceptual understanding of *reproduction numbers* and the *simple epidemic* is useful. Five minute epidemics MOOC introductions are:
Reproduction number https://www.youtube.com/watch?v=ju26rvzfFg4.
Closed epidemic https://www.youtube.com/watch?v=sSLfrSSmJZM.
The sir.app shinyApp provides an interactive interface as part of the epimdr2 package.

O. N. Bjørnstad, *Epidemics*, Use R!, https://doi.org/10.1007/978-3-031-12056-5_2

or less susceptible to the disease in question. The disease spreads from the affected to the unaffected by contact infection. Each infected person runs through the course of his sickness, and finally is removed from the number of those who are sick, by recovery or by death. The chances of recovery or death vary from day to day during the course of his illness. The chances that the affected may convey infection to the unaffected are likewise dependent upon the stage of the sickness. As the epidemic spreads, the number of unaffected members of the community becomes reduced [...] In the course of time the epidemic may come to an end. One of the most important problems in epidemiology is to ascertain whether this termination occurs only when no susceptible individuals are left, or whether the interplay of the various factors of infectivity, recovery and mortality, may result in termination, whilst many susceptible individuals are still present in the unaffected population.

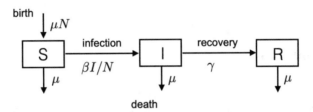

Fig. 2.1: The SIR flow diagram of transitions among Susceptibles (S), Infected and Infectious (I), and Recovered/Removed (R) compartments. Rates are per capita rates among compartments

Following a general mathematical exposé, they suggested a set of pragmatic assumptions that lead to the standard SIR model of ordinary differential equations (ODEs) for the flow of hosts between Susceptible, Infectious, and Recovered compartments. In modern notation, the simplest set of equations is (Fig. 2.1)

$$\frac{dS}{dt} = \underbrace{\mu N}_{\text{birth}} - \underbrace{\beta I \frac{S}{N}}_{\text{infection}} - \underbrace{\mu S}_{\text{death}} \tag{2.1}$$

$$\frac{dI}{dt} = \underbrace{\beta I \frac{S}{N}}_{\text{infection}} - \underbrace{\gamma I}_{\text{recovery}} - \underbrace{\mu I}_{\text{death}} \tag{2.2}$$

$$\frac{dR}{dt} = \underbrace{\gamma I}_{\text{recovery}} - \underbrace{\mu R}_{\text{death}} \tag{2.3}$$

The assumptions of Eqs. (2.1)–(2.3) are:

- The infection circulates in a population of size N, with a per capita baseline death rate, μ, which is balanced by a birth rate μN. From the sum of Eqs. (2.1)–(2.3), $dN/dt = 0$ and $N = S + I + R$ is thus constant. N is assumed to be large, so epidemics will unfold according to the predictable clockwork of the coupled deterministic differential equations. We will consider how to accommodate deviations from this assumption throughout the ensuing text, notably in Sects. 3.4, 8.2, and 9.2.

- The infection causes acute morbidity (not mortality); that is, in this version of the SIR model, we assume we can ignore disease-induced mortality. This is reasonable for certain infections like chickenpox, but certainly not for others like rabies, SARS, or Ebola (Sects. 3.7, 3.9, and 10.6 introduce models that relax on this assumption).
- Individuals are recruited directly into the susceptible class at birth (so ignore perinatal maternal immunity).
- Transmission of infection from infectious to susceptible individuals is controlled by a bilinear contact term $\beta I \frac{S}{N}$. This stems from the assumption that the I infectious individuals are independently and randomly mixing with all other individuals, so a fraction S/N of the encounters is with susceptible individuals; β is the contact rate times the probability of transmission given a contact between a susceptible and an infectious individual.
- Chances of recovery or death are assumed not to change during the course of infection.
- Infectiousness is assumed not to change during the course of infection.
- Infected individuals are assumed to move directly into the infectious class (as opposed to the SEIR model introduced in Sect. 3.7) and remain there for an average infectious period of $1/\gamma$ (assuming $\mu << \gamma$).[1]
- The model finally assumes that recovered individuals are immune from reinfection for life.[2]

The basic reproduction number (R_0), interchangeably also termed the basic reproductive ratio, is defined as the expected number of secondary infections from a single index case in a completely susceptible population. This is a pivotal quantity in the theory of infectious disease dynamics. Chapter 3 is entirely devoted to this quantity. For this particular model (Eqs. (2.1)–(2.3)), $R_0 = \frac{\beta}{\gamma + \mu}$, and thus $\beta = R_0(\gamma + \mu)$. The later relationship is useful because while β is one of the key rate parameters in the model, it is often more intuitive to think in terms of R_0 as it can be estimated from a variety of data using a variety of methods (Chap. 3).

---

[1] The implicit assumptions that stem from the use of deterministic, ordinary differential equation (ODE) are that the infectious periods (and resident times in all compartments) are exponentially distributed. This is a tractable approximation for exploring overall dynamics, but observed duration of infection periods is often much less variable—the *Eimeria*-gut parasite (a relative of the *Plasmodium* parasites that cause malaria) undergoes a fixed number of replication cycles before all parasites leave the host (Smith et al., 2002b) or much more variable. Section 2.9 discusses a practical approach to modeling disease dynamics when the exponential assumption is deemed too simplistic.

[2] Sections 10.5 and 11.4 visits on dynamics under transient immunity via the SIRS and SIRWS models.

2.3 Numerical Integration of the SIR Model

If there are no (or negligible) births and deaths during the duration of an epidemic ($\mu \simeq 0$), the dynamics are commonly referred to as a closed epidemic. While it is occasionally possible to derive analytical solutions to systems of ODEs like Eqs. (2.1)–(2.3), we generally have to resort to numerical integration to predict the numbers over time. The deSolve R package provides functions to numerically integrate such equations. Throughout this text numerical integration of a variety of different ODE models will be required. While the models differ, the basic recipe is generally the same: (1) define an R function for the general system of equations, (2) specify the time points at which we want the integrator to save the state of the system, (3) provide values for the parameters, (4) give initial values for all state variables, and finally (5) invoke the ode function.

```
require(deSolve)
```

STEP 1: Define the function (often called the gradient function) for the equation systems. The deSolve package requires the function to take the following parameters: time, t,[3] a vector with the values for the state variables (in this case S, I, and R), y, and parameter values (for β, μ, γ, and N), parameters:

```
sirmod = function(t, y, parameters) {
    # Pull state variables from y vector
    S = y[1]
    I = y[2]
    R = y[3]
    # Pull parameter values from the input vector
    beta = parameters["beta"]
    mu = parameters["mu"]
    gamma = parameters["gamma"]
    N = parameters["N"]
    # Define equations
    dS = mu * (N - S) - beta * S * I/N
    dI = beta * S * I/N - (mu + gamma) * I
    dR = gamma * I - mu * R
    res = c(dS, dI, dR)
    # Return list of gradients
    list(res)
}
```

STEPS 2–4: Specify the time points at which we want ode to record the states of the system (here we use a half year with weekly time increments as specified in the vector times), the parameter values (in this case as specified in the vector paras), and starting conditions (specified in start). If we model the fraction of individuals in each class, we set $N = 1$ (though we could do percentages with $N = 100$ or some other population size of relevance). Let us consider a disease with

---

[3] Though, in the case of the simple SIR model, there is no time dependence in any of the parameters, so this parameter is not called within the gradient function; this will change when we consider seasonality (Chap. 6).

an infectious period of 2 weeks ($\gamma = 365/14$ per year) for the closed epidemic (no births or deaths so $\mu = 0$). A reproduction number of 4 implies a transmission rate β of 2. For starting conditions, assume that 0.1% of the initial population is infected and the remaining fraction is susceptible.

```
times = seq(0, 0.5, by = 1/365)
paras = c(mu = 0, N = 1, R0 = 4, gamma = 365/14)
paras["beta"] = paras["R0"] * (paras["gamma"] + paras["mu"])
start = c(S = 0.999, I = 0.001, R = 0) * paras["N"]
```

STEP 5: Feed `start` values, `times`, the gradient function `sirmod`, and parameter vector `paras` to the `ode` function as suggested by `args(ode)`.[4] For convenience, we convert the output to a data frame (ode returns a `list`). The `head` function shows the first 5 rows of `out` and `round(,3)` rounds the number to three decimals.

```
out = ode(y = start, times = times, func = sirmod, parms = paras)
out = as.data.frame(out)
head(round(out, 3))

##     time     S     I     R
## 1  0.000 0.999 0.001 0.000
## 2  0.003 0.999 0.001 0.000
## 3  0.005 0.998 0.002 0.000
## 4  0.008 0.998 0.002 0.000
## 5  0.011 0.997 0.002 0.000
## 6  0.014 0.996 0.003 0.001
```

Figure 2.2 shows how the model predicts an initial exponential growth of the epidemic that decelerates as susceptibles are depleted and finally fade out as susceptible numbers are too low to sustain a chain of transmission.

```
plot(x = out$time, y = out$S, ylab = "Fraction", xlab = "Time",
     type = "l")
lines(x = out$time, y = out$I, col = "red")
lines(x = out$time, y = out$R, col = "green")
```

R allows for a lot of customization of graphics—Rseek.org is a useful resource to find solutions to all things R... Fig. 2.2 has some added features such as a right-hand axis for the effective reproduction number (R_E)—the expected number of new cases per infected individuals in a *not* completely susceptible population—and a legend so as to confirm that the turnover of the epidemic happens exactly when $R_E = R_0 s = 1$, where s is the fraction of remaining susceptibles. The threshold $R_0 s = 1 \Rightarrow s = 1/R_0$ results in the powerful rule of thumb for vaccine-induced elimination and herd immunity: if, through vaccination, the susceptible population is kept below a critical fraction, $p_c = 1 - 1/R_0$, then pathogen spread will dissipate and the pathogen will not be able to reinvade the host population (e.g., Anderson & May, 1982; Roberts & Heesterbeek, 1993; Ferguson et al., 2003). This rule of thumb appeared to work well for smallpox, the only vaccine-eradicated human disease; its R_0

---

[4] For further details on usage, do `?function` on the R command line, i.e., `?ode` in this instance.

was commonly around 5, and most countries saw elimination once vaccine cover exceeded 80% (Anderson & May, 1982). The actual code for Fig. 2.2 is:

```
R0 = paras["R0"]
# Adjust margins to accommodate a second right axis
par(mar = c(5, 5, 2, 5))
# Plot state variables
plot(x = out$time, y = out$S, ylab = "Fraction", xlab = "Time",
     type = "l")
lines(x = out$time, y = out$I, col = "red")
lines(x = out$time, y = out$R, col = "green")

# Add vertical line at turnover point
xx = out$time[which.max(out$I)]
lines(c(xx, xx), c(1/R0, max(out$I)), lty = 3)

# prepare to superimpose 2nd plot
par(new = TRUE)
# plot effective reproduction number  (w/o axes)
plot(x = out$time, y = R0 * out$S, type = "l", lty = 2,
     lwd = 2, col = "black", axes = FALSE, xlab = NA, ylab = NA,
     ylim = c(-0.5, 4.5))
lines(c(xx, 26), c(1, 1), lty = 3)
# Add right-hand axis for RE
axis(side = 4)
mtext(side = 4, line = 4, expression(R[E]))
# Add legend
legend("right", legend = c("S", "I", "R", expression(R[E])),
       lty = c(1, 1, 1, 2), col = c("black", "red", "green",
            "black"))
```

2.4 Final Epidemic Size

The closed epidemic model has two equilibria: the disease free equilibrium, $\{S = 1, I = 0, R = 0\}$, which is unstable when $R_0 > 1$ and the $\{S^*, I^*, R^*\}$ equilibrium which reflects the final epidemic size, R^*, for which $I^* = 0$ as the epidemic eventually self-extinguish in the absence of susceptible recruitment; S^* is the fraction of susceptibles that escape infection altogether. For the closed epidemic, there is an exact mathematical solution to the final epidemic size (below). It is nevertheless useful to consider computational ways of finding steady states in the absence of exact solutions.

The easiest approach is to use the ode function to integrate the system until it settles on a steady state (if it exists).[5]

---

[5] By varying initial conditions, we should be able to find multiple stable equilibria if there are more than one of them. This approach will not find unstable equilibria, for these we need to use other strategies. Section 10.3 considers in more depth how to find all equilibria whether stable or not.

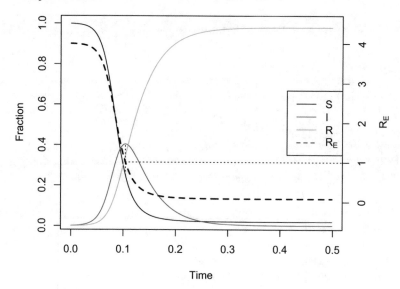

Fig. 2.2: The closed SIR epidemic with left and right axes and effective reproduction number, R_E. The epidemic turns over at $R_E = 1$

```
require(rootSolve)
equil = runsteady(y = c(S = 1 - 1e-05, I = 1e-05, R = 0),
    times = c(0, 1e+05), func = sirmod, parms = paras)
round(equil$y, 3)

##    S    I    R
## 0.02 0.00 0.98
```

So for these parameters, 2% of susceptibles are expected to escape infection alto-gether and 98%—the final epidemic size—are expected to be infected during the course of the epidemic.

The final epidemic size depends completely on R_0. For this specific SIR vari-ant, $\beta = R_0(\gamma + \mu)$ and for the closed epidemic $\mu = 0$. Continuing to assume an infectious period of 2 weeks (i.e., $\gamma = 1/2$), we may vary R_0 from 0.1 to 5. For mod-erate to large R_0, this fraction has been shown to be approximately $1 - \exp(-R_0)$ (e.g., Anderson & May, 1982). We can check how well this approximation holds (Fig. 2.3).[6]

```
# Candidate values for R0 and beta
R0 = seq(0.1, 5, length = 50)
```

---

[6] The `for` loop here calculates the final epidemic size for a range of values of R_0; a loop works by repeating calculations (in this case 50 times), and after each repeat, the value of the looping variable (in this case i) is changed to the next value in the looping vector. So in this example i will be 1 first, then 2, and then ... until the loop ends after i = 50.

```
betas = R0 * (paras["gamma"] + paras["mu"])
# Vector of NAs to be filled with numbers
fs = rep(NA, 50)
# Loop over 1 from 1, 2, ..., 50
for (i in seq(from = 1, to = 50, by = 1)) {
    equil = runsteady(y = c(S = 1 - 1e-05, I = 1e-05, R = 0),
        times = c(0, 1e+05), func = sirmod, parms = c(mu = 0,
            N = 1, beta = betas[i], gamma = 365/14))
    fs[i] = equil$y["R"]
}
plot(R0, fs, type = "l", xlab = expression(R[0]))
curve(1 - exp(-x), from = 1, to = 5, add = TRUE, col = "red")
```

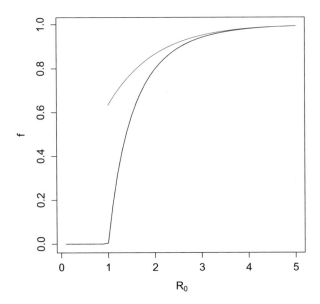

Fig. 2.3: The final epidemic size as a function of R_0. The black line is the solution based on numerically integrating the closed epidemic, the red line is the approximation $f \simeq 1 - \exp(-R_0)$

The approximation is good for $R_0 > 2.5$ but overestimates the final epidemic size for smaller R_0 (and is terrible for subcritical $R_0 < 1$).

For the closed epidemic SIR model, there is an exact mathematical solution to the fraction of susceptibles that escapes infection $(1 - f)$ given by the implicit equation $f = \exp(-R_0(1 - f))$ or equivalently $\exp(-R_0(1 - f)) - f = 0$ (Swinton, 1998). So we can also find the true expected final size by using the uniroot function to the equation. The uniroot function finds numerical solutions to equations with one unknown variable (which has to be named x).

```
# Define function
fn = function(x, R0) {
    exp(-(R0 * (1 - x))) - x
}
1 - uniroot(fn, lower = 0, upper = 1 - 1e-09, tol = 1e-09,
    R0 = 2)$root

  ## [1] 0.7968121

# check accuracy of approximation
exp(-2) - uniroot(fn, lower = 0, upper = 1 - 1e-09, tol = 1e-09,
    R0 = 2)$root

  ## [1] -0.06785259
```

So, for $R_0 = 2$, the final epidemic size is 79.6% and the approximation is off by around 6.7%-points. We will visit on stochastic aspects of the final epidemic size distribution in detail in Sect. 14.6.

2.5 The Open Epidemic

An open epidemic has recruitment of new susceptibles (i.e., $\mu > 0$). As long as $R_0 > 1$, the open epidemic has an endemic equilibrium were the pathogen and host coexist. If we use the SIR equations to model fractions (i.e., set $N = 1$), Eq. (2.2) of the SIR model implies that $S^* = (\gamma + \mu)/\beta = 1/R_0$ is the endemic S equilibrium, which when substituted into Eq. (2.1) gives $I^* = \mu(R_0 - 1)/\beta$, and finally, $R^* = N - I^* - S^*$ as the I and R endemic equilibrium values. We can study the predicted dynamics of the open epidemic using the sirmod function. In a stable host population with a life expectancy of 50 years, the per capita weekly birth/death rate is $\mu = 1/(50*52)$. For illustration, assume that 19.99% of the initial population is susceptible and 0.01% is infected, and numerically integrate the model for 50 years (Fig. 2.4).

```
times  = seq(0, 50, by=1/365)
paras  = c(mu = 1/50, N = 1, R0=4, gamma = 365/14)
paras["beta"]=paras["R0"]*(paras["gamma"]+paras["mu"])
start = c(S=0.1999, I=0.0001, R = 0.8)*paras["N"]
out = as.data.frame(ode(y=start, times=times,
      func=sirmod, parms=paras))
par(mfrow=c(1,2)) #Make room for side-by-side plots
#Prevalence in time
plot(times, out$I, ylab="Fraction", xlab="Time",
     type="l")
#S-I phase-plane
plot(out$S, out$I, type="l", xlab="Susceptible",
     ylab="Infected")
```

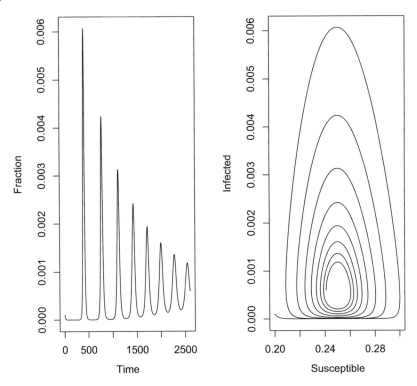

Fig. 2.4: The open SIR epidemic. (**a**) The fraction infected over time. (**b**) The joint time series of infecteds and susceptibles in the S–I phase plane. The trajectory forms a counterclockwise inward spiral in the S–I plane (note that the 50-year simulation is not long enough for the system to reach the steady-state endemic equilibrium at the center of the spiral)

2.6 Phase Analysis

When working with dynamical systems, one is often interested in studying the dynamics in the phase plane and deriving the isoclines that divide this plane into regions of increase and decrease of the various state variables. The phaseR package is a wrapper around ode that makes it easy to visualize 1- and 2-dimensional differential equation flows.[7] The *R* state in the SIR model does not influence the dynamics, so we can rewrite the SIR model as a 2D system.

---

[7] The phaseR package requires the gradient function to take the arguments t, y, and parameters.

```
simod = function(t, y, parameters) {
    S = y[1]
    I = y[2]

    beta = parameters["beta"]
    mu = parameters["mu"]
    gamma = parameters["gamma"]
    N = parameters["N"]

    dS = mu * (N - S) - beta * S * I/N
    dI = beta * S * I/N - (mu + gamma) * I
    res = c(dS, dI)
    list(res)
}
```

The isoclines (sometimes called the null-clines) in this system are given by the solution to the equations $dS/dt = 0$ and $dI/dt = 0$ and partition the phase plane into regions where S and I are increasing and decreasing. For $N = 1$, the I-isocline is $S = (\gamma + \mu)/\beta = 1/R_0$ and the S-isocline is $I = \mu(1/S - 1)/\beta$. We can draw these in the phase plane and add a simulated trajectory to the plot (Fig. 2.5). The trajectory cycles in a counterclockwise dampened fashion toward the endemic equilibrium (Fig. 2.5). To visualize the expected change to the system at arbitrary points in the phase plane, we can further use the function flowField in the phaseR package to superimpose predicted arrows of change.

```
require(phaseR)
#Plot vector field
fld = flowField(simod, xlim = c(0.2,0.3), ylim = c(0,.007),
    parameters = paras, system = "two.dim",
    add = FALSE, ylab = "I", xlab = "S")
#Add trajectory
out = as.data.frame(ode(y = c(S = 0.1999, I = 0.0001),
    times = seq(0, 52*100, by = 1/365), func = simod,
    parms = paras))
 lines(out$S, out$I, col = "red")
#Add S-isocline
curve(paras["mu"]*(1/x-1)/paras["beta"], 0.15, 0.35,
    xlab = "S", ylab = "I", add = TRUE)
#Add I-isocline
icline = (paras["gamma"] + paras["mu"])/paras["beta"]
lines(rep(icline, 2), c(0,0.01))
legend("topright", legend = c("Transient", "Isoclines"),
    lty = c(1, 1), col = c("red", "black"))
```

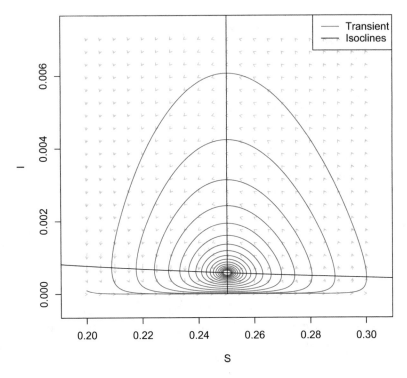

Fig. 2.5: The S–I phase plane with isoclines and the predicted counterclockwise trajectory toward the endemic equilibrium

2.7 Stability and Periodicity

As a preview of more detailed discussions in Chap. 10, this section is just a teaser. For continuous-time ODE models like the SIR, equilibria are locally stable if (and only if) all the real parts of the eigenvalues of the <u>Jacobian matrix</u> when evaluated at the equilibrium are smaller than zero. An equilibrium is (i) a node (i.e., all trajectories moves monotonically toward/away from the equilibrium) if the largest eigenvalue has only a real part and (ii) a focus (i.e., trajectories spiral toward or away from the equilibrium) if the largest eigenvalues are a conjugate pair of complex numbers $(a \pm bi)$.[8] For a focus, the imaginary part determines the dampening period of the cycle according to $2\pi/b$. We can thus use the Jacobian matrix to study the SIR model's equilibria. If we set $F = dS/dt = \mu(N - S) - \beta SI/N$ and $G = dI/dt = \beta SI/N - (\mu + \gamma)I$, the Jacobian of the SIR system is

---

[8] And (iii) a center, as is the case for the <u>Lotka–Volterra predator–prey</u> model, if the conjugate pair only has imaginary parts.

$$\mathbf{J} = \begin{pmatrix} \frac{\partial F}{\partial S} & \frac{\partial F}{\partial I} \\ \frac{\partial G}{\partial S} & \frac{\partial G}{\partial I} \end{pmatrix},$$

(2.4)

and the two equilibria are the disease free equilibrium and the endemic equilibrium as defined above.

R can help with all of this. The endemic equilibrium is:

```
# Pull values from paras vector
gamma = paras["gamma"]
beta = paras["beta"]
mu = paras["mu"]
N = paras["N"]
# Endemic equilibrium
Sstar = (gamma + mu)/beta
Istar = mu * (beta/(gamma + mu) - 1)/beta
eq1 = list(S = Sstar, I = Istar)
```

The elements of the Jacobian using R's differentiation D function are

```
# Define equations
dS = quote(mu * (N - S) - beta * S * I/N)
dI = quote(beta * S * I/N - (mu + gamma) * I)
# Differentiate w.r.t. S and I
j11 = D(dS, "S")
j12 = D(dS, "I")
j21 = D(dI, "S")
j22 = D(dI, "I")
```

Pass the values for S^* and I^* in the eq1 list to the Jacobian,[9] and use the eigen function to calculate the eigenvalues:

```
# Evaluate Jacobian at equilibrium
JJ = with(data = eq1, expr = matrix(c(eval(j11), eval(j12),
    eval(j21), eval(j22)), nrow = 2, byrow = TRUE))
# Calculate eigenvalues
eigen(JJ)$values
```

```
## [1] -0.04+1.250554i -0.04-1.250554i
```

For the endemic equilibrium, the eigenvalues are a pair of complex conjugates which real parts are negative, so it is a stable focus. The period of the inward spiral is:

---

[9] In previous coding of the sirmod function, parameter values were pulled from the input arguments inside the function to make the code as transparent as possible; while it makes the code easy to read, it makes for extra coding and can clutter up the workspace with variables that are defined in multiple locations. The with function allows the evaluation of an expression using variables defined in a data list.

```
2 * pi/(Im(eigen(JJ)$values[1]))
```

```
  ## [1] 5.024321
```

So with these parameters, the dampening period is predicted to be just over 5 years. Thus, during disease invasion, we expect this system to exhibit initial outbreaks every 5 years. A further significance of this number is that if the system is stochastically perturbed by environmental variability affecting transmission, the system will exhibit low-amplitude "phase-forgetting" cycles (Nisbet & Gurney, 1982) with approximately this period in the long run. We can make more accurate calculations of the stochastic system using transfer functions (Priestley, 1981; Nisbet & Gurney, 1982). We will visit on this more advanced topic in Sect. 10.8.

The same protocol can be used for the disease free equilibrium $\{S^* = 1, I^* = 0\}$.

```
eq2 = list(S = 1, I = 0)
JJ = with(eq2, matrix(c(eval(j11), eval(j12), eval(j21),
    eval(j22)), nrow = 2, byrow = TRUE))
eigen(JJ)$values
```

```
  ## [1] 78.27429 -0.02000
```

The eigenvalues are strictly real and the largest value is greater than zero, so it is an unstable node (a "saddle"); the epidemic trajectory is predicted to move monotonically away from this disease free equilibrium if infection is introduced into the system. This makes sense because with the parameter values used, $R_0 = 4$, which is greater than the invasion threshold value of 1.

Because we will require Jacobian matrices for a large number of different calculations regarding infectious disease dynamics, Sect. 6.8 will introduce a general-purpose `jacobian` function that is part of the `epimdr2` package.

2.8 Heterogeneities

The bare-bones SIR model makes many simplifying assumption. A lot of the theory in the subsequent chapters contends with making more realistic models by incorporating various heterogeneities. Important complications are age-dependence in susceptibility, infectiousness, contact rates and disease symptomology (Chaps. 4 and 5), a greater number of functionally distinct classes such as nosocomical (hospital associated) transmission being different from that in the community (Sect. 3.10), waning/boosting of immunity (Sect. 11.4), infections having multiple distinct outcomes (Sect. 10.6), seasonal changes in dynamics (Chap. 6), and spatial/social heterogeneities (Chaps. 12 and 14). The need to consider more elaborate models typically depends on the biology/ecology of the host and pathogen and the scientific problem in question.

2.9 Advanced: More Realistic Infectious Periods

As an initial illustrative example of added realism, we can consider how infectivity and removal rates are usually not constant during the course of infection. For acute pathogens, recently infected individuals are usually likely to be infected for a while longer, whereas individuals infected some time ago are likely to have a higher rate of removal either because the immunity is ramping up or increased risk of death or quarantining if disease severity increases over time. We can baby step toward solving the Kermack & McKendrick (1927) general equations of such time dependence by modifying the basic SIR model to consider more realistic infectious periods.

The S(E)IR-type differential equation models assume that the rate of exit from the infectious classes is constant, and the implicit assumption is thus that the infectious period is exponentially distributed among infected individuals. The average infectious period predicted from Eq. (2.2) is $1/(\gamma+\mu)$, but an exponential fraction is infectious much shorter/longer than this. The chain-binomial model, which will be discussed in Sect. 3.4, in contrast, assumes that everybody is infectious for a fixed period and then instantaneously recovers (or dies). These assumptions are mathematically convenient, but in reality neither are particularly realistic. Hope-Simpson (1952) traced the chains of transmission of measles in multi-sibling households. The timing of secondary and tertiary cases was analyzed in detail by Bailey (1956) and Bailey and Alff-Steinberger (1970). The average latent and infectious periods were calculated to be 8.58 and 6.57 days, respectively. While the distribution around each of these averages was not estimated separately (the latent period was assumed to be distributed and the infectious period assumed fixed), the variance around the roughly fortnight period of infection was estimated to be 3.13. The mean duration of infection is thus 15.15 days with a standard deviation of 1.77 (Fig. 2.6). So neither a fixed nor an exponential distribution is very accurate (Keeling & Grenfell, 1997; Lloyd, 2001).

Kermack and McKendrick's (1927) original model allows for arbitrary infectious period distributions. We can write Kermack and McKendrick's original equations as renewal equations (Breda et al., 2012), introducing the additional notation of $k(t)$ being the (instantaneous) incidence at time t (i.e., flux into the I class at time t).

$$\frac{dS}{dt} = \underbrace{\mu N}_{\text{birth}} - \underbrace{\mu S}_{\text{death}} - \underbrace{k(t)}_{\text{outflux}} \tag{2.5}$$

$$k(t) = \beta I(t)\frac{S(t)}{N} \tag{2.6}$$

$$\frac{dI}{dt} = \underbrace{k(t)}_{\text{influx}} - \underbrace{\mu I}_{\text{death}} - \underbrace{\int_0^\infty \frac{h(\tau)}{1-H(\tau)}k(t-\tau)d\tau}_{\text{distributed recovery}} \tag{2.7}$$

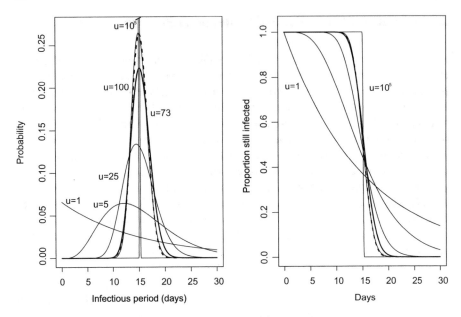

Fig. 2.6: Gamma distributed infectious periods. **(a)** The predicted infectious period distribution based on a gamma distribution with shape $u = 1, 5, 25, 100$, and
$100,000$; $u = 1$ corresponds to the exponential distribution implicit in the standard
SIR model. The bold line ($u = 73$) is the one corresponding to the variance observed
in Hope-Simpson's (1952) study of measles. The dotted line (virtually indistinguish-
able from the $u = 100$) is a Gaussian distribution intended to show that when u is
large the gamma distribution converges on the normal distribution. **(b)** The probability of still being infectious as a function of time for the different distributions. As
u becomes large, the distribution converges on a fixed infectious period. Note that
the empirical distribution (bold) is quite different from the exponential ($u = 1$)

$$\frac{dR}{dt} = \underbrace{\int_0^\infty \frac{h(\tau)}{1 - H(\tau)} k(t - \tau) d\tau}_{\text{distributed recovery}} - \underbrace{\mu R}_{\text{death}} , \qquad (2.8)$$

where $k(t - \tau)$ is the number of individuals that were infected τ time units ago,
$h(\tau)$ is the probability of recovering on infection day τ, and $H(\tau)$ is the cumulative
probability of having recovered by infection day τ; $k(t - \tau)/(1 - H(\tau))$ is thus the
fraction of individuals infected at time $t - \tau$ that still remains in the infected class on
day t and the integral is over all previous infections so as to quantify the total flux
into the removed class at time t. Though intuitive, these general integro-differential
equations (Eqs. (2.5)–(2.8)) are not easy to work with in general. For a restricted set
of distributions for the $h()$ function however—the Erlang distribution (the gamma
distribution with an integer shape parameter)—the model can be numerically inte-

grated using a gamma-chain model (referred to as "linear chain trickery" by Metz & Diekmann, 1991) of coupled ordinary differential equations (e.g., Blythe et al., 1984; Lloyd, 2001; Bjørnstad et al., 2016). The trick is to separate any distributed-delay compartment into u sub-compartments through which individuals pass at a rate of $x * u$. The resultant infectious period will have a mean duration of $1/x$ and a coefficient of variation of $1/\sqrt{u}$.

A chain SIR model to simulate $S \to I \to R$ flows with more realistic infectious period distributions is:[10]

```
sirChainmod = function(t, logx, parameters) {
    x = exp(logx)
    u = parameters["u"]
    S = x[1]
    I = x[2:(u + 1)]
    R = x[u + 2]
    with(as.list(parameters), {
        dS = mu * (N - S) - sum(beta * S * I)/N
        dI = rep(0, u)
        dI[1] = sum(beta * S * I)/N - (mu + u * gamma) *
            I[1]
        if (u > 1) {
            for (i in 2:u) {
                dI[i] = u * gamma * I[i - 1] - (mu + u *
                    gamma) * I[i]
            }
        }
        dR = u * gamma * I[u] - mu * R
        res = c(dS/S, dI/I, dR/R)
        list(res)
    })
}
```

We can compare the predicted dynamics of the simple SIR model with the $u = 2$ chain model, the $u = 500$ chain model (which is effectively the fixed-delay differential model), and the "measles-realistic" $u = 73$ model.

```
times = seq(0, 10, by = 1/52)
paras2 = c(mu = 1/75, N = 1, R0 = 18, gamma = 365/14, u = 1)
paras2["beta"] = paras2["R0"] * (paras2["gamma"] + paras2["mu"])
xstart2 = log(c(S = 0.06, I = c(0.001, rep(1e-04, paras2["u"] -
    1)), R = 1e-04))
out = as.data.frame(ode(xstart2, times, sirChainmod, paras2))
plot(times, exp(out[, 3]), ylab = "Infected", xlab = "Time",
    ylim = c(0, 0.003), type = "l")
```

---

[10] With a high number of compartments, this system of equations can become "stiff" with the computer potentially making rounding errors leading to erroneous negative numbers. We use a "log-trick" available for systems where all state variables are strictly positive: we solve the system in log-coordinates to smooth abrupt changes and force all states to be greater than zero. To employ this technique, log-transform all initial values in start, change the first line in the function to x = exp(logx) and the last line to return dS/S, etc. in place of dS which comes from the chain-rule of differentiation and the fact that $D(\log x) = 1/x$.

```
paras2["u"] = 2
xstart2 = log(c(S = 0.06, I = c(0.001, rep(1e-04/paras2["u"],
    paras2["u"] - 1)), R = 1e-04))
out2 = as.data.frame(ode(xstart2, times, sirChainmod, paras2))
lines(times, apply(exp(out2[, -c(1:2, length(out2))]), 1,
    sum), col = "blue")

paras2["u"] = 73
xstart2 = log(c(S = 0.06, I = c(0.001, rep(1e-04/paras2["u"],
    paras2["u"] - 1)), R = 1e-04))
out3 = as.data.frame(ode(xstart2, times, sirChainmod, paras2))
lines(times, apply(exp(out3[, -c(1:2, length(out3))]), 1,
    sum), col = "red", lwd = 2, lty = 2)

paras2["u"] = 500
xstart2 = log(c(S = 0.06, I = c(0.001, rep(1e-04/paras2["u"],
    paras2["u"] - 1)), R = 1e-04))
out4 = as.data.frame(ode(xstart2, times, sirChainmod, paras2))
lines(times, apply(exp(out4[, -c(1:2, length(out4))]), 1,
    sum, na.rm = TRUE), col = "green")

legend("topright", legend = c("SIR", "u=2", "u=500",
    "u=73 (H-S)"), lty = c(1, 1, 1, 2), lwd = c(1, 1, 1, 2),
    col = c("black", "blue", "green", "red"))
```

The more narrow the infectious period distribution, the more punctuated the predicted epidemics. However, infectious period narrowing alone cannot sustain recurrent epidemics. In the absence of stochastic or seasonal forcing, epidemics will dampen to the endemic equilibrium (though the damping period is slightly accelerated and the convergence on the equilibrium is slightly slower with narrowing infectious period distributions) (Fig. 2.7).

In the above we considered non-exponential infectious period distributions. However, the general gamma-chain method can be used for any compartment. Lavine et al. (2011), for example, used it to model non-exponential waning of natural and vaccine-induced immunity to whooping cough.

2.10 An SIR shinyApp

The following code will launch a shinyApp of the SIR model in a local browser. This App can also be launched by calling runApp(sir.app) from the epimdr2 package. Several of the subsequent chapters also have associated shinyApps. Those will be accessible from the epimdr2 package or the epimdr2 GitHub site, but not scripted in the text because the code is long and a bit tedious. The sir.app is presented here in full, so the interested readers can get a sense of shinyApp coding. Bjørnstad et al. (2020a) provide a more elaborate online accessible shinyApp to study the SIR model at https://shiny.bcgsc.ca/posepi1/.

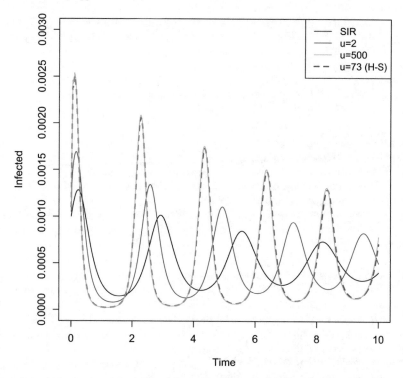

Fig. 2.7: Chain SIR models with different infectious period distributions

```
require(shiny)
require(deSolve)
require(phaseR)

# This creates the User Interface (UI)
ui <- pageWithSidebar(
headerPanel("The SIR model"),
#The sidebar for parameter input
sidebarPanel(
#Sliders
sliderInput("R0", "R0:", 2,
            min = 0.5, max = 20),
sliderInput("infper", "Infectious period (days)", 5,
            min = 1, max = 100),
sliderInput("mu", "birth rate (yr^-1):", 5,
            min = 0, max = 100),
sliderInput("T", "Time range:",
            min = 0, max = 1, value = c(0,1))
),
#Main panel for figures and equations
mainPanel(
```

```r
  #Multiple tabs in main panel
  tabsetPanel(
    #Tab 1: Time plot (plot1 from server)
    tabPanel("Time", plotOutput("plot1")),
    #Tab 2: Phase plot (plot2 from server)
    tabPanel("Phase plane", plotOutput("plot2",
      height = 500)),
    #Tab 3: MathJax typeset equations
    tabPanel("Equations",
      withMathJax(
        helpText("Susceptible $$\\frac{dS}{dt} =
          \\mu (N - S) - \\frac{\\beta I S}{N}$$"),
        helpText("Infecitous $$\\frac{dI}{dt} =
          \\frac{\\beta I S}{N} - (\\mu+\\sigma) I$$"),
        helpText("Removed $$\\frac{dR}{dt} =
          \\gamma I - \\mu R$$"),
        helpText("reproduction number $$R_0 =
          \\frac{1}{\\gamma+\\mu} \\frac{\\beta N}{N}$$")
      ))
  ))) #End of ui()


# This creates the 'behind the scenes' code (Server)
server <- function(input, output) {
  #Gradient function for SIR model
  sirmod=function(t, x, parameters){
    S=x[1]
    I=x[2]
    R=x[3]
    R0=parameters["R0"]
    mu=parameters["mu"]
    gamma=parameters["gamma"]
    N=parameters["N"]
    beta=R0*(gamma+mu)
    dS = mu * (N   - S)   - beta * S * I / N
    dI = beta * S * I / N - (mu + gamma) * I
    dR = gamma * I - mu * R
    res=c(dS, dI, dR)
    list(res)
  }

  #Plot1: renderPlot to be passed to UI tab 1
  output$plot1 = renderPlot({
  #input\$xx's are pulled from UI
  times  = seq(0, input$T[2], by=1/1000)
  paras  = c(mu = input$mu, N = 1, R0 =  input$R0,
    gamma = 365/input$infper)
  start = c(S=0.999, I=0.001, R = 0)
  paras["beta"] = with(as.list(paras), R0*(gamma+mu))
  #Resonant period
  AA=with(as.list(paras), 1/(mu*(R0-1)))
  GG=with(as.list(paras), 1/(mu+gamma))
  rp=round(2*pi*sqrt(AA*GG),2)
```

```r
#Integrate ode with parameters pulled from UI
out=ode(start,  times, sirmod, paras)
out=as.data.frame(out)

#Plot1
sel=out$time>input$T[1]&out$time<input$T[2]
plot(x=out$time[sel], y=out$S[sel], ylab="fraction",
xlab="time", type="l", ylim=range(out[sel,-c(1,4)]))
title(paste("R0=", paras["R0"], "Period=", rp))
lines(x=out$time[sel], y=out$I[sel], col="red")
lines(x=out$time[sel], y=out$R[sel], col="green")
legend("right",
     legend=c("S", "I", "R"),
     lty=c(1,1,1),
       col=c("black", "red", "green"))
})

#Plot2: renderPlot to be passed to UI tab 2
output$plot2 <- renderPlot({
times  = seq(0, input$T[2], by=1/1000)
paras  = c(mu = input$mu, N = 1, R0 =  input$R0,
  gamma = 365/input$infper)
paras["beta"] = with(as.list(paras), R0*(gamma+mu))

start = c(S=0.999, I=0.001, R = 0)

#Gradient function used for phaseR phase-plot
simod=function(t, y, parameters){
 S=y[1]
 I=y[2]
 beta=parameters["beta"]
 mu=parameters["mu"]
 gamma=parameters["gamma"]
 N=parameters["N"]
 dS = mu * (N  - S) - beta * S * I / N
 dI = beta * S * I / N - (mu + gamma) * I
 res=c(dS, dI)
 list(res)
}

#Integrate simod
out=ode(start[-3], times, simod, paras)
out=as.data.frame(out)

AA=with(as.list(paras), 1/(mu*(R0-1)))
GG=with(as.list(paras), 1/(mu+gamma))
rp=round(2*pi*sqrt(AA*GG),2)

plot(x=out$S, y=out$I, xlab="Fraction suceptible",
   ylab="Fraction infected", type="l")
title(paste("R0=", paras["R0"], "Period=", rp))
#Add vector field
fld=flowField(simod, xlim=range(out$S),
```

```
ylim=range(out$I), parameters=paras,
system="two.dim", add=TRUE,ylab="I", xlab="S")
#Add isoclines
abline(v=1/paras["R0"], col="green")
curve(paras["mu"]*(1-x)/(paras["beta"]*x), min(out$S),
  max(out$S), add=TRUE, col="red")
legend("topright",
      legend=c("S-isocline", "I-isocline"),
      lty=c(1,1),
    col=c("red", "green"))
 })
 } #End of server()

shinyApp(ui, server)
```

Chapter 3
R_0

3.1 Primacy of R_0

For directly transmitted pathogens, R_0 is per definition the expected number of secondary cases that arise from a typical infectious index case in a completely susceptible host population. R_0 plays a critical role for a number of aspects of disease
dynamics and is therefore the focus of much study in historical and contemporary
infectious disease dynamics (Heesterbeek & Dietz, 1996). For perfectly immunizing
infections in homogeneously mixing populations, these include:

- The threshold for pathogen establishment. When R_0 is greater than one, a
  pathogen can invade. When it is smaller than one, the chain of transmission will
  stutter and break (Lloyd-Smith et al., 2009, see Sect. 15.2). For directly transmitted wildlife diseases, there is often an associated critical host density for disease
  invasion. This has for example been estimated to be 1 red fox per km^2 for rabies
  in Europe (Anderson et al., 1981) and 17 mice per ha for *Sin nombre* hantavirus
  in Montana (Luis et al., 2015). Section 10.7 provides a worked example for raccoon rabies.
- The threshold for vaccine-induced herd immunity. If a sufficient number of individuals are vaccinated, the effective reproduction number (R_E, the expected
  number of secondary cases in a partially immune population) will be below
  one, and the population will be resistant to pathogen invasion. The threshold
  is $p_c = 1 - 1/R_0$. Thus, measles with an R_0 of up to 20 requires around 95%
  vaccine cover for elimination and smallpox ($R_0 \simeq 5$) around 80%.
- In a closed epidemic, the peak prevalence is $1 - (1 + \log R_0)/R_0$ (House & Keeling, 2011) and the early doubling time is $\log(2)V/\log R_0$, where V is the serial
  interval (the average infection-to-onward-transmission time).

This chapter uses the following R packages: bbmle and statnet.
A discussion of the reproduction number and epidemic curve can be found in two five minute
epidemics MOOC videos:
Reproduction number https://www.youtube.com/watch?v=ju26rvzfFg4.
Closed epidemic https://www.youtube.com/watch?v=sSLfrSSmJZM.

© The Author(s), under exclusive license to Springer Nature Switzerland AG 2023
O. N. Bjørnstad, *Epidemics*, Use R!, https://doi.org/10.1007/978-3-031-12056-5_3

- As discussed in Sect. 2.4, the final epidemic size is given by R_0 according to the approximate relationship $f \simeq 1 - \exp(-R_0)$ if there are no changes to host behavior in response to the epidemic.
- In a stable host population, the mean age of infection is approximately $\bar{a} \simeq L/(R_0 - 1)$, where L is host life expectancy (Dietz & Schenzle, 1985). In a changing population, a more accurate calculation is $\bar{a} \simeq 1/(\mu(R_0 - 1))$, where μ is the host birth rate.
- As derived in Sect. 2.6, the susceptible fraction at equilibrium is $S^* = 1/R_0$. A consequence of this is that for competing strains that elicit cross-protecting immunity R_0 will determine competitive dominance and strain replacement (Shrestha et al., 2014).[1] A recent illustration of this is the replacement among SARS-CoV-2 variants as evolution increases human-to-human transmission.

For these reasons and more, a lot of attention has been given to measuring R_0 for various infectious diseases as detailed below.

3.2 Rates and Probabilities

When working with data, models, and "models-and-data" for infectious disease dynamics, it is important to keep a cool head in terms of keeping track of which quantities are *probabilities* and which quantities are *rates* and how to move between these two mathematical currencies.[2] Confusion arises because the nomenclature of epidemiology and mathematical epidemiology is related but not always identical. In epidemiology, the "case-fatality rate" is sometimes used to denote the fraction of infections that ends in death, which from a mathematical/statistical point of view is not a rate but a probability: the probability that an infection will lead to death (Dietz & Heesterbeek, 2002). Likewise, in epidemiology, the seasonal influenza "attack rate" denotes the fraction of people that contracts the flu in a given influenza season. Again, from a mathematical/statistical/dynamical systems point of view, this quantity is not a rate but a probability representing the chance of any randomly chosen individual of unknown previous influenza infection history getting infected during the season.

When considering events in modeling terms, a rate x per time unit is defined on $[0, \infty]$ and $1/x$ is the average time to an event (if the rate remains constant). If events are random and independent, the probability of no events in a time interval Δt is $\exp(-x\Delta t)$ and the number of events in Δt follows a Poisson distribution with

---

[1] This result is parallel to Tilman's (1976) R^* theory of resource-based competition of free-living organisms; whichever species that can sustain positive growth at the lowest concentration of the limited resource will be competitively dominant. The `twostrain.app` in Sect. 3.12 allows further exploration of this.

[2] The disease dynamics literature has many example of how easy it is to confuse the two, which often becomes particularly apparent when grappling with acute crises such as the 2014 West Africa Ebola outbreak and the SARS-CoV-2 corona emergence in late 2019 through 2020.

mean $x\Delta t$ (if the rate remains constant). A probability, in contrast, is defined on $[0,1]$. If we observe a probability p of something happening in a time interval, we can back-calculate the associated (constant) rate as $x = -log(1-p)/\Delta t$.

If there are two competing processes, with rate x at which event one (e.g., recovery) happens and rate y at which event two (e.g., death) happens, the probability of ending up with outcome one is $x/(x+y)$ and the probability of ending up with outcome two is $y/(x+y)$. This scales such that with three competing rates the probability of outcome one is $x/(x+y+z)$, etc.

3.3 Estimating R_0 from a Simple Epidemic

A variety of methods have been proposed to estimate R_0 (or the effective reproduction number, R_E).[3] Some are purely model based, others involve very elaborate model fitting exercises, and some use fairly simple ideas based on the closed epidemic and analogies to the ecology of free-living organisms (Dietz, 1993).

The simplest idea is that during the initial spread phase susceptible depletion may be sufficiently negligible that the epidemic may be assumed to grow in a density-independent, exponential fashion. Basic ecology of free-living organisms tells us that the rate of exponential growth is $r = log(R_0)/V$, where V is the generation time; thus $R_0 = \exp(rV)$.[4] Moreover, since an exponentially growing population grows according to $N(t) = N(0)\exp(rt)$, the time for a population to double is $log(2)/r$. By analogy, we can apply these ideas to the early phase of an epidemic to estimate R_0.

For pathogens, the Ns above would represent the *prevalence* and V represents the *serial interval* which is the average time between infection and reinfection. This interval will normally be a little shorter than the latent plus infectious period. It is, again, important to clarify some additional nomenclature here. The *latent period* of an infectious disease is the typical time from being exposed to becoming infectious, and the *infectious period* is the typical time from becoming infectious to stop being infectious (through recovery or death).[5] These quantities differ sometimes mildly and sometimes by a lot from the clinical concepts of the *incubation period*, which is the time between exposure and overt symptoms of disease and *period of illness*. For influenza, for example, the infectious period has been estimated to be around 4 days (Carrat et al., 2008), the latent period around 1 day (Canini & Carrat, 2011), and the serial interval around 4 days (Cowling et al., 2009). For anyone who has had a bad bout of influenza, this contrasts with the often 10 days to 2 weeks of

---

[3] Recall that the effective reproduction number is the expected number of secondary cases in a partially immune population: $R_E = sR_0$, where s is the fraction of the population that is susceptible.

[4] Unless explicitly stated otherwise, log will always be taken to mean the natural logarithm in this text.

[5] Though for certain infections like anthrax, Ebola, and entomopathic viruses, a cadaver can be infectious and in the case of anthrax for a very long time.

feeling miserable. It is also important to keep in mind that latent and infectious periods vary wildly among pathogens. For example, for influenza, the latent period and infectious period are very short. For tuberculosis, in contrast, the latent period can span decades (Dye, 2015).

Disease data most often represent incidence, i.e., the number of new infections not the number of current infections. However, the nature of exponential growth is such that incidence also grows at the same exponential rate as prevalence. Initial growth is $\exp(r)$, where $r = (R_0 - 1)/V$ (e.g., Ferguson et al., 2003). The simplest way to estimate R_0 is thus to regress log(cumulative incidence) on time to estimate the rate of exponential increase (r) and then back-calculate $R_0 = Vr + 1$ (e.g., Anderson & May, 1991).

One can explore using the weekly measles data from the 2003 outbreak in Niamey, Niger (Grais et al., 2008). The data is available as `niamey`. The `tot_cases` column represents the total incidence across the city for each week of the outbreak.

```
data(niamey)
head(niamey[, 1:5])
```

```
##     absweek week tot_cases tot_mort lethality
## 1         1   45        11        0  0.000000
## 2         2   46        12        1  8.333333
## 3         3   47        15        0  0.000000
## 4         4   48        14        1  7.142857
## 5         5   49        30        0  0.000000
## 6         6   50        41        1  2.439024
```

The following provides a visual inspection to identify the initial period of exponential growth.

```
par(mar = c(5, 5, 2, 5))
plot(niamey$absweek, niamey$tot_cases, type = "b", xlab = "Week",
    ylab = "Incidence")
par(new = TRUE)
plot(niamey$absweek, niamey$cum_cases, type = "l", col = "red",
    axes = FALSE, xlab = NA, ylab = NA, log = "y")
axis(side = 4)
mtext(side = 4, line = 4, "Cumulative incidence")
legend("topleft", legend = c("Cases", "Cumulative"), lty = c(1,
    1), pch = c(1, NA), col = c("black", "red"))
```

The cumulative incidence looks pretty log-linear for the first 6 weeks or so (Fig. 3.1). The data is weekly and the serial interval for measles is around 10–12 days, and thus V is around 1.5–1.8 weeks. We can calculate R_0 assuming either 1.5 or 1.8:

```
fit = lm(log(cum_cases) ~ absweek, subset = absweek <
    7, data = niamey)
r = fit$coef["absweek"]
V = c(1.5, 1.8)
V * r + 1
```

```
## [1] 1.694233 1.833080
```

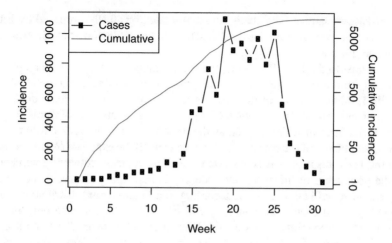

Fig. 3.1: Weekly incidence of measles in Niamey, Niger during the 2003–2004 out-break

So a fast-and-furious estimate of the reproduction number for this outbreak places it in the 1.5–2 range. Measles exhibits recurrent epidemics in the presence of various vaccination campaigns in Niger, so this number represents an estimate of the *effective* reproduction number, R_E, at the beginning of this epidemic.

In their analysis of the SARS-CoV-1 emergence, Lipsitch et al. (2003) showed that for an infection with distinct latent and infectious periods, a more refined estimate is given by $R = Vr + 1 + f(1 - f)(Vr)^2$, where f is the ratio of infectious period to serial interval. For measles, the infectious period is around 5 days.

```
V = c(1.5, 1.8)
f = (5/7)/V
V * r + 1 + f * (1 - f) * (V * r)^2

## [1] 1.814450 1.999198
```

Lipsitch et al.'s (2003) refined calculations thus produce slightly higher estimates of R_E in the range of 1.8–2. These simple methods based on initial growth are very handy because they are simple. However, they only use a portion of the data, and as pointed out by King et al. (2015a), it may be desirable to carry out more rigorous estimation.

3.4 The Chain-Binomial Model

Ferrari et al. (2005) proposed a maximum likelihood removal method for estimating R_0 for the closed epidemic based on the so-called chain-binomial model of infectious disease dynamics. The chain-binomial model, originally proposed by Bailey (1957), is a discrete-time stochastic alternative[6] to the continuous-time deterministic SIR model introduced in Chap. 2.

In contrast to the S(E)IR models, the chain-binomial assumes that an epidemic is formed from a succession of discrete generations of infectious individuals in a coin-flip fashion. Just like in the SIR, we assume that infectious individuals exert a force of infection on susceptibles of $\beta I/N$. In a generation, t, of duration given by the serial interval which is used as the basic time unit, the probability that any given susceptible will escape an infectious contact will be $\exp(-\beta I/N)$. This comes from the basic result that if some event—such as contacts between a susceptible and the population of infectious individuals—is happening at rate, x, the number of events in Δt will be distributed according to a Poisson$(x\Delta t)$ distribution, so the probability of no events (no contacts) will be $e^{-x\Delta t}$. The converse outcome will happen with a probability $1 - \exp(-\beta I/N)$, and thus if there are S_t susceptibles we expect $S_t(1 - \exp(-\beta I_t/N))$ new infecteds in generation $t+1$. The assumption that contacts happen at random leads to the stochastic chain-binomial model:

$$I_{t+1} \sim \text{Binomial}(S_t, 1 - \exp(-\beta I_t/N)) \tag{3.1}$$

$$S_{t+1} = S_t - I_{t+1} = S_0 - \sum_{i=1}^{t} I_i \tag{3.2}$$

If we ignore observational error, we thus have two unknown parameters: the initial number of susceptibles, S_0, and the transmission rate, β. The reproduction number is a composite of these two as $R_0 = S_0(1 - \exp(-\beta/N))$, which for large populations is approximately $\beta S_0/N$ because $1 - \exp(-x) \simeq x$ for $x << 1$. Thus, in the case of the chain-binomial, β is approximately the reproduction number at the beginning of the epidemic, which makes sense since infectious individuals are expected to transmit for exactly a time unit before recovering.[7]

If we make the assumption that each epidemic generation depends only on the state of the system in the previous time step ("conditional independence"), the removal method estimates β and S_0 from a sequence of binomial likelihoods. The advantage of this method relative to the earlier methods is that we can use all the data and not just a few observations from the beginning of an epidemic.

We employ a standard recipe, for doing a "nonstandard" maximum likelihood analysis (see Bolker 2008 for an excellent discussion of this). The first step is to write a function for the likelihood. Conditional on some parameters, the function returns the negative log-likelihood of observing the data given the model. The likelihood, which is the probability of observing data given a model and some parameter values, is the working-horse of a large part of statistics. R has inbuilt dxxxx-functions to calculate the likelihood for any conceivable probability distribution.

---

[6] This model also forms the foundation for the TSIR model (Bjørnstad et al., 2002a; Grenfell et al., 2002) which is the focus of Chap. 8.

[7] This is comparable with previous SIR calculations of $R_0 = \beta/(\gamma + \mu)$ from Sect. 2.2 since when the time unit is scaled by the serial interval the denominator is typically quite close to unity.

The function to calculate a binomial likelihood is `dbinom`. We can thus define a likelihood function for the chain-binomial model:[8]

```
llik.cb = function(S0, beta, I) {
    n = length(I)
    S = floor(S0 - cumsum(I[-n]))
    p = 1 - exp(-beta * (I[-n])/S0)
    L = -sum(dbinom(I[-1], S, p, log = TRUE))
    return(L)
}
```

For the proper statistical analysis (below), the two parameters will be estimated simultaneously. However, in order to ease into the idea of likelihood estimation, we will consider the two sequentially and visualize the likelihood by plotting it over a grid of potential values. We can illustrate these ideas with the data on measles from one of the three different reporting centers in Niamey, Niger from 2003 (Grais et al., 2008). The data first needs to be aggregated into 2-week intervals which is roughly the serial interval for measles. The epidemic in district 1 lasted for 30 weeks (the 31st week is a zero). The function `split` divides a vector into a list based on some grouping variable and `sapply` applies a function, in this case `sum`, to the list to return a new vector.

```
twoweek = rep(1:15, each = 2)
y = sapply(split(niamey$cases_1[1:30], twoweek), sum)
sum(y)
```

```
## [1] 5920
```

In district 1, there were 5920 cases during the epidemics, so S_0 needs to be at least that number. In the above parameterization $R_E \simeq \beta$, let us initially assume a candidate value of 6500 for S_0 and calculate the likelihood for each candidate value of β between 1 and 10 by 0.1 (Fig. 3.2):

```
S0cand = 6500
betacand = seq(0,10, by = 0.1)
ll = rep(NA, length(betacand))
for(i in 1:length(betacand)) {
    ll[i] = llik.cb(S0 = S0cand, beta = betacand[i],
    I = y)}
plot(ll ~ betacand, ylab = "Neg log-lik",
    xlab = expression(beta))
betacand[which.min(ll)]
```

```
## [1] 2.3
```

---

[8] Note that the `[-x]` subsetting in R means "drop the x'th observation," and thus the `[-n]` and `[-1]` make sure that adjacent pairs of observations are aligned correctly. We use the `floor` function for the vector of S's because `dbinom` requires the denominator and numerator to be integers.

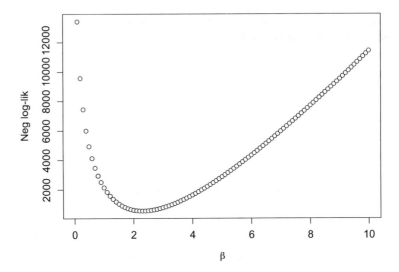

Fig. 3.2: The conditional profile log-likelihood of β for Niamey's district 1 assuming $S_0 = 6500$

The convention is to consider the negative log-likelihood to profile over the parameter.[9] Intuitively, one may think that it would be more natural to consider the *likelihood* itself (i.e., the probability of observing the data given particular parameter values). However, since this would be a product of numbers (one for each observation) smaller than 1, computers are not precise enough to distinguish the joint probability from zero if the dataset is large. Since logarithms of products are sums of logarithms ($\log(a * b) = \log a + \log b$), the change of scale solves this problem.

If the S_0 guess is right, then β should be around 2.3. We can do a similar check for S_0 (assuming β is 2.3). The grid value associated with the highest likelihood value is 7084.8 (Fig. 3.3), so the original S_0 guess was good but not perfect.

```
betacand = 2.3
S0cand = seq(5920, 8000, length = 101)
ll = rep(NA, length = 101)
for (i in 1:101) {
    ll[i] = llik.cb(S0 = S0cand[i], beta = betacand, I = y)
}
plot(ll ~ S0cand, ylab = "Neg log-lik", xlab = expression(S[0]))
S0cand[which.min(ll)]

## [1] 7084.8
```

---

[9] Section 9.4 will summarize basic likelihood theory in more detail.

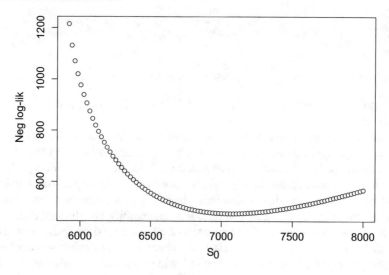

Fig. 3.3: The conditional profile log-likelihood of S_0 for Niamey's district 1 assuming $\beta = 2.3$

For a proper analysis, we minimize the negative log-likelihood by varying both parameters simultaneously. We can do this using the generic `optim` function or the `mle2` function in the `bbmle` package. The `mle2` function not only uses `optim` to find maximum likelihood estimates but also provides confidence intervals, profile likelihoods, and a variety of other useful measures (Bolker, 2008).

```
require(bbmle)
fit = mle2(llik.cb, start = list(S0 = 7085, beta = 2.3),
    method = "Nelder-Mead", data = list(I = y))
summary(fit)

## Maximum likelihood estimation
##
## Call:
## mle2(minuslogl = llik.cb, start = list(S0 = 7085,
##      beta = 2.3), beta = 2), data = list(I = y))
##
## Coefficients:
##          Estimate Std. Error z value      Pr(z)
## S0     7.8158e+03 1.3022e+02  60.019 < 2.2e-16 ***
## beta   1.8931e+00 3.6968e-02  51.209 < 2.2e-16 ***
## ---
## Signif:  0 '***' 0.001 '**' 0.01 '*' 0.05 '.' 0.1 ' ' 1
##
## -2 log L: 841.831

confint(fit)
```

```
## Profiling...
```

```
##              2.5 %        97.5 %
## S0    7577.967212  8088.641095
## beta     1.820943     1.966336
```

So the joint MLE estimates are $S_0 = 7816$ (CI: $\{7578, 8088\}$) and $\beta = 1.89$ (CI: $\{1.82, 1.97\}$).

Applying statistical tools to biological models, like the chain-binomial, can usefully highlight uncertainties due to parametric interdependencies. In the case of a closed epidemic like the measles outbreak considered here, for example, it is conceivable that similar epidemic trajectories can arise from having a large number of initial susceptibles and a low transmission rate or a more moderate number of susceptibles and a higher transmission rate. We can quantify this through considering the correlation matrix among the parameters of our likelihood analysis; vcov calculates their variance–covariance matrix from which we can calculate standard errors according to sqrt(diag(vcov(fit))) and cov2cor converts this to a correlation matrix. As intuition suggested there is a strong negative correlation between the estimates of the β and S_0 parameters.

```
cov2cor(vcov(fit))
```

```
##                 S0         beta
## S0       1.0000000  -0.7444261
## beta    -0.7444261   1.0000000
```

3.5 Stochastic Simulation

The chain-binomial is both a statistical model for estimation and a stochastic model for dynamics. We can thus write a function to simulate dynamics using the estimated parameters.[10] The function takes 3 parameters representing the initial number of susceptibles (S0), the transmission rate (beta), and the initial number of infectious (I0).

```
sim.cb = function(S0, beta, I0) {
    I = I0
    S = S0
    i = 1
    while (!any(I == 0)) {
        i = i + 1
        I[i] = rbinom(1, size = S[i - 1], prob = 1 - exp(-beta *
            I[i - 1]/S0))
        S[i] = S[i - 1] - I[i]
```

---

[10] In contrast to the loop introduced in Sect. 2.4, where the number of iterations is constant and known, the number of epidemic generations may vary among realizations because disease extinction is a stochastic process. We therefore use while instead of for when looping; ! means "not" in R.

```
    }
    out = data.frame(S = S, I = I)
    return(out)
}
```

We can superimpose 100 stochastic simulations on the observed epidemic. The simulations from the chain-binomial model brackets the observed epidemic nicely (Fig. 3.4), suggesting that the model is a reasonable first approximation to the underlying dynamics. We will revisit on this case study in the context of outbreak response vaccination in Sect. 9.8.

```
plot(y, type="n", xlim=c(1,18), ylab="Predicted/observed",
     xlab="Week")
for(i in 1:100){
    sim=sim.cb(S0=floor(coef(fit)["S0"]),
           beta=coef(fit)["beta"], I0=11)
    lines(sim$I, col=grey(.5))
}
points(y, type="b", col=2)
```

3.6 Further Examples

Example 1: The flu dataset represents the number of children confined to bed each day during a 1978 outbreak of the reemerging influenza A/H1N1 strain in a boarding school in North England (Fig. 3.5). This subtype of influenza had been absent from human circulation after the A/H2N2 pandemic of 1957 but reemerged (presumably from some laboratory freezer) in 1977. The school had 763 boys of which 512 boys were confined to bed sometime during the outbreak. None of the boys would have had previous exposure to A/H1N1.

The typical time of illness was 5–7 days. Since the data is the number confined to bed each day, the data is not incidence but a proxy for *prevalence*. The data looks pretty log-linear for the first 5 days. Family studies have been used to estimate the serial interval for flu between two and four days (most between two and three; Cowling et al., 2009; Vink et al., 2014). Volunteer studies show the mean infectious period around 5 days (Carrat et al., 2008).

```
data(flu)
plot(flu$day, flu$cases, type = "b", xlab = "Day", ylab = "sick",
     log = "y")
tail(flu)

##      day cases
## 9      9   192
## 10    10   126
## 11    11    70
## 12    12    28
```

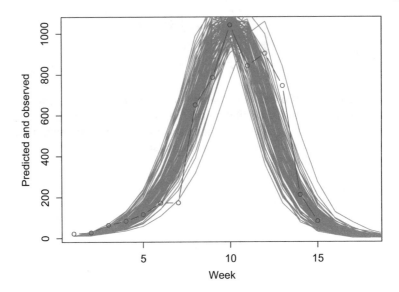

Fig. 3.4: Observed (red) and 100 simulated (gray) epidemics using the chain-binomial model and ML parameters for S_0 and β from Niamey's district 1 data

```
## 13    13        12
## 14    14         5
```

The "fast-and-furious" estimate of R_0 is thus:

```
fit = lm(log(cases) ~ day, subset = day <= 5, data = flu)
r = fit$coef["day"]
V = c(2, 3)
V * r + 1

   ## [1] 3.171884 4.257827
```

This is higher than most estimates of R_0 of pandemic flu (which typically lies in the 1.5–2.5 interval). However, contact rates within a boarding school are likely to be higher than average across human populations as a whole.

Example 2: The CDCs record for the 2014–2015 Ebola outbreak in Sierra Leone is in the ebola dataset. The serial interval for Ebola is estimated at around 15 days with an incubation period of 11 days. The mean time to hospitalization was 5 days and the mean time to death or dismissal was 5 and 11 days, respectively (WHO Ebola Response Team, 2014; White & Pagano, 2008). The data is the back-calculated incidence as the difference of the cumulative cases reported by the CDC. Because of the complexities of reporting and revisions of case load through time,

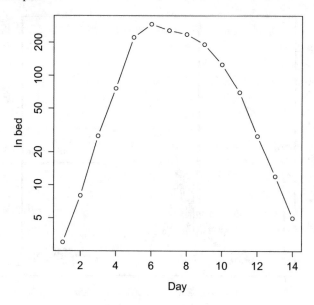

Fig. 3.5: The daily number of children confined to bed (on a log-10 scale) in a boarding school in North England during an outbreak in 1978 of the reemerging A/H1N1 strain

this leads to some negative numbers for certain dates. These are set to zero as a crude fix (Fig. 3.6).

```r
data(ebola)
par(mar = c(5, 5, 2, 5))
plot(ebola$day, ebola$cases, type = "b", xlab = "Week",
    ylab = "Incidence")
par(new = T)
plot(ebola$day, ebola$cum_cases, type = "l", col = "red",
    axes = FALSE, xlab = NA, ylab = NA, log = "y")
axis(side = 4)
mtext(side = 4, line = 4, "Cumulative incidence")
legend("right", legend = c("Cases", "Cumulative"), lty = c(1,
    1), pch = c(1, NA), col = c("black", "red"))
tail(ebola)

##           date day cum_cases cases
## 98      7/8/15 468     13945    34
## 99     7/15/15 475     13982    37
## 100    7/22/15 482     14001    19
## 101    7/29/15 489     14061    60
## 102     8/5/15 496     14089    28
## 103    8/12/15 503     14122    33
```

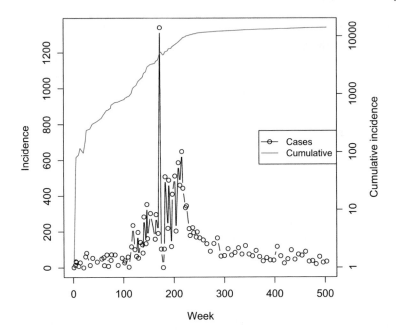

Fig. 3.6: Incidence and cumulative incidence of Ebola during the 2014–2015 outbreak in Sierra Leone

We first use the regression method with Lipsitch's correction:

```
fit = lm(log(cum_cases) ~ day, subset = day < 100, data = ebola)
r = fit$coef["day"]
V = 15
f = 0.5
V * r + 1 + f * (1 - f) * (V * r)^2

  ##        day
  ## 1.698811
```

We next aggregate the data in 2 week increments roughly corresponding to the serial interval, so we can apply the removal method.

```
# Data aggregation
cases = sapply(split(ebola$cases, floor((ebola$day - 0.1)/14)),
    sum)
sum(cases)

  ## [1] 14721
```

```
# Removal MLE
fit = mle2(llik.cb, start = list(S0 = 20000, beta = 2),
    method = "Nelder-Mead", data = list(I = cases))
```

```
summary(fit)

  ## Maximum likelihood estimation
  ##
  ## Call:
  ## mle2(minuslogl = llik.cb, start = list(S0 = 20000,
  ##     beta = 2), data = list(I = cases))
  ##
  ## Coefficients:
  ##          Estimate Std. Error    z value      Pr(z)
  ## S0    2.7731e+04 2.5949e-07 1.0687e+11 < 2.2e-16 ***
  ## beta  1.4237e+00 1.1783e-02 1.2083e+02 < 2.2e-16 ***
  ## ---
  ## Signif:   0 '***' 0.001 '**' 0.01 '*' 0.05 '.' 0.1 ' ' 1
  ##
  ## -2 log L: 5546.683
```

Because of the difference in magnitude of the estimates of S_0 (in the ten thousands) and R_0 (around 1.4), the numerical method used to calculate confidence intervals struggles, so we need to suggest starting standard errors for the confint function.

```
confint(fit, std.err = c(100, 0.1))

## Profiling...

  ##              2.5 %       97.5 %
  ## S0    26393.579452 29287.725327
  ## beta      1.384683     1.463184
```

The removal and Lipsitch methods provide comparable estimates that are somewhat lower than those concluded by more elaborate analyses by the WHO team for the Sierra Leone outbreak (WHO Ebola Response Team, 2014). The meaning of S_0 from this analysis is a bit amorphous because Sierra Leone is a country of 8M people virtually none of which were likely to have been exposed to EBOV previous to the 2014 outbreak. Probably the best way to think of it is as under the chain-binomial assumptions this is the most plausible number of people within the eventual sphere of spread of the virus across the country. Some such considerations should become more clear in the discussions of spatial and social networks in Chaps. 12 and 14.

Example 3: The ferrari dataset holds the incidence data for a number of outbreaks—Ebola DRC '95, Ebola Uganda '00, SARS Hong Kong '03, SARS Singapore '03, Hog Cholera Netherlands '97 and Foot-and-mouth UK '00—aggregated by disease-specific serial intervals (Table 3.1; Ferrari et al., 2005). As a further example we can look at the DRC Ebola outbreak in Kikwit, Democratic Republic of Congo between January and June 1995.

Disease	Serial interval	Location	Year
Ebola	14d	DRC	1995
		Uganda	2000
SARS	5d	Hong Kong	2003
		Singapore	2003
Hog cholera	7d	Netherlands	1997
FMD	21d	UK	2000

Table 3.1: Serial interval for each outbreak in the `ferrari` dataset

```
names(ferrari)
```

```
## [1] "Eboladeaths00" "Ebolacases00"  "Ebolacases95"
## [4] "FMDfarms"      "HogCholera"    "SarsHk"      "SarsSing"
```

```
ferrari$Ebolacases95
```

```
## [1]   4   6   5  18  36  99  40  17   4   1 NA NA NA NA NA
```

```
sum(ferrari$Ebolacases95, na.rm = TRUE)
```

```
## [1] 230
```

```
y = c(na.omit(ferrari$Ebolacases95))
```

The number of initial susceptibles must be larger than the summed incidence, so we make an initial guess of 300.

```
fit = mle2(llik.cb, method = "Nelder-Mead", start = list(S0 = 300,
    beta = 2), data = list(I = y))
fit
```

```
##
## Call:
## mle2(minuslogl = llik.cb, start = list(S0 = 300,
##     beta = 2), data = list(I = y))
##
## Coefficients:
##          S0       beta
## 241.118108    3.181465
##
## Log-likelihood: -48.3
```

```
confint(fit, std.err = 2)
```

```
## Profiling...
##             2.5 %      97.5 %
## S0     233.973778 254.051292
## beta     2.692505   3.718357
```

The estimated R_0 is 3.2. It thus appears that the Ebola outbreak in DRC in 1995 was more explosive than in Sierra Leone in 2014. This could be due to aggregation across a larger geographic area for the latter and/or the more intensive public health interventions. The interpretation of the S_0 estimate, here, is a bit easier; Kikwit is a city of almost 500k inhabitants, but by early May 1995 most cases were isolated in a quarantine ward of the Kikwit central hospital. In the removal estimator, S_0 is again accommodating overall social clique size within the sphere of spread. Perhaps the best way to think of the S_0 parameter when applied to data from larger areas is as a flexible accommodation to best use all available data to estimate the reproduction number.

We will revisit on R_0 calculations for the DRC outbreak using the next-generation matrix method in Sect. 3.10.

3.7 R_0 from S(E)IR Flows

As discussed in Sect. 2.2, $R_0 = \beta/(\gamma + \mu)$ for the simple SIR model. This is the correct quantity assuming that the force of infection (the rate at which susceptibles are infected) is $\beta I/N$, there is no latent period and no disease-induced mortality, so the index case is expected to be infectious for a period of $1/(\gamma + \mu)$ time units during which it will transmit at a rate of $\beta * N/N$. The numerator comes about because all the N individuals in the population are by definition susceptible when we consider the basic reproduction number, and thus initial $S = N$.

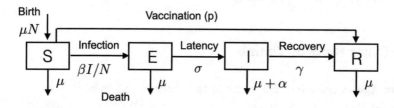

Fig. 3.7: The SEIR flow diagram. Apart from vaccination, parameters represent per capita rates of flow from the donor compartment. Vaccination is assumed to be a fraction of children vaccinated at birth

Different SIR-like flows will produce different quantifications of R_0, but we can use the same logic for all linear flows. Consider, for example, the case when infections have a latent period leading to the SEIR model (Fig. 3.7) of the flow of hosts between **S**usceptible, **E**xposed (but not yet infectious), **I**nfectious, and **R**emoved (either recovered with immunity or dead) compartments in a randomly mixing population:

$$\frac{dS}{dt} = \underbrace{\mu N(1-p)}_{\text{recruitment}} - \underbrace{\beta I \frac{S}{N}}_{\text{infected}} - \underbrace{\mu S}_{\text{dead}} \qquad (3.3)$$

$$\frac{dE}{dt} = \underbrace{\beta I \frac{S}{N}}_{\text{infected}} - \underbrace{\sigma E}_{\text{infectious}} - \underbrace{\mu I}_{\text{dead}} \tag{3.4}$$

$$\frac{dI}{dt} = \underbrace{\sigma E}_{\text{infectious}} - \underbrace{\gamma I}_{\text{recovered}} - \underbrace{(\mu + \alpha)I}_{\text{dead}} \tag{3.5}$$

$$\frac{dR}{dt} = \underbrace{\gamma I}_{\text{recovered}} - \underbrace{\mu R}_{\text{dead}} + \underbrace{\mu Np}_{\text{vaccinated}} . \tag{3.6}$$

Here susceptibles are assumed either vaccinated at birth (fraction p) or infected at a rate $\beta I/N$. Infected individuals will remain in the latent class for an average period of $1/(\sigma + \mu)$ and subsequently (if they escape natural mortality at a rate μ) enter the infectious class for an average time of $1/(\gamma + \mu + \alpha)$; α is the *rate* of disease-induced mortality (*not* case fatality rate). By the rules of competing rates (Sect. 3.2), the case fatality rate is $\alpha/(\gamma + \mu + \alpha)$ because during the time an individual is expected to remain in the infectious class the disease is killing at a rate α. By a similar logic, the probability of recovering with immunity (for life in the case of the SEIR model) is $\gamma/(\gamma + \mu + \alpha)$. Putting all these pieces together and assuming no vaccination, the expected number of secondary cases in a completely susceptible population is the probability of making it through latent stage without dying * expected infectious period * transmission rate while infectious. Thus, $R_0 = \frac{\sigma}{\sigma + \mu} \frac{1}{\gamma + \mu + \alpha} \frac{\beta N}{N} = \frac{\sigma}{\sigma + \mu} \frac{\beta}{\gamma + \mu + \alpha}$.

3.8 Other Rules of Thumb

Mean Age of Infection: For endemic fully immunizing infections in a constant-sized host population, R_0 is related to mean age of infection, $\bar{a}$, according to $R_0 \simeq 1 + L/\bar{a}$, where L is the life expectancy of the host (e.g., Dietz & Schenzle, 1985). This rule of thumb is often used in conjunction with seroprevalence-by-age profiles to get estimates of R_0. Chapter 5 discusses age-incidence patterns in more detail.

Final Epidemic Size: In principle, the reproduction number can be estimated from the final epidemic size according to the equations discussed in Sect. 2.4. If there is some preexisting immunity and there is homogeneous mixing, then R_0 can be quantified according to $\frac{\log(s_0) - \log(s_\infty)}{s_0 - s_\infty}$, where s_0 and s_∞ are the fractions of the population that is susceptible at the beginning and end of the epidemic, respectively (Heesterbeek & Dietz, 1996). However, this is unlikely to be very reliable because the final epidemic size calculations assume that the epidemic is progressing according to the deterministic model (and all its assumptions) including no changes in host behavior in the face of the epidemic (Funk et al., 2010). For example, Ebola is thought to have an R_0 in the 2–3.5 range, which is what lead CDC to warn that the West-African outbreak could result in millions of cases. In the end, the total number of cases in Guinea, Liberia, and Sierra Leone was a far lower number, around 25,000, because of extensive public health interventions and changes to dangerous contacts and funeral practices. The outbreak of a novel coronavirus in 2020 saw extensive changes to behavior through movement bans within 4 weeks of recognition of the pathogen (e.g., Tian et al., 2020; Inglesby, 2020). Interventions and social distancing will thus generally stop epidemics reaching their logical conclusion based on the R_0. Bjørnstad et al. (2020a) provide a web-based interactive shinyApp to study how social distancing and vaccination affect the shape of an SIR epidemic.

For certain common infections like seasonal influenza, the rule of thumb regarding the final epidemic size may hold; the historical annual attack rate for the flu is around 10–15%, which is probably close to that expected from its R_0 (around 1.5–2) and the typical fraction of susceptibles of around 25% (prevaccination, assuming immunity following infection lasting around 4 years; Koelle et al., 2006).

Contact Tracing: Contact tracing can provide direct estimates of R_0. Blumberg and Lloyd-Smith (2013a) showed that this together with size distributions of subcritical transmission chains can provide estimates in important low R_0 ("subcritical") settings, such as human monkey pox in the face of eroding smallpox herd immunity. They estimated the human-to-human reproduction number to be 0.32. Given that the smallpox vaccine is likely to be cross-protective against monkey pox, the worry is that this effective reproduction number will increase over time since smallpox vaccination is no longer carried out. Contact tracing was also used to estimate R_0 during the early spread of SARS during the 2003 outbreak (Riley et al., 2003). The type of branching process models used by, for example, Lloyd-Smith et al. (2005) and Blumberg and Lloyd-Smith (2013a) will be discussed further in Sect. 15.2.

De et al. (2004) did a contact tracing study of the spread of gonorrhea across a sexual network in Alberta, Canada. The directional transmission graph among the 89 individuals is in the gonnet dataset. The initial cluster of 17 cases all frequented the same bar, each infected between 0 and 7 other partners with 2.17 as the average. The subsequent infections, in turn, infected between 0 and 6 partners with an average of 0.62. The drop is (i) due to the sexual network being depleted of susceptibles and (ii) because infection across heterogenous networks will differentially infect individuals according to their number of contacts (Ferrari et al., 2006a). Epidemics across social networks is the topic of Chap. 14, and we will revisit on this network therein. The statnet package has great tools for visualizing chains of transmission on networks (Fig. 3.8).

```
require(statnet)
data(gonnet)
nwt = network(gonnet, directed = TRUE)
plot(nwt, vertex.col = c(0, rep(1, 17), rep(2, 71)))
```

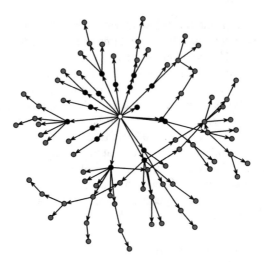

Fig. 3.8: Network of spread of gonorrhea as studied by De et al. (2004). The initial 17 cases (in black) frequented the same bar (white) were ultimately responsible for a cluster of 89 cases identified through contact tracing

3.9 Advanced: The Next-Generation Matrix

For epidemics that are not simple linear chains, it is less straightforward to calculate R_0 from parameterized models using the "logical method." The next-generation matrix is the general approach that works for all compartmental models of any complexity (Diekmann et al., 1990). It is done in a sequence of steps:

1. Identify all n infected compartments.
2. Construct an $n \times 1$ matrix, **F**, that contains expressions for all *completely new* infections entering each infected compartment.
3. Construct an $n \times 1$ matrix, $\mathbf{V}^-$, that contains expressions for all losses out of each infected compartment.
4. Construct an $n \times 1$ matrix, $\mathbf{V}^+$, that contains expressions for all gains into each infected compartment that does *not* represent *new* infections but transfers among infected classes.
5. Construct an $n \times 1$ matrix, $\mathbf{V} = \mathbf{V}^- - \mathbf{V}^+$.
6. Generate two $n \times n$ Jacobian matrices, **f** and **v**, that are the partial derivatives of **F** and **V** with respect to the n infectious state variables.
7. Evaluate the matrices at the disease free equilibrium (dfe).
8. Finally, R_0 is the greatest eigenvalue of $\mathbf{f}\mathbf{v}^{-1}|_{dfe}$.

This is quite an elaborate scheme, so we will try it out first for the SEIR model for which we already know the answer. Unfortunately, R is not naturally designed to do vectorized *symbolic* calculations, so we need to do this, one matrix element at a time.[11] Chapter 2 introduced how to use `quote` to do symbolic differentiation in R. The `substitute` function allows for some simple symbolic additional manipulations.

STEP 1: Infected classes are E and I; let us label them 1 and 2. STEP 2: All new infections: $dE/dt = \beta SI/N, dI/dt = 0$

```
F1 = quote(beta * S * I/N)
F2 = 0
```

STEP 3: All losses: $dE/dt = (\mu + \sigma)E, dI/dt = (\mu + \alpha + \gamma)I$

```
Vm1 = quote(mu * E + sigma * E)
Vm2 = quote(mu * I + alpha * I + gamma * I)
```

STEP 4 : All gained transfers: $dE/dt = 0, dI/dt = (\sigma)E$

```
Vp1 = 0
Vp2 = quote(sigma * E)
```

STEP 5: Subtract Vp from Vm

```
V1 = substitute(a - b, list(a = Vm1, b = Vp1))
V2 = substitute(a - b, list(a = Vm2, b = Vp2))
```

STEP 6: Generate the partial derivatives for the two Jacobians

```
f11 = D(F1, "E")
f12 = D(F1, "I")
f21 = D(F2, "E")
f22 = D(F2, "I")

v11 = D(V1, "E")
v12 = D(V1, "I")
v21 = D(V2, "E")
v22 = D(V2, "I")
```

STEP 7: Assuming N=1, the disease free equilibrium (dfe) is $S = 1, E = 0, I = 0$, $R = 0$. We also need values for other parameters. Assuming a weekly time step and something chickenpox-like, we may use $\mu = 0, \alpha = 0, \beta = 5, \gamma = 0.8, \sigma = 1.2$, and $N = 1$.

```
paras = list(S = 1, E = 0, I = 0, R = 0, mu = 0, alpha = 0,
    beta = 5, gamma = 0.8, sigma = 1.2, N = 1)
f = with(paras, matrix(c(eval(f11), eval(f12), eval(f21),
    eval(f22)), nrow = 2, byrow = TRUE))
v = with(paras, matrix(c(eval(v11), eval(v12), eval(v21),
    eval(v22)), nrow = 2, byrow = TRUE))
```

---

[11] Though Sect. 3.10 will introduce a `nextgenR0` function that shows how it is possible to do calculations more compactly using a `list` of equations and some acrobatic combinations of D, `lapply`, and `attr`.

STEP 8: Calculate the largest eigenvalue of $f \times$ inverse(v). The function for invert-
ing matrices in R is `solve`.

```
max(eigen(f %*% solve(v))$values)
```

```
  ## [1] 6.25
```

Let us check that the next-generation method and the logical method are in agreement recalling that for the SEIR flow $R_0 = \frac{\sigma}{\sigma+\mu} \frac{\beta}{\gamma+\mu+\alpha}$.

```
with(paras, sigma/(sigma + mu) * beta/(gamma + mu + alpha))
```

```
  ## [1] 6.25
```

3.10 SEIHFR

Legrand et al. (2007) form the foundation for many of the recent Ebola models. The
model has five compartments corresponding to Susceptible, Exposed, Infectious in
community, infectious in Hospital, dead but not yet buried (at Funeral rites), and
Removed (either buried or immune). The model is more complex than previous
compartmental models and cannot be represented by a simple linear chain (Fig. 3.9).
The parameterization used here is motivated by the original formulation by Legrand
et al. (2007), but the notation conforms to the other sections of this book; each
infectious compartment contributes to the force of infection through their individual

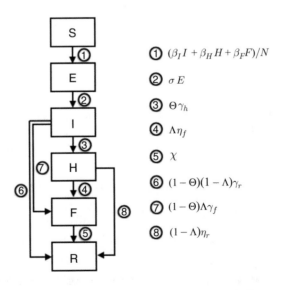

Fig. 3.9: The SEIHFR flow diagram for Ebola dynamics

Table 3.2: Parameters for Legrand et al. (2007)'s Ebola model using the data from the 1995 DRC epidemic

Parameter	Meaning	Value
N	Population size	
$1/\sigma$	Incubation period	7d
$1/\gamma_h$	Onset to hospitalization	5d
$1/\gamma_f$	Onset to death	9.6d
$1/\gamma_r$	Onset to recovery	10d
$1/\eta_f$	Hospitalization to death	4.6d
$1/\eta_r$	Hospitalization to recovery	5d
$1/\chi$	Death to burial	2d
Θ	Proportion hospitalized	80%
Λ	Case fatality ratio	81%
β_i	Transmission rate in community	0.588
β_h	Transmission rate in hospital	0.794
β_f	Transmission rate at funeral	7.653

For clarity lowercase Greek are rates and uppercase are probabilities/fractions

βs. There are two branching points in the flow: the hospitalization of a fraction Θ of the infectious cases after an average time of $1/\gamma_h$ days following onset of symptoms and the death of a fraction Λ of the I and H classes after an average time of $1/\gamma_f$ days and $1/\eta_f$ days, respectively. For the 1995 DRC outbreak, Legrand et al. (2007) assumed that hospitalization affected transmission rates but not duration of infection or probability of dying. Model parameters are given in Table 3.2, and the model equations are

$$\frac{dS}{dt} = -\underbrace{(\beta_i I + \beta_h H + \beta_f F)S/N}_{\text{transmission}} \tag{3.7}$$

$$\frac{dE}{dt} = \underbrace{(\beta_i I + \beta_h H + \beta_f F)S/N}_{\text{transmission}} - \underbrace{\sigma E}_{\text{end of latency}} \tag{3.8}$$

$$\frac{dI}{dt} = \sigma E - \underbrace{\Theta \gamma_h I}_{\text{hospitalization}} - \underbrace{(1-\Theta)(1-\Lambda)\gamma_r I}_{\text{recovery}} - \underbrace{(1-\Theta)\Lambda \gamma_f I}_{\text{death}} \tag{3.9}$$

$$\frac{dH}{dt} = \underbrace{\Theta \gamma_h I}_{\text{hospitalization}} - \underbrace{\Lambda \eta_f H}_{\text{death}} - \underbrace{(1-\Lambda)\eta_r H}_{\text{recovery}} \tag{3.10}$$

$$\frac{dF}{dt} = \underbrace{(1-\Theta)(1-\Lambda)\gamma_r I + \Lambda \eta_f H}_{\text{dead}} - \underbrace{\chi F}_{\text{burial}} \tag{3.11}$$

$$\frac{dR}{dt} = \underbrace{(1-\Theta)(1-\Lambda)\gamma_r I + (1-\Lambda)\eta_r H}_{\text{recovered}} + \underbrace{\chi F}_{\text{buried}} . \tag{3.12}$$

There are four infected compartments (E, I, H, and F), thus $\mathbf{F}$, $\mathbf{V}^-$, and $\mathbf{V}^+$ will be 4×1 matrices, and $\mathbf{f}$ and $\mathbf{v}$ will be 4×4 matrices.

STEP 1: Infected classes are E, I, H, and F; let us label them 1–4.

STEP 2: All new infections: $dE/dt = \beta SI/N$, $dI/dt = 0$, $dH/dt = 0$, $dF/dt = 0$

```
F1 = quote(betai * S * I/N + betah * S * H/N + betaf *
     S * F/N)
F2 = 0
F3 = 0
F4 = 0
```

STEP 3: All losses

```
Vm1 = quote(sigma * E)
Vm2 = quote(Theta * gammah * I + (1 - Theta) * (1 - Lambda) *
      gammar * I + (1 - Theta) * Lambda * gammaf * I)
Vm3 = quote(Lambda * etaf * H + (1 - Lambda) * etar *
      H)
Vm4 = quote(chi * F)
```

STEP 4: All gained transfers

```
Vp1 = 0
Vp2 = quote(sigma * E)
Vp3 = quote(Theta * gammah * I)
Vp4 = quote((1 - Theta) * (1 - Lambda) * gammar * I +
      Lambda * etaf * H)
```

STEP 5: Subtract Vp from Vm

```
V1 = substitute(a - b, list(a = Vm1, b = Vp1))
V2 = substitute(a - b, list(a = Vm2, b = Vp2))
V3 = substitute(a - b, list(a = Vm3, b = Vp3))
V4 = substitute(a - b, list(a = Vm4, b = Vp4))
```

STEP 6: Generate the partial derivatives for the two Jacobians

```
f11 = D(F1, "E"); f12 = D(F1, "I"); f13 = D(F1, "H")
     f14 = D(F1, "F")
f21 = D(F2, "E"); f22 = D(F2, "I"); f23 = D(F2, "H")
     f24 = D(F2, "F")
f31 = D(F3, "E"); f32 = D(F3, "I"); f33 = D(F3, "H")
     f34 = D(F3, "F")
f41 = D(F4, "E"); f42 = D(F4, "I"); f43 = D(F4, "H")
     f44 = D(F4, "F")

v11 = D(V1, "E"); v12 = D(V1, "I"); v13 = D(V1, "H")
     v14 = D(V1, "F")
v21 = D(V2, "E"); v22 = D(V2, "I"); v23 = D(V2, "H")
     v24 = D(V2, "F")
v31 = D(V3, "E"); v32 = D(V3, "I"); v33 = D(V3, "H")
     v34 = D(V3, "F")
v41 = D(V4, "E"); v42 = D(V4, "I"); v43 = D(V4, "H")
     v44 = D(V4, "F")
```

STEP 7: Disease free equilibrium: the dfe is $S = 1, E = 0, I = 0, H = 0, F = 0, R = 0$.
We also need values for other parameters. We use the estimates from the DRC 1995
outbreak scaled as weekly rates from tables and appendices of Legrand et al. (2007).

```
gammah = 1/5 * 7
gammaf = 1/9.6 * 7
gammar = 1/10 * 7
chi = 1/2 * 7
etaf = 1/4.6 * 7
etar = 1/5 * 7
paras = list(S = 1, E = 0, I = 0, H = 0, F = 0, R = 0,
    sigma = 1/7 * 7, Theta = 0.81, Lambda = 0.81, betai = 0.588,
    betah = 0.794, betaf = 7.653, N = 1, gammah = gammah,
    gammaf = gammaf, gammar = gammar, etaf = etaf, etar = etar,
    chi = chi)

f = with(paras, matrix(c(eval(f11), eval(f12), eval(f13),
        eval(f14), eval(f21), eval(f22), eval(f23), eval(f24),
        eval(f31), eval(f32), eval(f33), eval(f34), eval(f41),
        eval(f42), eval(f43), eval(f44)), nrow = 4, byrow = T))

v = with(paras, matrix(c(eval(v11), eval(v12), eval(v13),
        eval(v14), eval(v21), eval(v22), eval(v23), eval(v24),
        eval(v31), eval(v32), eval(v33), eval(v34), eval(v41),
        eval(v42), eval(v43), eval(v44)), nrow = 4, byrow = T))
```

STEP 8: Calculate the largest eigenvalue of $f \times \text{inverse}(v)$

```
max(eigen(f %*% solve(v))$values)

## [1] 2.582429
```

3.11 A Next-Generation R_0 Function

Among programmers in general and R enthusiasts in particular, there is often a
bizarre obsession with compact "elegant" code (where elegant usually translates
to incomprehensible). While developing this text, I wasted a day of work finding
that for the SEIR model steps 6–8 can also be done with:

```
Flist = c(F1, F2)
f1 = lapply(lapply(Flist, deriv, "E"), eval, paras)
f2 = lapply(lapply(Flist, deriv, "I"), eval, paras)
f = matrix(c(attr(f1[[1]], "gradient")[1, ], attr(f1[[2]],
    "gradient")[1, ], attr(f2[[1]], "gradient")[1, ],
    attr(f2[[2]], "gradient")[1, ]), nrow = 2)
Vlist = c(V1, V2)
v1 = lapply(lapply(Vlist, deriv, "E"), eval, paras)
v2 = lapply(lapply(Vlist, deriv, "I"), eval, paras)
v = matrix(c(attr(v1[[1]], "gradient")[1, ], attr(v1[[2]],
```

```
    "gradient")[1, ], attr(v2[[1]], "gradient")[1, ],
    attr(v2[[2]], "gradient")[1, ]), nrow = 2)
max(eigen(f %*% solve(v))$values)
```

```
## [1] 6.25
```

The utility of this is that it leads to a general-purpose function nextgenR0 to do the final calculations for arbitrarily complex compartmental flows that takes five arguments:

1. Istates is a vector naming all Infected classes.
2. Flist is a list that contains equations (as quotes) for completely new infections entering each infected compartment for each class.
3. Vlist is a list that contains the equations (as quotes) for losses out of each infected compartment minus the equations (as quotes) for all gains into each infected compartment that does not represent new infections but transfers among infectious classes.
4. parameters is a labeled vector of parameters.
5. dfe is a labeled vector of all states at the disease free equilibrium.

```
nextgenR0 = function(Istates, Flist, Vlist, parameters, dfe) {
    paras = as.list(c(dfe, paras))
    k = 0
    vl = fl = list(NULL)
    for(i in 1:length(Istates)) {
        assign(paste("f", i, sep = "."), lapply(lapply(Flist,
            deriv, Istates[i]), eval, paras))
        assign(paste("v", i, sep = "."), lapply(lapply(Vlist,
            deriv, Istates[i]), eval, paras))
        for(j in 1:length(Istates)){
            k=k+1
            fl[[k]] = attr(eval(as.name(paste("f", i,
                sep = ".")))[[j]], "gradient")[1, ]
            vl[[k]] = attr(eval(as.name(paste("v", i,
                sep = ".")))[[j]], "gradient")[1, ]
        }
    }
    f = matrix(as.numeric(as.matrix(fl)[ ,1]),
        ncol = length(Istates))
    v = matrix(as.numeric(as.matrix(vl)[ ,1]),
        ncol = length(Istates))
    R0 = max(eigen(f %*% solve(v))$values)
    return(R0)
}
```

For the SEIHFR model, the modified calculations are:

```
istates=c("E", "I", "H", "F")

flist=c(dEdt=quote(betai * S * I / N +
```

```
        betah * S * H / N + betaf * S * F / N),
        dIdt = quote(0), dHdt = quote(0), dFdt = quote(0))

Vm1 = quote(sigma * E)
Vm2 = quote(Theta * gammah * I + (1 - Theta) * (1 -
    Lambda) * gammar * I + (1 - Theta) * Lambda *
    gammaf * I)
Vm3 = quote(Lambda * etaf * H + (1 - Lambda) * etar * H)
Vm4 = quote(chi * F)

Vp1 = 0
Vp2 = quote(sigma * E)
Vp3 = quote(Theta * gammah * I)
Vp4 = quote((1 - Theta) * (1 - Lambda) * gammar * I +
    Lambda * etaf * H)

vlist = c(substitute(a - b, list(a = Vm1, b = Vp1)),
    substitute(a - b, list(a = Vm2, b = Vp2)),
    substitute(a - b, list(a = Vm3, b = Vp3)),
    substitute(a - b, list(a = Vm4, b = Vp4)))

df = list(S = 1,E = 0, I = 0, H = 0, F = 0,R = 0)

paras=c(sigma = 1/7*7, Theta = 0.81, Lambda = 0.81,
    betai = 0.588, betah = 0.794, betaf = 7.653, N = 1,
    gammah = 1/5 * 7, gammaf = 1/9.6 * 7, gammar = 1/10 * 7,
    etaf = 1/4.6 * 7, etar = 1/5 * 7, chi = 1/2 * 7)

nextgenR0(Istates = istates, Flist = flist, Vlist = vlist,
    parameters=paras, dfe=df)

## [1] 2.582429
```

3.12 A Two-Strain shinyApp

Section 3.1 alluded to how strains that elicit cross-immunity R_0 determine their competitive dominance. This is a plausible explanation for why there were historically very few cases of monkey pox, but increasing incidence in West and Central Africa in recent decades after small pox was eradicated and vaccination seized (Rimoin et al., 2010). A parallel question is whether canine distemper virus may begin to circulate in humans if measles is eradicated and mass vaccination is stopped (Yoshikawa et al., 1989); just like many pox viruses, morbilliviruses induce cross-protective immunity and recent data indicates substantial infection of cattle by the pest-de-petite-ruminant virus (PPRV) in goat/sheep endemic areas following rinderpest eradication (Herzog et al., 2019). The historical decline of leprosy caused by *Mycobacteria leprae* long before antibiotics has been suggested to be related to immune-mediated interactions with the more transmissible Tb causing *M. tuber-*

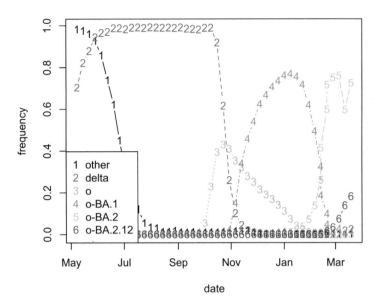

Fig. 3.10: Variant replacement during the second year (2021–2022) of the SARS-CoV-2 pandemic. "Other" represents wild type plus alpha through gamma. The other traces represent delta and the various surging omicron variants

culosis (Lietman et al., 1997; Donoghue et al., 2005). The "variant" displacement dynamics currently being played out by SARS-CoV-2 is a striking contemporary example. The `variant` dataset represents the time series of variant dominance between May 2021 and March 2022 (Fig. 3.10):

```
data(variants)
matplot(variants$date, variants[, 2:7], type = "b",
    xlab = "date", ylab = "frequency")
legend("bottomleft", legend = c("other", "delta", "o",
    "o-BA.1", "o-BA.2", "o-BA.2.12"), pch = as.character(1:6),
    col = 1:6, bg = "white")
```

The extended two-strain SIR model to cover various scenarios of cross-immunity whereby prior infection by one strain may reduce shedding (Θ) or susceptibility (Ξ) of another is detailed below.[12] The extended model also allows for the possibility that a fraction ($1 - \Pi$) of the hosts becomes completely immune following primary exposure by either strain (Fig. 3.11). A simple strategic model that assumes no co-infections is:

---

[12] Note: There are only so many Greek symbols, so the Θ in Fig. 3.11 has a different meaning than in the model of Eqs. (3.7)–(3.12) and Fig. 3.9.

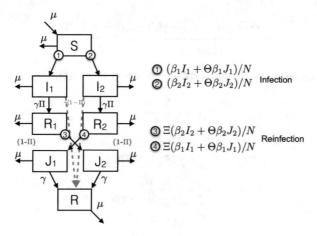

Fig. 3.11: The flowchart for a competing two-strain SIR model assuming no co-infections

$$\frac{dS}{dt} = \underbrace{\mu N}_{\text{birth}} - \underbrace{\mu S}_{\text{death}} - \underbrace{\frac{\beta_1 S I_1}{N}}_{1° \text{ infection by 1}} - \underbrace{\frac{\beta_2 S I_2}{N}}_{1° \text{ infection by 2}} \tag{3.13}$$

$$\frac{dI_1}{dt} = \underbrace{\frac{\beta_1 S I_1}{N}}_{1° \text{ infection by 1}} - \underbrace{\gamma I_1}_{\text{recovery 1}} - \underbrace{\mu I_1}_{\text{death}} \tag{3.14}$$

$$\frac{dI_2}{dt} = \underbrace{\frac{\beta_2 S I_2}{N}}_{1° \text{ infection by 2}} - \underbrace{\gamma I_2}_{\text{recovery 2}} - \underbrace{\mu I_2}_{\text{death}} \tag{3.15}$$

$$\frac{dR_1}{dt} = \underbrace{\Pi \gamma I_1}_{\text{susceptible to 2}} - \underbrace{\frac{(\beta_2 I_2 + \Theta \beta_2 J_2)\Xi R_1}{N}}_{2° \text{ infection by 2}} - \underbrace{\mu R_1}_{\text{death}} \tag{3.16}$$

$$\frac{dR_2}{dt} = \underbrace{\Pi \gamma I_2}_{\text{susceptible to 1}} - \underbrace{\frac{(\beta_1 I_1 + \Theta \beta_1 J_1)\Xi R_2}{N}}_{2° \text{ infection by 1}} - \underbrace{\mu R_2}_{\text{death}} \tag{3.17}$$

$$\frac{dJ_1}{dt} = \underbrace{\frac{(\beta_1 I_1 + \Theta \beta_1 J_1)\Xi R_2}{N}}_{2° \text{ infection by 1}} - \underbrace{\gamma J_1}_{\text{recovery}} - \underbrace{\mu J_1}_{\text{death}} \tag{3.18}$$

$$\frac{dJ_2}{dt} = \underbrace{\frac{(\beta_2 I_2 + \Theta \beta_2 J_2)\Xi R_1}{N}}_{2° \text{ infection by 2}} - \underbrace{\gamma J_2}_{\text{recovery}} - \underbrace{\mu J_2}_{\text{death}} \tag{3.19}$$

$$\frac{dR}{dt} = \underbrace{(1 - \Pi)\gamma(I_1 + I_2) + \gamma(J_1 + J_2)}_{\text{immune}} - \underbrace{\mu R}_{\text{death}} . \tag{3.20}$$

In the absence of a competitor, the R_0 and endemic equilibrium of strain 1 are:

$$R_{0,1} = \frac{\beta}{\gamma + \mu} \frac{N}{N} \tag{3.21}$$

$$S_1^* = 1/R_0 \tag{3.22}$$

$$I_1^* = \mu(R_0 - 1)/\beta \tag{3.23}$$

$$R_1^* = \frac{\gamma I_1^*}{(1 - \Pi) + mu} \tag{3.24}$$

$$R^* = (1 - \Pi) * R_1^*/\mu. \tag{3.25}$$

The invasion equations for a second strain are:

$$\frac{dS}{dt} = \underbrace{\mu N}_{\text{birth}} - \underbrace{\mu S}_{\text{death}} - \underbrace{\frac{\beta_1 S I_1^*}{N}}_{1° \text{ infection by } 1} - \underbrace{\frac{\beta_2 S I_2}{N}}_{1° \text{ infection by } 2} \tag{3.26}$$

$$\frac{dI_2}{dt} = \underbrace{\frac{\beta_2 S I_2}{N}}_{1° \text{ infection by } 2} - \underbrace{\gamma I_2}_{\text{recovery } 2} - \underbrace{\mu I_2}_{\text{death}} \tag{3.27}$$

$$\frac{dR_2}{dt} = \underbrace{\Pi \gamma I_2}_{\text{susceptible to } 1} - \underbrace{\frac{(\beta_1 I_1^* + \Theta \beta_1 J_1) \Xi R_2}{N}}_{2° \text{ infection by } 1} - \underbrace{\mu R_2}_{\text{death}} \tag{3.28}$$

$$\frac{dJ_2}{dt} = \underbrace{\frac{\beta_2 I_2 \Xi R_1^*}{N}}_{2° \text{ infection by } 2} - \underbrace{\gamma J_2}_{\text{recovery}} - \underbrace{\mu J_2}_{\text{death}} \tag{3.29}$$

$$\frac{dR}{dt} = \underbrace{(1 - \Pi)\gamma(I_1^* + I_2) + \gamma(J_1^8 + J_2)}_{\text{immune}} - \underbrace{\mu R}_{\text{death}} \tag{3.30}$$

$$R_{0,2} = \frac{\beta_2}{\gamma + \mu} \tag{3.31}$$

$$Q_{0,2} = \frac{\beta_2}{\gamma + \mu} \frac{S^*}{N} + \frac{\Xi \beta_2 R_1^* I_2}{N(\gamma + \mu)}. \tag{3.32}$$

The R_0s represents the single-strain situations and the $Q_{0,2}$ is the invasion number of strain 2 assuming strain 1 is at its endemic equilibrium $\{S_1^*, I_1^*, R_1^*\}$. The doubling time of the invader is $T_d = \frac{\log(2)}{\log(Q_0)/(\gamma + \mu)}$ by the logic that during disease invasion the doubling time is $\log(2)/r$ where $r = \log(R_E)/\text{serial interval}$. The coded gradient functions for Eqs. (3.13)–(3.20) are:

```
twostrain = function(t, y, parameters) {
    S = ifelse(y[1] < 0, 0, y[1])
    I1 = ifelse(y[2] < 0, 0, y[2])
    I2 = ifelse(y[3] < 0, 0, y[3])
    R1 = ifelse(y[4] < 0, 0, y[4])
    R2 = ifelse(y[5] < 0, 0, y[5])
    J1 = ifelse(y[6] < 0, 0, y[6])
    J2 = ifelse(y[7] < 0, 0, y[7])
    R = ifelse(y[8] < 0, 0, y[8])

    with(as.list(parameters), {
        phi = (beta1 * I1 + beta2 * I2 + Theta * (beta1 *
            J1 + beta2 * J2))/N
        dS = mu * N - phi * S - mu * S
        dI1 = (beta1 * I1 + Theta * beta1 * J1) * S/N -
            (gamma + mu) * I1
        dI2 = (beta2 * I2 + Theta * beta2 * J2) * S/N -
            (gamma + mu) * I2
        dR1 = Pi * gamma * I1 - (beta2 * I2 + Theta *
            beta2 * J2) * Xi * R1/N - mu * R1
        dR2 = Pi * gamma * I2 - (beta1 * I1 + Theta *
            beta1 * J1) * Xi * R2/N - mu * R2
        dJ1 = (beta1 * I1 + Theta * beta1 * J1) * Xi *
            R2/N - gamma * J1 - mu * J1
        dJ2 = (beta2 * I2 + Theta * beta2 * J2) * Xi *
            R1/N - gamma * J2 - mu * J2
        dR = (1 - Pi) * gamma * (I1 + I2) + gamma * (J1 +
            J2) - mu * R
        res = c(dS, dI1, dI2, dR1, dR2, dJ1, dJ2, dR)
        return(list(res))
    })
}
```

The reason R_0 uniquely determines competitive dominance in the presence of perfect cross-immunity is that the equilibrium fraction of susceptible is $s^* = 1/R_0$. Recalling the effective reproduction number $R_E = sR_0$, whichever strain has the greatest R_0 will force all other strains into their subcritical territory ($R_E < 1$) and thus drive them extinct. By analogy to Tilman's (1976) theory of resource-based competition of free-living organisms, we may coin this as the S^* theory of strain dominance. For illustration, we may consider a scenario with imperfect but strong cross-immunity ($\theta = 0.15, \Xi = 0.15, \Pi = 0.8$), wild type $\beta_1 = 500$/year and a 50% transmission advantage of a mutant, an infectious period of 5 days, and an annual host birth rate of 0.02/year. With these parameters, the respective R_0s are 6.9 and 10.3, and the invasion number ($Q_{0,2}$) when the original strain is at its endemic equilibrium is 2.8 predicting an initial doubling time (T_d) of around 5 days.

```
paras = c(mu = 0.02, N = 1, beta1 = 500, beta2 = 750,
    gamma = 365/5, Theta = 0.15, Xi = 0.15, Pi = 0.8)
R01 = with(as.list(paras), beta1/(gamma + mu))
R01
```

```
## [1] 6.847439
```

```
R02 = with(as.list(paras), beta2/(gamma + mu))
R02
```

```
  ## [1] 10.27116
```

```
# Q02:
Q02 = with(as.list(paras), {
    S1star = 1/R01
    I1star = mu * (R01 - 1)/beta1
    R1star = 1 - (S1star + I1star)
    Q02 = (beta2 * S1star)/(mu + gamma) + (beta2) * Xi *
        R1star/(mu + gamma)
    Q02
})
# Invasion number
Q02
```

```
  ## [1] 2.815313
```

```
# Strain 2 doubling time (in days) at invasion
365 * log(Q02)/(paras["mu"] + paras["gamma"])
```

```
  ##      mu
  ## 5.17395
```

For the assumed parameters, we can visualize the S^* idea by considering a scenario in which the mutant appears in year 15 at which time the original strain has drawn down the susceptible fraction to 26% with 59% being in the R_1 compartment of the flow depicted in Fig. 3.11. Since $Q_{0,2}$ is greater than 1, the mutant can invade and add to the depletion of susceptibles. At some point, the susceptible fraction is so low as to push $R_{E,1}$ permanently below zero and at the new endemic equilibrium (with these parameters S^* is about 10%), the original strain will be driven extinct (Fig. 3.12).

```
require(deSolve)
times = seq(0, 30, by = 1/200)
start = c(S = 0.999, I1 = 0.001, I2 = 0, R1 = 0, R2 = 0,
    J1 = 0, J2 = 0, R = 0)
out1 = as.data.frame(ode(start, times, twostrain, paras))

ta = out1[out1[, 1] > 15, ]
start2 = c(S = ta[1, 2], I1 = ta[1, 3], I2 = 0.001, R1 = ta[1,
    5], R2 = ta[1, 6], J1 = ta[1, 7], J2 = ta[1, 8], R = ta[1,
    9])
out2 = as.data.frame(ode(start2, times, twostrain, paras))

R01 = with(as.list(paras), beta1/(gamma + mu))
R02 = with(as.list(paras), beta2/(gamma + mu))
plot(out1$S, R01 * out1$S, ylim = c(0, R01), type = "l",
    xlab = "S", ylab = "Re")
lines(out2$S, R02 * out2$S, col = 2)
abline(h = 1)
points(1/R01, 1, pch = "X")
```

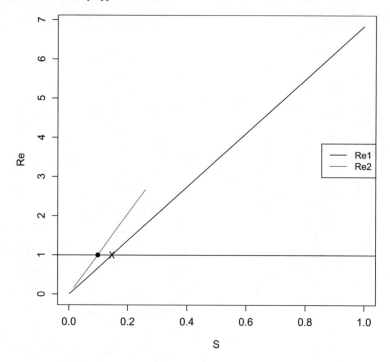

Fig. 3.12: An illustration of the S^* theory of competitive dominance. The original strain will draw down the susceptible fraction toward its endemic equilibrium (at which point $R^*_{E,1} = 1$, marked X. The higher R_0 emergent strain will continue to draw down the susceptibles to its equilibrium ($S^*_2 = 1/R_{0,2}$, marked ●) at which point $R_{E,1} = S^*_2 R_{0,1}$ is held below one, so the original strain is outcompeted and permanently prevented from reemerging

```
points(1/R02, 1, pch = 19)
legend("right", legend = c("Re1", "Re2"), lty = c(1, 1),
    col = c("black", "red"))
```

The twostrain.app contains an interactive interface to study this model of competitive displacement versus coexistence of strains with various scenarios of R_0 dominance and partial-to-complete cross-immunity. The shinyApp can be launched from R through:

```
require(epimdr2)
runApp(twostrain.app)
```

Chapter 4
FoI and Age-Dependence

4.1 Force of Infection

The force of infection (FoI) is the per capita rate at which susceptibles are exposed to infection. The FoI in the S(E)IR compartmental model (Eqs. (2.1)–(2.3) and (3.3)–(3.3)) is $\phi = \beta I/N$ because each susceptible is assumed to contact other individuals in the population at some rate, the fraction of those contacts that are with infected individuals is I/N, and β is by definition the contact rate times the probability of infection upon contact.[1]

An important basic and applied question is how the FoI scales with population density/size (de Jong et al., 1995), i.e., how the transmission rate parameter should be considered to be a function of N, $\beta(N)$. The literature suggests two extreme situations termed: density-dependent transmission for which the FoI scales linearly with density and frequency-dependent transmission for which the FoI is independent of density. Roberts and Heesterbeek (1993) point out that there is some significant confusion in the literature about the meaning of these terms, as the denominator N in the SEIR formulations is by some wrongly interpreted as Eqs. (3.3)–(3.6) being a frequency-dependent model. Roberts and Heesterbeek (1993) clarify that this is a mistaken interpretation; the I/N simply stems from the idea that only this fraction of random contacts is with infectious individuals (as opposed to the complimentary fraction which is with noninfectious individuals). The issue of density- versus frequency-dependence should be thought of in terms of how β (= contact rate $*$ transmission probability) and therefore R_0 scale with density (Roberts & Heesterbeek, 1993; Bjørnstad et al., 2002a; Ferrari et al., 2011). For the strictly density-

---

This chapter uses the following R packages: `splines`, `fields`, and `scatterplot3d`. A discussion of the force of infection can be found in two five minute epidemics MOOC videos: Force of Infection https://www.youtube.com/watch?v=dj1DiqA4Lvg. Pathogens and Extinction https://www.youtube.com/watch?v=v67gtiACBTY.

[1] The theoretical FoI is model specific, so more complicated models may have more complicated FoIs. The FoI for the Ebola SEIHFR model of Sect. 3.10, for example, is given by rate ① in Fig. 3.9.

© The Author(s), under exclusive license to Springer Nature Switzerland AG 2023   67
O. N. Bjørnstad, *Epidemics*, Use R!, https://doi.org/10.1007/978-3-031-12056-5_4

dependent model, numbers of contacts are proportional to density, so $\beta(N) \propto N$, and thus transmission and R_0 scale linearly with density, so the FoI eventually simplifies to βI. In contrast, the strictly frequency-dependent model assumes that contact rates are independent of N and, therefore, so is R_0 and thus the compound FoI remains $\beta I/N$. It is easy to envisage intermediate phenomenological models, say, contact rates scaling with some decelerating power q of population size $(0 < q < 1)$ (Smith et al., 2009b) leading to an FoI of $\beta I/N^q$.[2]

The frequency-dependent model is often used for sexually transmitted diseases (STDs) and vector-borne infections with the logic that the number of sexual partners does not scale with density and neither does the feeding requirements of mosquitoes; the female mosquito vectors of many vector-borne pathogens—including dengue, yellow fever, zika, and malaria causing *Plasmodium* parasites—have to take a blood meal to complete the gonotrophic cycle to lay a new batch of eggs every handful of days (the exact timeline of which depend on temperature; Delatte et al., 2009). With fewer hosts available, the vectors will increase their search radius to meet their need, and, thus, transmission rate will not decrease with decreasing host density.

An interesting ecological implication is that in the absence of an alternative host, a deadly density-dependently transmitted pathogen is less likely to drive a host extinct because as the pathogen decimates the host, the reproduction number is expected to eventually decrease below one, at which time the chain of transmission will falter and break.[3] Frequency-dependent pathogens, in contrast, may be able to sustain the chain of transmission to a bitter end as the reproduction number may remain supercritical even as the host population size dwindles (De Castro & Bolker, 2005).

4.2 Burden of Disease

Various time, space, and host heterogeneities are important forces in shaping epidemic curves and changing epidemiological patterns. In humans, age-related differences in susceptibility, exposure, and disease are among the most important such heterogeneities.

In everyday conversation about contagious maladies, disease and infection are sometimes used interchangeably. Often this imprecision does not matter. It is however useful to keep in mind that disease strictly speaking refers to symptomology and infection to chains of transmission and pathogen/parasite colonization status. The latent period—the time between a pathogen colonizes a host and the host can pass the infection on—is different from the incubation period—the time from colonization to onset of symptoms. Such distinctions are obvious for certain infections; all recognize the distinction between HIV positive and AIDS. The latter refers to disease status and the former to infection status. For influenza, the virus is typically

---

[2] Liu et al. (1986) proposed that spatial clustering can be modeled by a transmission term $\beta S^p I^q/N$, with p and q between zero and one.

[3] The notion of a critical host density is discussed in more detail in Sect. 10.7.

cleared in less than a week, but non-contagious cough and discomfort can last for another week or more. Thus, clinical relevance is not always the same as dynamic relevance.

The severity of disease of many infections depends on age. The very young are often prone to more severe disease. Both measles and whooping cough, for example, cause highest morbidity and mortality in children under one (e.g., Miller & Fletcher, 1976; Grais et al., 2007). Other diseases are more severe in the elderly. Mortality from influenza-like illness (ILI) is a common example and more recently SARS-CoV-2 (Verity et al., 2020). Teratogenic diseases are those that cause complications during pregnancies. Rubella, chickenpox, and Zika are important examples (Metcalf & Barrett, 2016). For these, infections of reproductive age women are the most pressing public health concern. It is important to understand determinants of age-prevalence curves for two reasons: first, because of such age-specificity in burden of disease and second because age-structure can mold infectious disease dynamics in important ways. Age-dependence in incidence arises through the interacting forces of age-specific susceptibility as molded by the past exposure and the age-specific force of infection.

4.3 WAIFW

Age-structured FoIs result from age-varying contact rates and assortative mixing among different age groups. The so-called Who-Acquires-Infection-From-Whom (WAIFW) matrix is used to describe the patterns of non-homogeneous mixing among different age groups (Grenfell & Anderson, 1989). Mossong et al. (2008) conducted a diary-based social study to map age-stratified contact rates for various countries in Europe as part of the polymod project. The contact rates by `contactor` and `contactee` are provided in the `mossong` dataset. We can visualize the diary data using an image plot with contours superimposed (Fig. 4.1).

```
data(polymod)
head(polymod)

##   contactor contactee contact.rate
## 1         1         1    120.37234
## 2         2         1     33.45833
## 3         3         1     23.13380
## 4         4         1     24.33333
## 5         5         1     29.00662
## 6         6         1     14.50331

x = y = polymod$contactor[1:30]
z = matrix(polymod$contact.rate, ncol = 30, nrow = 30)
image(x = x, y = y, z = z, xlab = "Contactor", ylab = "Contactee",
    col = gray((12:32)/32))
contour(x = x, y = y, z = z, add = TRUE)
```

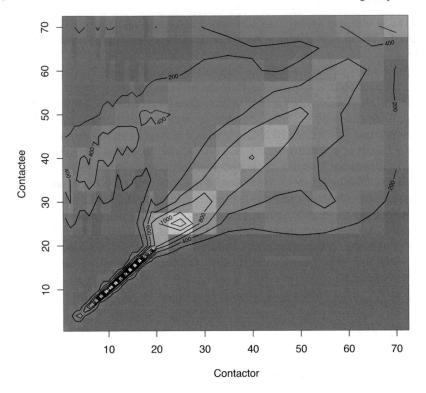

Fig. 4.1: The contact rates reported in the diary study of Mossong et al. (2008)

The reported contact rates are not symmetrical, which a WAIFW matrix will necessarily be, because of age-specific biases in diary entry rates as well as the age-profile of the contactors vs contactees. Before we symmetrize the matrix, we can look at the reported marginal contact rate for each age group. Most contacts are among same-aged individuals and school-aged children have the greatest number of contacts (Fig. 4.2). There are, however, important off-diagonal ridges resulting from, for example, parent/offspring or pupil/teacher interactions.

```
plot(apply(z, 1, mean) ~ x, ylab = "Total contact rate",
    xlab = "Age")
```

4.4 A RAS Model

Schenzle (1984) emphasized the importance of age-structured mixing and age-structured FoIs when modeling infectious disease dynamics. Bolker and Grenfell (1993) extended this model to the "realistic age-structured (RAS) model," which in

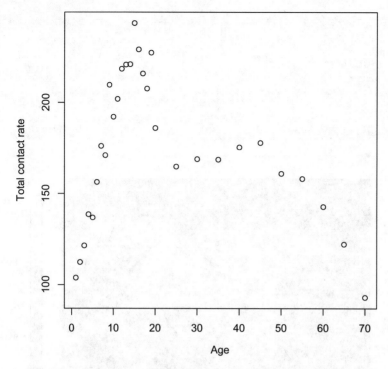

Fig. 4.2: The age-specific contact rates reported by the diary study of Mossong et al. (2008)

its full elaboration is an age-structured compartmental model with discrete aging of each birth cohort (at the beginning of each school year) and seasonality in transmission. Seasonality is the topic of Chap. 6. Here we can incorporate the `polymod` contact matrix in a simpler age-structured compartmental model making the simplifying assumption that individuals age exponentially (i.e., aging in and out are constant within each age group with rates set such that they will on average spend the right amount of time in each age-bracket). This allows the formulation of a RAS model using chains of differential equations. In the below example, the upper age cut-offs and age-progression rates for the $n = 70$ age categories are a. One can in principle use the raw symmetric contact matrix in the model, but here we use a thin-plate spline[4] smoothed matrix using the `Tps` function in the `fields` package. The smoothing protocol allows interpolation to use different age-brackets, in this case annual brackets to age 70, for the model projections (Fig. 4.3).

---

[4] A thin-plate spline is a spline-based technique that produces smooth surfaces in 2 (or higher) dimensions (Wood, 2003).

```
require(fields)
n = length(x)
# symmetrize
z2 = (z + t(z))/2
z3 = as.vector(z2)
xy = data.frame(x = rep(x[1:n], n), y = rep(y[1:n], each = n))
# smooth
polysmooth = Tps(xy, z3, df = 100)
surface(polysmooth, xlab = "", ylab = "", col = gray((12:32)/32))
```

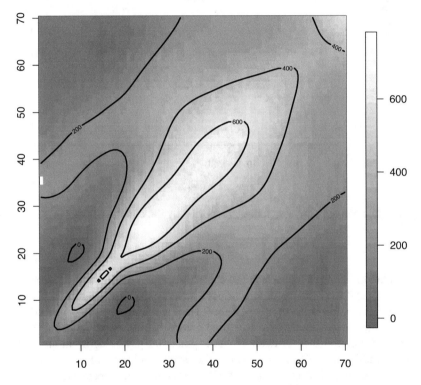

Fig. 4.3: The thin-plate spline smooth estimate of the WAIFW matrix

For the age-structured SIR model, first annualize and normalize the WAIFW matrix:

```
n = 70
ra = rep(1, 70)   #aging rates
x = cumsum(1/ra)  #age brackets
# annualize & symmetrize
ps = predict(polysmooth, x = expand.grid(1:70, 1:70))
ps2 = matrix(ps, ncol = 70)
ps2 = ps2 + t(ps2)
# normalize
```

```
W = ps2/mean(ps2)
```

An age-structured SIR model assuming all children are born into the first susceptible class (S_1; so ignoring maternal immunity), that aging through the a'th age-class
happens a rate r_a (so average time in age-bracket a is $1/r_a$) and allowing for the
possibility of age-specific vaccination rate v_a ($= -log(1-p)r_a$, where p is vaccine
cover; *cf.* discussion on rate/probability conversions of Sect. 3.2) is:

$$\frac{dS_1}{dt} = \underbrace{\mu N}_{\text{birth}} - \underbrace{\phi_1 S_1}_{\text{infection}} - \underbrace{v_1 S_1}_{\text{vaccination}} - \underbrace{r_1 S_1}_{\text{aging}} - \underbrace{\mu S_1}_{\text{death}} \tag{4.1}$$

$$\frac{dS_a}{dt} = \underbrace{r_{a-1} S_{a-1}}_{\text{aging in}} - \underbrace{\phi_a S_a}_{\text{infection}} - \underbrace{v_a S_a}_{\text{vaccination}} - \underbrace{r_a S_a}_{\text{aging out}} - \underbrace{\mu S_a}_{\text{death}} \tag{4.2}$$

$$\frac{dI_a}{dt} = \underbrace{r_{a-1} I_{a-1}}_{\text{aging in}} + \underbrace{\phi_a S_a}_{\text{infection}} - \underbrace{\gamma I_a}_{\text{recovery}} - \underbrace{r_a I_a}_{\text{aging out}} - \underbrace{\mu I_a}_{\text{death}} \tag{4.3}$$

$$\frac{dR_a}{dt} = \underbrace{r_{a-1} R_{a-1}}_{\text{aging in}} + \underbrace{\gamma I_a}_{\text{recovery}} - \underbrace{r_a R_a}_{\text{aging out}} + \underbrace{v_a S_a}_{\text{vaccination}} - \underbrace{\mu R_a}_{\text{death}} \tag{4.4}$$

$$\phi_a = \underbrace{\sum_{j=1}^{A} \beta W_{aj} I_j / N}_{\text{force of infection}} , \tag{4.5}$$

where ϕ_a is the FoI on the a'th age class. In matrix notation (see Sect. 4.7 for a gentle
introduction to matrix calculations in biology), the age-specific FoI is $\phi = \beta \mathbf{WI}/N$.
The age-structured SIR model is thus (in log-coordinates)[5]

```
sirAgemod = function(t, logx, parameters) {
    n = length(parameters$r)
    xx = exp(logx)
    S = xx[1:n]
    I = xx[(n + 1):(2 * n)]
    R = xx[(2 * n + 1):(3 * n)]
    with(as.list(parameters), {
        phi = (beta * W %*% I)/N
        dS = c(mu, rep(0, n - 1)) * N - (phi + r) * S +
            c(0, r[1:(n - 1)] * S[1:(n - 1)]) - mu * S -
            v * S
        dI = phi * S + c(0, r[1:(n - 1)] * I[1:(n - 1)]) -
            (gamma + r) * I - mu * I
        dR = v * S + c(0, r[1:(n - 1)] * R[1:(n - 1)]) +
            gamma * I - r * R - mu * R
        res = c(dS/S, dI/I, dR/R)
```

[5] Recall that the `with(as.list(...))` allows evaluation of the equations using the definitions
in the `parameters` vector and `%*%` denotes matrix multiplication.

```
        list((res))
    })
}
```

where S, I, and R are vectors of length n, phi is the age-specific force of infection
predicted from the WAIFW matrix, and v is a vector of length n that allows for age-
specific vaccination rates. The r vector sets appropriate aging rates if age groups
vary in duration. The below illustration assumes that the initial population is 9.9%
susceptible and 0.1% infected and assumes an infectious period of 14 days, a life
expectancy of 50 years, and a base transmission rate of 100/year:

```
v.pre = rep(0, n)
paras = list(N = 1, gamma = 365/14, mu = 0.02, beta = 100,
    W = W, v = v.pre, r = ra)
ystart = log(c(S = rep(0.099/n, n), I = rep(0.001/n, n),
    R = rep(0.9/n, n)))
```

Following integration, Fig. 4.4a shows the age-specific prevalence and equilibrium
age-specific prevalence (Fig. 4.4b) using the polymod contact matrix. Figure 4.4b
also shows the predicted age-prevalence curve for the age-structured model with
homogenous mixing.

```
require(deSolve)
times = seq(0, 500, by = 1/52)
# polymod mixing
out = as.data.frame(ode(ystart, times, sirAgemod, paras))
par(mfrow = c(1, 2))   #Room for side-by-side plots
# Time series of infecteds
matplot(times/52, exp(out[, (n + 2):(2 * n + 1)]), type = "l",
    xlab = "Year", ylab = "Prevalence")
# homogenous mixing:
paras$W = matrix(1, ncol = n, nrow = n)
out2 = as.data.frame(ode(ystart, times, sirAgemod, paras))
# Final age-prevalence curve
plot(x, t(exp(out2[2608, (n + 2):(2 * n + 1)]))/sum(exp(out2[2608,
    (n + 2):(2 * n + 1)])), ylab = "Prevalence", xlab = "Age",
    col = 2, pch = "*")
points(x, t(exp(out[2608, (n + 2):(2 * n + 1)]))/sum(exp(out[2608,
    (n + 2):(2 * n + 1)])))
legend("topright", c("polymod", "homogenous"), col = 1:2,
    pch = c("o", "*"))
```

In contrast to the model with homogenous mixing which predicts that age-intensity
curves decay exponentially with age (as expected for a process with constant rates),
the RAS model can lead to a variety of age-incidence curves including the hump-
shaped curve with a mode at around 15 years given the parameters employed
(Fig. 4.4b).

The RAS model is useful in clarifying how age-incidence curves will change
under realistic mixing and various vaccination regimes. For simplicity, consider the
above parameterization and vaccine delivered with a 60% cover during the second year of life and study the effect on the mean age of infection. A 60% vaccine

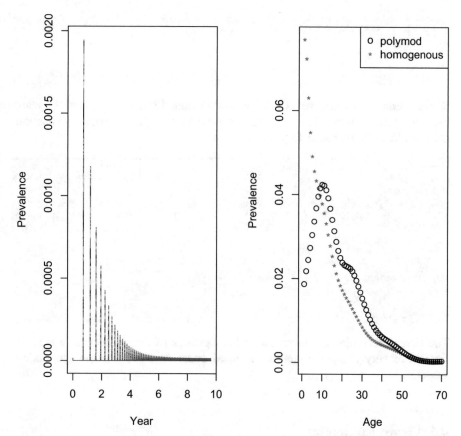

Fig. 4.4: The age-specific prevalences from the age-structured SIR model. (**a**) Trajectory through time. (**b**) Equilibrium age-incidence curves for the polymod matrix (o) vs homogenous mixing (∗)

cover will reduce R_0 from 3.5–4 to around 1.5 and implies a vaccination rate of $v = -log(1 - 0.6) = 0.91$ year^{-1} for the 12–23 month target group.

```
# polymod matrix
paras$W = W
# 60\% vaccination  of second age-class
paras$v = c(0, -log(1 - 0.6) * ra[2], rep(0, n - 2))
out3 = as.data.frame(ode(ystart, times, sirAgemod, paras))
# Mid-point for each age-bracket
x2 = x - (1/ra/2)
# Equilibrium age-prevalence and MAI
pv3 = t(exp(out3[2608, (n + 2):(2 * n + 1)]))
sum(x2 * pv3)/sum(pv3)

## [1] 27.55307
```

```
# Prevaccination
pv = t(exp(out[2608, (n + 2):(2 * n + 1)]))
sum(x2 * pv)/sum(pv)

  ## [1] 17.55689
```

So the mean age of infection (MAI) is shifted from 17 years to around 27 years because of the reduction in susceptible recruitment. With homogenous mixing, the shift would be from around 13 years to 22 years:

```
paras$W = matrix(1, ncol = n, nrow = n)
out4 = as.data.frame(ode(ystart, times, sirAgemod, paras))
# Equilibrium MAI
pv4 = t(exp(out4[2608, (n + 2):(2 * n + 1)]))
sum(x2 * pv4)/sum(pv4)

  ## [1] 22.09802
```

```
# Prevaccination
pv2 = t(exp(out2[2608, (n + 2):(2 * n + 1)]))
sum(x2 * pv2)/sum(pv2)

  ## [1] 13.01221
```

The lower prevaccination mean under homogenous mixing is because a smaller fraction of very young children are exposed under the more realistic age-mixing scenario.

4.5 Virgin Epidemics

At the time of revising this chapter for the 2nd edition, the SARS-CoV-2 2020/21 pandemic is unfolding, one of only a few true global virgin epidemics in a long time. In 2009, influenza A/H1N1pmd was a new recombinant strain (Smith et al., 2009a), but subsequent evidence indicates that prior exposure to the already circulating A/H1N1 strain provided substantial cross-immunity to reduce disease symptoms and transmission (Chowell et al., 2011). Looking at historical age-mortality patterns, the 1918 Spanish influenza A/H1N1 pandemic also testified to the critical importance of both age and prior exposure on burden of disease and mortality. While not serologically confirmed, historical records suggest that the elderly in 1918 were protected by immunity from an A/H1N1-related strain replaced during a mid/late nineteenth-century pandemic (Simonsen et al., 1998). Sero-archaeology suggests that the curiously limited excess mortality in older age groups may be due to the 1847 pandemic being an influenza A virus of an H1 and/or N1 variant (Dowdle, 1999; Morens & Fauci, 2007). Such sero-archaeological studies have suggested that the Russian pandemic of 1889 was possibly due to an influenza A/H3 variant. Intriguingly, however, Vijgen et al. (2005) used genomic tools to trace the probable date of origin of the OC43 coronavirus to the late 1880s to suggest that the deadly pandemic that killed millions of people could alternatively have been caused, not by an influenza virus, but by what is today a harmless winter cold.

Both the 1918 and 2009 influenza A pandemics were associated with very different temporal patterns from subsequent seasonal endemics, both exhibiting three waves during the initial year of invasion (Gog et al., 2014; Bjørnstad & Viboud, 2016). History further shows that age-structure and mortality during virgin epidemics are often very different from subsequent endemic age-circulation, whether looking at transiently immunizing viruses like the 1918 Spanish flu pandemic or viruses that resulted in sterilizing immunity for survivors such as was the case when Europeans brought measles and smallpox to the Americas at the end of the fifteenth century. Such changes can shift patterns of morbidity and mortality over time even in the absence of any pathogen evolution. The changing public health burden is governed by factors at the intersection between incidence at age, disease at age, and possible complete or partial protection due to prior exposure. During the period of establishment toward long-term endemism, incidence at age will change because of contact patterns and early removal of high contact people (oftentimes of school and college age) as per the discussion in Sect. 4.3 and further discussed in a social network context by Ferrari et al. (2006a). Later disease at age profiles may shift because over time re-exposed at-risk individuals may suffer lower burden of disease because of residual partial immune protection (Lavine et al., 2021; Li et al., 2021b).

The RAS model can be used to investigate plausible transitions by assuming a completely susceptible initial population[6] and study how age-specific risk may change over time. Figure 4.5 shows one scenario of changes in age-incidence patterns during a transition from emergence to endemicity of an immunizing pathogen.

```
n = 70
a = rep(1, 70)
ystart2 = log(c(S = rep(0.9989/n, n), I = rep(0.001/n,
    n), R = rep(1e-04/n, n)))
paras = list(N = 1, gamma = 365/14, mu = 0.02, beta = 100,
    W = W, v = v.pre, r = ra)
out5 = as.data.frame(ode(ystart2, times, sirAgemod, paras))

# year 1 relative risk
y1 = apply(t(exp(out5[1:52, (n + 2):(2 * n + 1)])), 1,
    sum)
y1 = y1/sum(y1)

# year 2 relative risk
y10 = apply(t(exp(out5[(1:52) + 10 * 52, (n + 2):(2 *
    n + 1)])), 1, sum)
y10 = y10/sum(y10)

# endemic relative risk
yT = apply(t(exp(out5[(1:52) + 499 * 52, (n + 2):(2 *
```

---

[6] The tiny non-zero fraction of initials in the R group in the code is because integrating the model in log-coordinates for numerical stability requires non-zero state variables, so $\log(0) = -\infty$ would break the numerical integrator.

```
      n + 1)])), 1, sum)
yT = yT/sum(yT)

plot(x, y10, lty = 2, type = "l", ylab = "Relative risk",
    xlab = "Age")
points(x, yT, type = "b", col = 2, pch = "*")
points(x, y1, type = "b", pch = 1)

legend("topright", c("Virgin", "10yr", "Endemic"), col = c(1,
    1, 2), pch = c("o", NA, "*"), lty = c(NA, 2, NA))
```

Lavine et al. (2021) and Li et al. (2021b) provide discussion of how such calculations can be used to project plausible scenarios toward endemicity for the ongoing SARS-CoV-2 pandemic.

4.6 Vaccination by Age-Dependent Risk

Section 4.2 discussed how burden of disease may be strongly age-specific. Verity et al. (2020) showed that infection–mortality ratios from the SARS-CoV-2 virus were $<0.5\%$ in the young but $>10\%$ in the elderly during the first months of the 2020/21 pandemic. Accordingly, most countries instituted an age-based priority ranking for vaccine deployment (Li et al., 2021a) with a goal to broaden age-brackets once target cover of high-risk groups is reached (e.g., 85% of the 70+ bracket). To model plausible switch times for expanding age-targeting, we can use the rate/fraction conversion discussed in Sect. 3.2. Recalling that a rate, x, is related to the fraction, p, in a time interval Δt according to the quantile function for the exponential distribution: $x = -log(1-p)/\Delta t$. The time Δt to reach the target cover is $\Delta t = -log(1-p)/x$. So, for example, given a rate of $2N$ vaccines per year (i.e., a vaccine capacity where on average everyone can be vaccinated twice in a year), the length of time in years until 75% of the target population is vaccinated is

```
-log(1 - 0.75)/2

  ## [1] 0.6931472
```

which is 8.3 months.

Assuming a population where 30% of the population is in the high-risk age group (N_1) and the other 70% is in age group N_2, and assuming an 85% target cover of N_1 before vaccination is opened up for all, the duration of targeted vaccination will be $-log(1-0.85)/(0.69/N_1) = -log(1-0.85)/(0.69/0.3)$ years.

```
-log(1 - 0.85)/(0.69/0.3)

  ## [1] 0.8248348
```

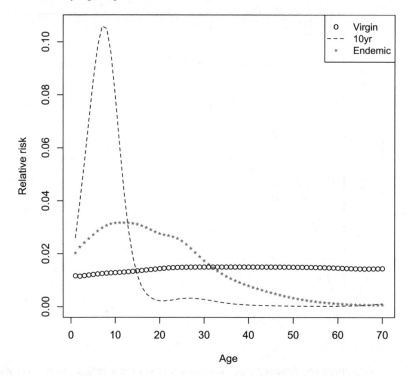

Fig. 4.5: The relative age-specific prevalences from the age-structured SIR model during the first year of invasion (the virgin epidemic), after 10 years and long-term endemism for an immunizing pathogen with a 14-day infectious period, an R_0 of 3.8, and a polymod mixing matrix. The risk during the virgin epidemic is broadly age-invariant, the endemic risk is strongly shifted toward high contact younger age groups after a decade, then flattens, and drifts slightly upward as community immunity lowers the force of infection

The 0.82 years is around 10 months. In order to project vaccine dynamics into the future, we can consider coverage over time in the two groups given this target and switch point (Fig. 4.6):

```
# N1 cover with time before switch
p1 = seq(0, 0.85, by = 0.01)
T1 = -log(1 - p1)/(0.69/0.3)
plot(T1, p1, type = "l", xlim = c(0, 2), ylim = c(0, 1),
    xlab = "year", ylab = "cover")
# After switch
T2 = seq(0, 2 - max(T1), length = 100)
p2 = 1 - exp(-0.69 * T2)
# N1 cover
lines(T2 + max(T1), p2 * 0.15 + 0.85)
# N2 cover
```

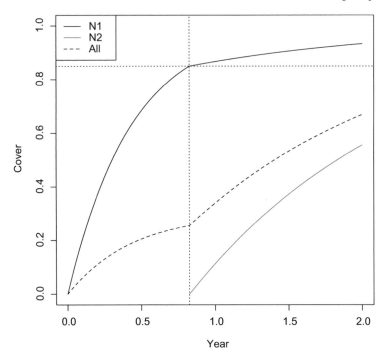

Fig. 4.6: The predicted trajectory of vaccination cover for a target group (N_1) with 30% of the population and the remainder 70% (N_2) given a vaccination capacity of 2N/year and target to 85% cover of the target group before broader dissemination

```
lines(T2 + max(T1), p2, col = 2)
# total cover
lines(c(T1, T2 + max(T1)), c(p1 * 0.3, (p2 * 0.15 + 0.85) *
    0.3 + p2 * 0.7), lty = 2)
abline(v = max(T1), lty = 3)
abline(h = 0.85, lty = 3)
legend("topleft", c("N1", "N2", "All"), lty = c(1, 1,
    2), col = c(1, 2, 1))
```

4.7 Projecting Host Age-Structure

As discussed in Sects. 4.3 and 4.4, age-dependent contact rates are important determinants of infectious disease dynamics. As a consequence, the host age-structure is critical. Moreover, as will be particularly well illustrated in Sect. 6.6 with respect to fully immunizing infections, the rate of susceptible recruitment (*viz.* vaccine-discounted birth rates) can greatly influence recurrence patterns. The most common framework to predict host age-structure and future birth numbers is the Leslie matrix model (Leslie, 1945; Caswell, 2001). While this theme is a bit tangential to the main focus of this monograph, it is a useful way to start thinking about matrix algebra for biology—a mathematical toolset that will be used frequently in the next chapters. The model projects the number of individuals of age a, n_a in discrete (often annual) time steps according to

$$n_{0,t+1} = f_1 n_{1,t} + f_2 n_{2,t} + \ldots + f_A n_{A,t} \tag{4.6}$$

$$n_{1,t+1} = s_0 n_{0,t} \tag{4.7}$$

$$n_{2,t+1} = s_1 n_{1,t} \tag{4.8}$$

$$\vdots \tag{4.9}$$

where f_a represents age-specific fecundities, A is the maximum life span, and s_a are age-specific survival probabilities. In matrix form, these equations can be written as $N_{t+1} = LN_t$, where N represents the vector of number of individuals in each age class and L is the Leslie matrix that has fecundities along the first row and survivals on the sub-diagonal:

$$L = \begin{pmatrix} f_0 & f_1 & f_2 & \cdots & f_A \\ s_0 & 0 & 0 & \cdots & 0 \\ 0 & s_1 & 0 & \cdots & 0 \\ \vdots & 0 & \ddots & \vdots & \vdots \\ 0 & 0 & \cdots & s_{A-1} & 0 \end{pmatrix} \tag{4.10}$$

The Leslie theory of population growth shows that if fecundities and survivorships are constant over time, then the host population will grow if the dominant eigenvalue (λ) of L is greater than 1 and decline otherwise. Moreover, in the long term, the population will reach a stable age-distribution (an unchanging fraction of individuals in each age-class) proportional to the dominant eigenvector of L. The theory further predicts that once the stable distribution is reached, the population will have a geometric rate of growth of λ. Thus, in the long run, the matrix calculation LN_t simplifies to λN_t. To illustrate, it is convenient to use a simple hypothetical population with three age classes:

```
fa <- c(0, 0.5, 1.2)
sa <- c(0.8, 0.8, 0)
L <- matrix(0, nrow = 3, ncol = 3)
# inserting fa vector in first row
L[1, ] <- fa
# inserting sa in the subdiagonal:
L[row(L) == col(L) + 1] <- sa[1:2]
```

A forward simulation and visualization using `scatterplot3d` shows the population growth and age-structure over time (Fig. 4.7):

```
Na = matrix(0, nrow = 65, ncol = 3)
Na[1, ] = c(10, 0, 0)
for (i in 2:65) {
    Na[i, ] = L %*% Na[i - 1, ]
```

```
}
scatterplot3d(Na[1:30, ], type = "b", xlab = expression(n[0]),
    ylab = expression(n[1]), zlab = expression(n[2]))
```

The simulation confirms the mathematical postulate that long-term growth of an age-structured host population converges on the dominant eigenvalue, λ, and thereafter the asymptotic age-structure is proportional to the dominant eigenvector of **L**:

```
Tot = apply(Na, 1, sum)
# growth during last years
tail(Tot[2:65]/Tot[1:64])
```

```
## [1] 1.060331 1.060331 1.060332 1.060331 1.060331 1.060331
```

```
# First EV is dominant and real only
Re(eigen(L)$values[1])
```

```
## [1] 1.060331
```

```
# Simulated age-structure for year 65
Na[65, ]/sum(Na[65, ])
```

```
## [1] 0.4303442 0.3246858 0.2449700
```

```
# Normalized dominant eigen vector
Re(eigen(L)$vector[, 1])/sum(Re(eigen(L)$vector[, 1]))
```

```
## [1] 0.4303438 0.3246864 0.2449698
```

After 65 years of population growth, the predictions are clearly borne out.

Advanced: Leslie Sensitivity and Elasticity

The f_a's and s_a's are the so-called vital rates of population growth. For a variety of reasons, we may be interested in understanding which vital rates are contributing most strongly to population growth and thus susceptible recruitment. Caswell (2001) defines two key quantities for such an analysis: the sensitivity and the elasticity. Both of these detail how the long-term (asymptotic) growth rate, λ, of age-structured populations depends sensitively on each fecundity/survival element (conventionally denoted by α)[7] of the Leslie matrix. The sensitivity is the derivative of λ with respect to each of the elements, α_{ij}, according to

$$s_{ij} = \frac{\partial \lambda}{\partial \alpha_{ij}} = \frac{v_i w_j}{<\mathbf{w}, \mathbf{v}>}, \tag{4.11}$$

---

[7] This is another unfortunate case of notation conventions in different fields pertinent to infectious disease dynamics that adds confusion to the Greek alphabet soup; this text generally adheres to mathematical epidemiology conventions for which α is commonly used for rate of infection-induced mortality, but in mathematical demography α_{ij} conventionally refers to the i'th row and j'th column of the Leslie matrix.

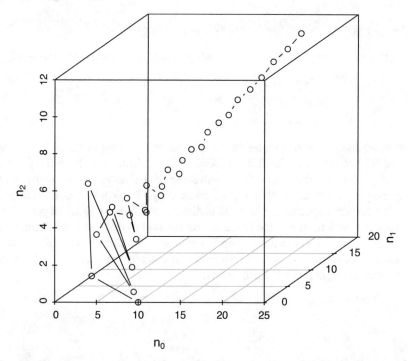

Fig. 4.7: The predicted number of individuals in each of the three age classes for the hypothetical host population for the first 30 years of simulation, starting with 10 newborn individuals. Initially, age-structure changes rapidly, but the increasingly straightened line shows the convergence on the stable age-distribution. Once reached, the total population size and each age group is growing by a factor of λ each time step

where $\mathbf{w}$ and $\mathbf{v}$ are the dominant right and left eigenvectors of $\mathbf{L}$, v_i and w_j are the i'th and j'th element of the of the $\mathbf{v}$ and $\mathbf{w}$ vectors, respectively, and $< \mathbf{w}, \mathbf{v} >$ is the scalar product of the two vectors:

$$< \mathbf{w}, \mathbf{v} >= w_1 v_1 + w_2 v_2 + \ldots + w_n v_n. \qquad (4.12)$$

The eigen function calculates all the central quantities:

```
Ex = eigen(L)
# The dominant eigenvalue
lambda = Ex$values[1]
lambda

  ## [1] 1.060331+0i

# The dominant (right) eigenvector is
w = Ex$vectors[, 1]
w
```

```
## [1] 0.7267629+0i 0.5483290+0i 0.4137040+0i
```

The left dominant eigenvector is calculated by transposing **L** and then decomposing:

```
v = eigen(t(L))$vectors[, 1]
v
```

```
## [1] 0.4976716+0i 0.6596208+0i 0.5632259+0i
```

Before proceeding in completing the calculations outlined in Eq. (4.11), it may be useful to make some clarifications about *eigen* calculations; from the point of view of general matrix theory, the eigenvectors and eigenvalues of matrices can have complex solutions involving $\sqrt{-1}$ denoted by ι (which will, as alluded to in Sect. 2.7, be very important for later calculations of stability and resonant periodicity in Chap. 10). As it turns out, the Leslie matrix always has real dominant eigenvalues and eigenvectors. However, the eigen function that solves for the general case does not know this, so the use of Re() strips the 0ι complex parts from the dominant eigenvalue and right and left eigenvectors.

```
sens = Re((v %*% t(w))/sum(v * w))
sens
```

```
##             [,1]       [,2]       [,3]
## [1,] 0.3781828 0.2853319 0.2152776
## [2,] 0.5012488 0.3781828 0.2853319
## [3,] 0.4279978 0.3229163 0.2436343
```

The *elasticity* (Caswell, 2001) is the proportional change in the population growth rate resulting from a proportional change in the transitions according to $e_{ij} = \alpha_{ij} s_{ij}/\lambda$. To simplify further calculations, a function to do all these calculations is:

```
leslie = function(L){
    Ex = eigen(L)        #Eigendecompostition of matrix
    w = Re(Ex$vectors[, 1]) #right eigenvector
    lambda = Re(Ex$values[1])  #dominant eigenvalue
    v = Re(eigen(t(L))$vectors[, 1])     #left eigenvector
    sens = (v %*% t(w))/sum(v * w)   #sensitivities
    elast = L * sens/lambda       #elasticities
    #list of results
    res = list(lambda = lambda, right.eigenvector = w,
        left.eigenvector = v, elasticity = elast,
        sensitivity = sens)
    return(res)
}
```

For the hypothetical three age-group population, the projected annual growth rate is 6% and the elasticities show that survival of the young of the year (α_{21}) is the most important contributor to population growth:

```
leslie(L)$lambda

  ## [1] 1.060331

leslie(L)$elasticity

  ##               [,1]        [,2]        [,3]
  ## [1,] 0.0000000 0.1345485 0.2436343
  ## [2,] 0.3781828 0.0000000 0.0000000
  ## [3,] 0.0000000 0.2436343 0.0000000
```

The us dataset contains age-specific survival and fecundities for the USA in 2005 in 5-year age brackets (Arias et al., 2010). Employing the above methodology and focusing on the 0–40 year group the life table predicts an annual growth of 2.3% which is higher than the US census data of 0.9% at the time. The analysis further shows that survival through childbearing age (e_{21}, e_{32}, and e_{43}) is the most influential contributor to growth:

```
L2 <- matrix(0, nrow = 8, ncol = 8)
L2[1, ] <- us$fa[1:8]
L2[row(L2) == col(L2) + 1] <- us$sa[1:7]
# Annualized growth rate
(leslie(L2)$lambda)^(1/5)

  ## [1] 1.023346

# Elasticities
round(leslie(L2)$elasticity, 2)

  ##        [,1] [,2] [,3] [,4] [,5] [,6] [,7] [,8]
  ## [1,] 0.00 0.00 0.00 0.02 0.05 0.05 0.04 0.02
  ## [2,] 0.17 0.00 0.00 0.00 0.00 0.00 0.00 0.00
  ## [3,] 0.00 0.17 0.00 0.00 0.00 0.00 0.00 0.00
  ## [4,] 0.00 0.00 0.17 0.00 0.00 0.00 0.00 0.00
  ## [5,] 0.00 0.00 0.00 0.15 0.00 0.00 0.00 0.00
  ## [6,] 0.00 0.00 0.00 0.00 0.10 0.00 0.00 0.00
  ## [7,] 0.00 0.00 0.00 0.00 0.00 0.05 0.00 0.00
  ## [8,] 0.00 0.00 0.00 0.00 0.00 0.00 0.02 0.00
```

Engen et al. (2021) provide an example of how the Leslie framework can further be applied to infectious disease dynamics, for example, in the case where "age" refers to time since infection.

Chapter 5
The Catalytic Model

5.1 Immune Memory

While immunobiology is not the focus of this text, some basic underpinnings are useful for motivating the so-called catalytic model to study how immunity may build up with age, how age-specific heterogeneities may affect this, and how we can use immune data to back-calculate key dynamic quantities. There are two main branches of the adaptive immune system—the part of the immune system that helps to build a repertoire for protection against reinfection. The T lymphocyte cells develop in the thymus where they are trained to recognize "self." The training is that cells with affinity for any cells encountered in this organ are culled so that only those with non-self affinity are released for general circulation. T effector cells are key to recognizing intracellular pathogens via the self-/non-self MHC pathways (Harty & Badovinac, 2008). A simplified caricature of this pathway is that most cells cut some small fraction of intracellular proteins into short amino acid sequences (usually of a length of 9–16 amino acids) and present them on the cell surface. T cells that bind to what they consider non-self proteins will multiply and trigger the killing of the infected cell. Following clearance of infection, some of the T cells will produce long-lived lineages that henceforth generate memory of past infection.

B lymphocyte cells that develop in the bone marrow are responsible for the second important branch of immune memory. Upon being stimulated and maturing (Kurosaki et al., 2015), they produce arsenals of antigen-specific antibodies, each mature lineage able to recognize a specific bit of a surface protein (an epitope) of a particular pathogen such as the hemagglutinin of the influenza virus or specific antigens of pathogenic bacteria (e.g., *Neisseria gonorrhoeae*), protists (e.g., malaria-causing *Plasmodium spp*), or any number of intestinal or systemic parasitic worms. When analyzed correctly, antigen-specific antibodies in blood or mucus contain powerful epidemiological information about the force of infection (FoI) in a population, the current prevalence, and the type of age-specific transmission heterogeneities discussed in Chap. 4. Ignoring all molecular and immunological

---

This chapter uses the following R package: splines.

© The Author(s), under exclusive license to Springer Nature Switzerland AG 2023
O. N. Bjørnstad, *Epidemics*, Use R!, https://doi.org/10.1007/978-3-031-12056-5_5

details, an important bit of biology is that B cells from any given linage will over time differentiate to produce different antibody isotypes (Duarte, 2016); isotypes means that they react to the same epitope but have a different structure and subtly varying purpose. A primary infection will result in the production of plasma B cells that produce antibodies (immunoglobulines) of type M (IgM). Once the infection is cleared, some cells will result in long-lived memory B lineages that produce IgG antibodies. In caricature, IgG looks like a Y where the top of the Y is the antigen-binding region, whereas IgM are five Y's anchored together in a circle at the base.[1] IgA that in caricature looks like two hinged Y's is secreted into mucus and is important for blocking pathogen reentry and also for fighting intestinal parasites. Depending on pathogen characteristics, such as what organs/tissues/cells they interact with, some memory lineages last for life to produce permanent infection-blocking "sterilizing" immunity following a primary infection. Examples of such are many of the vaccine-preventable childhood viruses such as measles, mumps, and rubella. For these, IgG-positivity-at-age data presents records of past infection that can be analyzed via the catalytic model framework. Measures of antigen-specific IgM flag current or recent primary exposure/infection. Lavine et al. (2021) provide an illustrative discussion w.r.t. human coronaviruses.

An important caveat for correct analysis of age-seroprevalence profiles is the presence of maternal antibodies in newborns. IgGs, but not their B cell generators, are actively transferred across the placenta prior to birth to protect infants until their immune system matures (Niewiesk, 2014). To a lesser extent, maternal IgAs are transferred through breast milk. Thus, high IgG titers in the very young generally reflect the mother's prior exposure to the pathogen. Such maternal antibodies protect newborns but increase the probability of primary vaccine failure because they limit antigen presentation, which is why most childhood vaccination protocols start in the 6–12 months age-window after maternal IgGs have decayed to no longer block stimulation and maturation of a child's B cells (Niewiesk, 2014).

5.2 The Catalytic Model

Age-incidence patterns are shaped by the intersections between the overall force of infection (Sect. 4.1), the age-specific mixing patterns (Sect. 4.3), and the population-level susceptibility-at-age profile. Muench (1959) proposed a catalytic model to study how immunity may build up with age, how age-specific heterogeneities may affect this, and how age-seroprevalence data can be used to estimate intensity of circulation of any given pathogen in any given population. Many subsequent refinements (e.g., Grenfell & Anderson, 1985; Hens et al., 2010; Long et al., 2010) show how such data can also help elucidate the important age-related heterogeneities discussed in Sects. 4.3 and 4.4.

---

[1] There are other isotypes. Duarte (2016) and Nature Immunology Milestones provides a series of short synopses for readers interested in digging deeper into immunobiology.

The force of infection ϕ is a rate, thus if age-invariant in a randomly mixing population the waiting time to first infection is exponentially distributed with a mean age of infection of $1/\phi$ (Fig. 4.4b). For endemic, fully immunizing infections in a constant-sized host population, the basic reproduction number (R_0) relates to the mean age of infection ($\bar{a}$) according to $R_0 \simeq 1 + L/\bar{a}$, where L is the life expectancy of the host. Thus the mean age of infection will be $\bar{a} \simeq L/(R_0 - 1)$ allowing easy back-of-the-envelope calculations of both ϕ and R_0 (Dietz & Schenzle, 1985). The reason why L enters into the calculation is that in a stable host population, host birth rates have to balance death rates, so susceptible recruitment will be $1/L$.[2]

The general rate, $\phi(a,t)$, posits that susceptible infection rates may depend on age (a) and time (t). Ignoring time-dependence (but see Ferrari et al., 2010, for dealing with deviations from this), the cumulative FoI to age a is $\int_0^a \phi(a)da$, and thus the probability of not having been infected by age a is $1 - p(a) = \exp(-\int_0^a \phi(a)da)$ and the probability of being infected on or before age a is (much by the same logic as laid out in Sect. 3.2):

$$p(a) = 1 - e^{-\int_0^a \phi(a)\,da}. \tag{5.1}$$

Equation (5.1) is the standard catalytic model (Muench, 1959; Hens et al., 2010).[3] Age-intensity curves and age-seroprevalence curves are important data sources for fitting the model estimating the FoI in any given population. For nonlethal, persistent infections and nonlethal, fully immunizing infections, the former/latter provides important data for estimating $\phi(a)$. In the simplest case where the FoI is independent of both age and time, the probability of having been infected by age a is $1 - \exp(-\phi a)$. If we have data on the number of infected individuals by age, we can then use the standard generalized linear model (glm) framework to estimate the FoI for the age-invariant FoI model.

Generalized linear models (McCullagh & Nelder, 1989) have two components: an error distribution (such as binomial, Poisson, negative binomial, normal, etc.) and a "link" function that specifies how the expected (predicted) values $\hat{y}$ are linked to the linear predictors $x = c_0 + c_1 x_1 + c_1 x_2 \cdots$. Common link functions are (depending on error distributions): "identity," "log," "logit" (= "log-odds" = $\log(\hat{y}/(1-\hat{y}))$), and "complimentary log-log" (= $\log(-\log(1-\hat{y}))$). The link functions are associated with inverse link functions which for the aforementioned are "identity," $\exp(x)$, $\frac{\exp(x)}{1+\exp(x)}$, and $1 - \exp(-x)$, respectively.

Assuming that some n_a individuals of age a reveal from serology that y_a individuals have been previously infected, inferring the average ϕ turns out to be a standard generalized linear binomial regression problem: $p(a) = 1 - exp(-\phi a)$ is the expected fraction infected (or seropositive) by age a. Thus $\log(-\log(1-p(a))) = \log(\phi) + \log(a)$, so we can estimate the age-invariant log-FoI as the intercept from a glm with binomial error, a complimentary log-log link and log-age as a regression

---

[2] In populations of changing size, a more accurate calculation is $\bar{a} \simeq 1/(\mu(R_0 - 1))$, where μ is the host birth rate (Dietz & Schenzle, 1985).

[3] If immunity wanes at a rate ω, the reversible catalytic model is $p(a) = \frac{\phi(a)}{\phi(a)+\omega}(1 - e^{-\int_0^a \phi(a)+\omega da})$ (see e.g., Pomeroy et al., 2015, for an example). Heisey et al. (2006) discuss corrections needed if infection causes significant disease-induced mortality.

"offset." An offset is a covariate that has a fixed coefficient of unity in a regression. The R call will be of the form:[4]

```
glm(cbind(inf, notinf) ~ offset(log(a)),
    family = binomial(link = "cloglog"))
```

The prevaccination measles antibody data of Black (1959) represent seroprevalence by age of some 300 people from New Haven, Connecticut from blood drawn in the summer of 1957:

```
data(black)
black
```

```
##      age   mid    n pos neg          f
## 1    <1   0.75   10    8   2  0.8000000
## 2   1-4   2.50   21    4  17  0.1904762
## 3   5-9   7.00   41   31  10  0.7560976
## 4 10-14  12.00   52   50   2  0.9615385
## 5 15-19  17.00   30   28   2  0.9333333
## 6 20-29  25.00   38   37   1  0.9736842
## 7 30-39  35.00   51   49   2  0.9607843
## 8 40-49  45.00   35   31   4  0.8857143
## 9   >50  60.00   30   26   4  0.8666667
```

The age profile of seroprevalence takes the characteristic shape of many prevaccination childhood diseases: high seroprevalence of the very young (< 1 year) due to the presence of maternal antibodies that wanes with age, followed by buildup of immunity to almost 100% seroprevalence by age 20 (Fig. 5.1). In these data, there is perhaps some evidence of loss of immunity in the elderly, so we use the binomial regression scheme to estimate the log-FoI based on the data for people in the 1–40 year groups and compare predicted and observed seroprevalence by age (Fig. 5.1):

```
b2 = black[-c(1, 8, 9), ]  #subsetting age brackets
#Estimate log-FoI
fit = glm(cbind(pos,neg) ~ offset(log(mid)),
    family = binomial(link = "cloglog"), data = b2)
#Plot predicted and observed
phi = exp(coef(fit))
curve(1 - exp(-phi * x), from = 0, to = 60,
    ylab = "Seroprevalence", xlab = "Age")
points(black$mid, black$f, pch = "*", col = "red")
points(x = b2$mid, y = b2$f, pch = 8)
phi
```

```
## (Intercept)
##   0.1653329
```

```
1/phi
```

```
## (Intercept)
##    6.048405
```

---

[4] Binomial regression using `glm` takes either a binary 0/1 variable as the response or a matrix with two columns representing number of successes and failures for each covariate level.

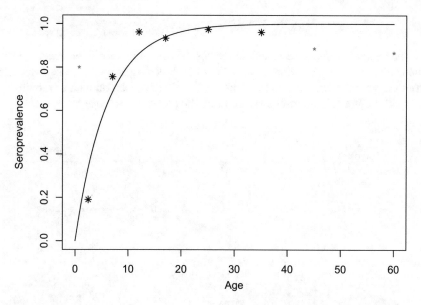

Fig. 5.1: Seroprevalence by age from the measles antibody study of Black (1959) from prevaccination Connecticut. The solid line is the predicted age-prevalence curve for the subset of the data used for estimation (black stars). The smaller red stars are data excluded from estimates due to maternal antibodies in the young and possibly waning titers in the elderly

The estimated FoI is 0.16/year, giving a predicted mean age of infection of 6 years.

5.3 More Flexible ϕ-Functions

The assumption of a constant, age-invariant FoI is usually too simplistic because of age- or time-varying patterns of mixing (Sect. 4.3). Long et al.'s (2010) data on prevalence of the bacterium *Bordetella bronchiseptica* in a rabbit breeding facility provides an illustration. *B. bronchiseptica* is a non-immunizing, largely avirulent (though it can cause snuffles), persistent infection of rabbits. The motivation for the study was to better understand which age groups are most involved in the circulation of the pathogen. Two hundred and fourteen rabbits of known age (in months) were swabbed nasally and tested for the bacterium.

```
data(rabbit)
head(rabbit)

##       a  n inf
## 1 1.0 59   3
## 2 2.0  8   7
## 3 2.5  4   4
## 4 3.0  2   1
## 5 3.5  5   1
```

```
## 6 4.0  2    0
```

The average FoI can be calculated using the binomial regression scheme introduced above. In the breeding facility, the older breeding animals are kept separate
from the younger animals, so the below estimation is based on data of rabbits < 1
year old. Figure 5.2 superimposes the fit on the plot of prevalence by age.

```
rabbit$notinf = rabbit$n - rabbit$inf
#Binomial regression
fit = glm(cbind(inf, notinf) ~ offset(log(a)),
    family = binomial(link = "cloglog"),
    data = rabbit, subset = a < 12)
#Plot data
symbols(rabbit$inf/rabbit$n ~ rabbit$a, circles = rabbit$n,
    inches = 0.5, xlab = "Age", ylab = "Prevalence")
#Predicted curves for <1 yr and all rabbits
phi = exp(coef(fit))
curve(1 - exp(-phi * x), from = 0, to = 12, add = TRUE)
curve(1 - exp(-phi * x), from = 0, to = 30, add = TRUE,
    lty = 2)
1/phi

    ## (Intercept)
    ##     5.918273
```

The predicted median age of infection is just under 6 months. The constant FoI
model seems to do well for up to about 15 months of age, but the model overpredicts
the prevalence in older individuals. To allow for the scenario that the FoI varies with
age, we need to implement our own framework (as opposed to using glm) using
the more general maximum likelihood ideas introduced in Sect. 3.4. One model for
age-specific FoI assumes a piecewise constant model (Grenfell & Anderson, 1985),
where individuals are classified into discrete age classes. For a piecewise constant
model, the integrand in Eq. (5.1) integrates to $\int \phi(a)da = \phi_a(a - c_a) + \sum_{k<a} \phi_k d_k$,
where ϕ_a is the FoI of individuals in the a'th age bracket, and c_a and d_a are the lower
cut-off age and duration of that bracket, respectively. A function for the integrand
takes the argument a for age, up is a vector of the upper cut-offs for each age
bracket, and foi is the vector of age-specific FoIs according to:

```
integrandpc = function(a, up, foi) {
    # Find which interval a belongs to
    wh = findInterval(a, sort(c(0, up)))
    # Calculate duration of each interval
    dur = diff(sort(c(0, up)))
    # Evaluate integrand
    inte = ifelse(wh == 1, foi[1] * a, sum(foi[1:(wh -
        1)] * dur[1:(wh - 1)]) + foi[wh] * (a - up[wh -
        1]))
    return(inte)
}
```

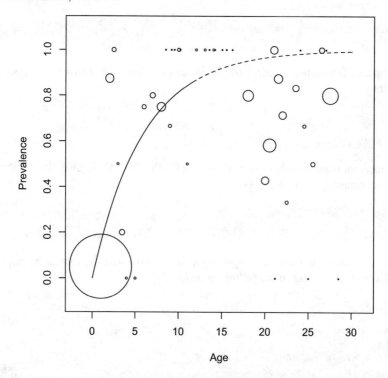

Fig. 5.2: Age-prevalence of *B. bronchiseptica* in a rabbit breeding facility. Circle size is proportional to the number of animals tested in each age group. The solid line is the predicted age-prevalence curve for the subset of the data used for estimation (up to 1-year old animals). The dotted line is the extrapolation to older individuals

The negative log-likelihood function for the piecewise model takes arguments corresponding to log-FoI (par), age (age), the number of positives (num), the number tested in each age group (denom), and age class cut-offs (up). Estimating the FoI on a log-scale (foi=exp(par)) ensures that all rates will be positive:

```
llik.pc = function(par, age, num, denom, up) {
    ll = 0
    for (i in 1:length(age)) {
        p = 1 - exp(-integrandpc(a = age[i], up = up,
            foi = exp(par)))
        ll = ll + dbinom(num[i], denom[i], p, log = TRUE)
    }
    return(-ll)
}
```

For this example, upper cut-off ages are taken as 1, 4, 8, 12, 18, 24, and 30 months and arbitrary initial values of 0.1 are assigned for each piece of the FoI function prior to optimization:

```
x = c(1, 4, 8, 12, 18, 24, 30)
para = rep(0.1, length(x))
```

The optim function will search for the maximum likelihood estimates for each age
bracket:

```
est = optim(par = log(para), fn = llik.pc, age = rabbit$a,
    num = rabbit$inf, denom = rabbit$n, up = x,
    method = "Nelder-Mead")
```

The resultant maximum likelihood estimates for the log-FoI are given in est$par.
The associated age-specific FoIs are:

```
round(exp(est$par), 4)
```

```
## [1] 0.0626 0.3712 0.0573 0.0000 0.0000 0.0000 0.0027
```

Figure 5.3 shows the predicted age-prevalence curve from the estimated stepwise
FoI function according to the following code:

```
#Make space for left and right axes
par(mar = c(5, 5, 2, 5))
#Add beginning and ends to x and y for step plot
xvals = c(0, x)
yvals = exp(c(est$par, est$par[7]))
plot(xvals, yvals, type = "s", xlab = "age", ylab = "FoI")

#Superimpose predicted curve
par(new = T)
p = rep(0, 28)
for (i in 1:28) {
    p[i] = 1 - exp(-integrandpc(a = i, up = x,
        foi = exp(est$par)))
}
plot(p ~ c(1:28), ylim = c(0, 1), type = "l", col = "red",
    axes = FALSE, xlab = NA, ylab = NA)

#Add right axis and legend
axis(side = 4)
mtext(side = 4, line = 4, "Prevalence")
legend("right", legend = c("FoI", "Prevalence"),
    lty = c(1, 1), col = c("black", "red"))
```

The FoI peaks perinatally and then falls to zero after the 8-month age class. This
is likely due to the older breeder females being housed separately and only having
contact with their kittens. Long et al. (2010) used this (in combination with some
other analyses; see Sect. 18.5) to conclude that most infections happen at a young
age from infected mothers to their offspring and then among litter mates.

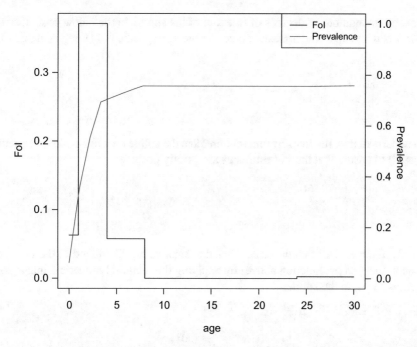

Fig. 5.3: The piecewise constant age-specific FoI of *B. bronchiseptica* in a rabbit breeding facility and the associated predicted age-prevalence curve

5.4 A Log-Spline Model

An alternative nonparametric approach to the piecewise constant model is to use smoothing splines. A regression spline is a smooth curve that can take an arbitrary shape except that it is constrained to be continuous and with continuous first and second derivatives (Härdle, 1990; Hastie & Tibshirani, 1990). The popularity of splines in nonparametric regression stems from its computational tractability; a spline can be fit by multiple regression on a set of basis function decompositions of a covariate. The gam and mgcv packages offer automated ways to fit a variety of spline variants to binomial data (and any other error distribution within the exponential family). Unfortunately, as with the case of the piecewise constant model, fitting the log-spline model is a bit more involved because of the integration step in Eq. (5.1). The splines package has functions to create various spline bases that can be used with the lm function; predict.lm can predict values for the spline given regression coefficients.

The approach taken here is a bit cheeky in that it hijacks a spline regression object created using the bs spline basis functions in combination with lm and uses optim to update/override the regression coefficients of the lm object via a binomial maximum likelihood until a solution is found. The smoothness of the age-FoI curve is set by the number of degrees of freedom of the spline. In the below code, the dl object will end up as the hijacked object for the age-specific FoI (Long et al., 2010).

```
require(splines)
# Degrees-of-freedom
df = 7
# Construct dummy lm object
dl = lm(inf ~ bs(a, df), data = rabbit)
```

To undertake this, the tmpfn function predicts the spline on a log-scale (to be anti-logged) to ensure that the FoI estimates are strictly positive:

```
tmpfn = function(x, dl) {
    x = predict(dl, newdata = data.frame(a = x))
    exp(x)
}
```

Finally, the tmpfn2 function calculates the negative log-likelihood of the FoIs (as done in the foipc function above) by applying the inbuilt R numerical integrator, integrate, to the spline:

```
tmpfn2 = function(par, data, df) {
    # Dummy lm object
    dl = lm(inf ~ bs(a, df), data = data)
    # Overwrite spline coefficients with new values
    dl$coefficients = par
    # Calculate log-likelihood
    ll = 0
    for (i in 1:length(data$a)) {
        p = 1 - exp(-integrate(tmpfn, 0, i, dl = dl)$value)
        ll = ll + dbinom(data$inf[i], data$n[i], p, log = T)
    }
    return(-ll)
}
```

As per previously, arbitrary initial values are optimized through the minimization of the negative log-likelihood using optim.

```
para = rep(-1, df + 1)
dspline = optim(par = para, fn = tmpfn2, data = rabbit,
    df = df, method = "Nelder-Mead", control = list(trace = 2,
        maxit = 2000))
```

Figure 5.4 shows the resultant maximum likelihood fits.

```
par(mar = c(5, 5, 2, 5))  #Room for two axes
# Overwrite dummy object coefficients with MLEs
dl$coefficients = dspline$par
# Age-prevalence plot
plot(tmpfn(rabbit$a, dl) ~ rabbit$a, type = "l", ylab = "FoI",
    xlab = "Age (mos)", las = 1)
# Overlay FoI
par(new = TRUE)
```

```
p = rep(0, 28)
for (i in 1:28) {
    p[i] = 1 - exp(-integrate(tmpfn, 0, i, dl = dl)$value)
}
plot(p ~ c(1:28), ylim = c(0, 1), type = "l", col = "red",
    axes = FALSE, xlab = NA, ylab = NA)
axis(side = 4, las = 1)
mtext(side = 4, line = 4, "Prevalence")
legend("topright", legend = c("FoI", "Prevalence"), lty = c(1,
    1), col = c("black", "red"))
```

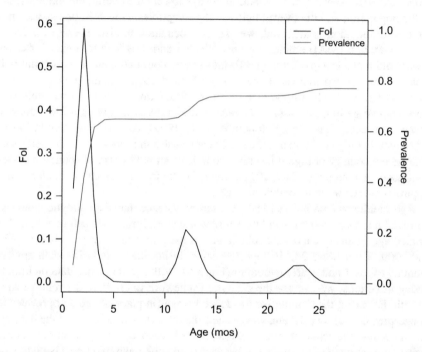

Fig. 5.4: The spline estimate of the age-specific FoI of *B. bronchiseptica* in a rabbit breeding facility

Both the piecewise (Fig. 5.3) and spline (Fig. 5.4) models show strong evidence of age-specificity in the FoI with a peak in transmission somewhere between 1 and 5 months of age, suggesting that circulation is mainly among the young and among litter mates (Long et al., 2010). We revisit this case study in Sect. 18.5.

5.5 Rubella

Rubella is a relatively mild, vaccine-preventable viral infection that causes fever and rash in children, but infection during pregnancy leads to stillbirths or congenital rubella syndrome (CRS). It is thus one of the classic teratogenic diseases. The main public health objective is therefore to minimize the FoI in women of childbearing age. As discussed in Sect. 5.2, being a rate of infection of susceptibles, the FoI governs not only the mean but also the full distribution of the age of first infection, which in the case of fully immunizing infection like rubella is the only infection an individual will experience. Vaccination always lowers the overall circulation (FoI) in the population and the overall number of susceptibles. However, unless vaccine-induced elimination is achieved, we expect vaccination to also increase the mean age of infection (MAI) among the unvaccinated and thus lead to a skew of cases toward older age groups. Knox (1980) thus pointed out that there is a potential risk that vaccination can increase burden of CRS (and other vaccine-preventable teratogenic diseases). The importance of this consideration is clearly illustrated by a surprising surge in CRS cases in Greece in the mid-90s following a low-intensity vaccination campaign (Panagiotopoulos et al., 1999). As a rule of thumb, WHO subsequently only recommends the use of the measles–mumps–rubella (MMR) vaccine once a country or region has reached at least an 80% cover of routine measles childhood vaccination (WHO, 2011). The catalytic framework can help clarify the tipping point for when to switch strategies.

Age-incidence data is less ideal than seroprevalence data for catalytic analysis; however, it is more common and therefore worth considering. Metcalf et al. (2011c) studied age-intensity curves for rubella across the provinces of Peru between 1997 and 2009. There were 24,116 reported cases during the period. The data are ½-monthly to age 1 and yearly thereafter (Fig. 5.5). With age-incidence data on immunizing infections, we can use the catalytic framework to estimate the relative age-specific FoI using the cumulative incidence by age (in place of age-seroprevalence or age-prevalence). For the analysis, we use the total number of cases as the denominator because the actual number of susceptibles in each age group is not monitored. Hence, the estimate is a *relative* FoI because of the unknown baseline. Using the total cases as a denominator leads to sever biases of the FoI at old age classes (because exactly all of the assumed susceptibles in the final age class will be presumed to be infected at the time), so it should only be applied to the younger portion of the data.[5]

```
data(peru)
head(peru)

##          age incidence cumulative      n
## 2 0.01095890         1         56  24116
## 3 0.01369863         1         57  24116
## 4 0.01643836         1         58  24116
## 5 0.01917808         2         60  24116
```

---

[5] Its application also assumes a uniform age distribution, so a correction for the age-pyramid may be necessary for a more refined analysis (Ferrari et al., 2010).

```
## 6 0.03561644              1              61 24116
## 7 0.03835616              2              63 24116

# Calculate cumulative incidence
peru$cumulative = cumsum(peru$incidence)
# Define denominator
peru$n = sum(peru$incidence)
par(mar = c(5, 5, 2, 5))   #Make room for two axes and plot
# Plot incidence with cumulative overlaid
plot(peru$incidence ~ peru$age, type = "b", xlab = "Age",
    ylab = "Incidence")
par(new = T)
plot(peru$cumulative ~ peru$age, type = "l", col = "red",
    axes = FALSE, xlab = NA, ylab = NA)
axis(side = 4)
mtext(side = 4, line = 4, "Cumulative")
legend("right", legend = c("Incidence", "Cumulative"),
    lty = c(1, 1), col = c("black", "red"))
```

The first analysis applies the piecewise model assuming a separate FoI for each year up to age 20 and 10 year classes thereafter. Convergence of the piecewise model with this many segments is very slow, so the actual figure (Fig. 5.6) was produced by doing repeat calls to optim using different optimization methods (Nelder-Mead, BFGS, and SANN), feeding the estimates from each call as starting values for the next. However, the basic analysis is:

```
#Upper age cut-offs
up = c(1:20, 30, 40, 50, 60, 70, 80)
para = rep(0.1, length(up)) #Inital values
#Minimize log-likelihood
est2 = optim(par = log(para), fn = llik.pc, age = peru$age,
    num = peru$cumulative, denom = peru$n, up = up,
    method = "Nelder-Mead", control =
    list(trace = 2, maxit = 2000))
#Step plot
x = c(0, up)
y = exp(c(est2$par, est2$par[26]))
plot(x, y, ylab = "Relative FoI", xlab = "Age", type = "s",
    ylim = c(0, 0.25), xlim = c(0, 80))
```

There is a clear peak in FoI in the 8–10 age group (Fig. 5.6). The pattern makes sense given the biology of rubella and the assortative mixing commonly seen in the human host with most contacts being among the same-aged individuals (Sect. 4.3). Peru has a life expectancy of around 75 years, and the R_0 of rubella is typically quoted in the 4–10 range, so according to $\bar{a} \simeq L/(R_0 - 1)$, the peak in circulation would be expected to be in an interval around 10 years of age.

More refined scenario analyses regarding consequences of vaccination can be done using the spline model introduced in Sect. 5.4. The focus is on the 0–45 year age range as this spans the pre- to post-childbearing age:

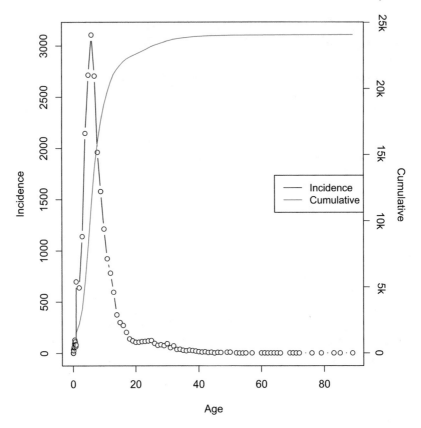

Fig. 5.5: Age-specific incidence and cumulative incidence of rubella in Peru 1997–2009

```
data3 = peru[peru$age < 45, ]
df = 5
para = rep(0.1, df + 1)
```

The analysis follows the above by using a log-transformation to constrain the FoI to be positive, create a dummy lm object, and define the function to evaluate the negative log-likelihood of the FoI curve given the data:

```
# Prediction function
tmpfn = function(x, dl) {
    x = predict(dl, newdata = data.frame(age = x))
    exp(x)
}
# Dummy lm object
dl = lm(cumulative ~ bs(age, df), data = data3)
# Log-likelihood function
tmpfn2 = function(par, data, df) {
```

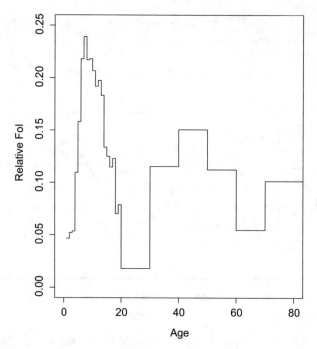

Fig. 5.6: The relative age-specific FoI of rubella in Peru as estimated using the piecewise-constant model

```
dl = lm(cumulative ~ bs(age, df), data = data)
dl$coefficients = par
ll = 0
for (a in 1:length(data$age)) {
    p = ((1 - exp(-integrate(tmpfn, 0, data$age[a],
        dl = dl)$value)))
    ll = ll + dbinom(data$cumulative[a], data$n[a],
        p, log = T)
}
return(-ll)
}
```

Getting a good fit is computationally expensive but reveals an interesting two-peaked force of infection (Fig. 5.7): A dominant peak just under 10 years and a subdominant peak around 35. A plausible scenario is that most people get infected in school, but the fraction that escapes this dominant age of infection is most likely to contract the virus when their children get infected during schooling age.

```
#Fit model
dspline.a45.df5 = optim(par = log(para), fn = tmpfn2,
    data = data3, df = df, method = "Nelder-Mead",
    control = list(trace = 4, maxit = 5000))
```

```
#Overwrite dummy object coefficients with MLEs
dl$coefficients = dspline.a45.df5$par
plot(exp(predict(dl)) ~ data3$age, xlab = "Age",
     ylab = "Relative FoI", type = "l")
```

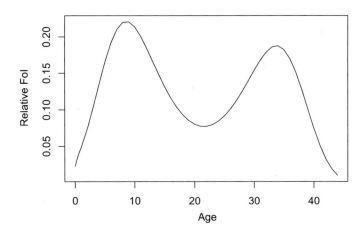

Fig. 5.7: The relative age-specific FoI of rubella in Peru as estimated using the spline model

The fraction of cases that is predicted to occur in the childbearing age-bracket is the joint probability of not being infected by age 15 and thence being infected before age 40:

$$\exp\left(-\int_0^{15} \phi(a)\,da\right)\left(1 - \exp\left(-\int_{15}^{40} \phi(a)\,da\right)\right). \tag{5.2}$$

We can predict this fraction from the spline model.

```
(exp(-integrate(tmpfn, 0, 15, dl = dl)$value)) * (1 -
    exp(-integrate(tmpfn, 15, 40, dl = dl)$value))

  ## [1] 0.08815273
```

Thus, with the current pattern of circulation, just over 9% of the cases are predicted to occur in the at-risk age group. With a flat 50% reduction in FoI, this fraction would change to:

```
redn = 0.5
(exp(-redn * integrate(tmpfn, 0, 15, dl = dl)$value)) *
    (1 - exp(-redn * integrate(tmpfn, 15, 40, dl = dl)$value))

  ## [1] 0.2376147
```

The reduction in FoI is a predicted increase in the mean age of infection (in reality, this will also likely lead to a change in the age-specific FoI curve; see Sect. 4.4), so that almost 24% of cases are predicted to fall in the at-risk group. For simplicity, assuming an associated 50% reduction in cases, the total number in the age-bracket of concern would thus *increase* given this intervention, predicting an intervention-induced enhancement of the public health problem as suggested by Knox (1980) and as was seen in Greece during the 1990s (Panagiotopoulos et al., 1999).

Metcalf and Barrett (2016) discuss public health issues related to the possible introduction of vaccines against the recent teratogenic Zika virus that can cause microcephaly in children of mothers infected during pregnancy in light of the lessons learnt from rubella. Whooping cough is another vaccine preventable disease that causes significant morbidity and mortality in young children. Lavine et al. (2011) discuss how a waning vaccine could increase circulation among people of childbearing age and thus increase the risk of parent–newborn transmission. They recommended that cocoon vaccination of expecting parents should be considered if the current acellular vaccine is as leaky as is feared (Warfel et al., 2014). Althouse and Scarpino (2015) provide further discussion of the utility of cocoon vaccination and other interventions.

Chapter 6
Seasonality

6.1 Environmental Drivers

Host behavior and environmental factors influence disease dynamics in a variety of ways through affecting the pathogen such as the survival of infective stages outside the host and via host demographies from changing birth rates, carrying capacities, social organization, etc. Sometimes such influences have relatively subtle consequences (e.g., slight changes in R_0) as is likely the effect of absolute humidity on influenza transmission (Lowen et al., 2007; Bjørnstad & Viboud, 2016). Other times the consequences are substantial by changing the dynamics qualitatively such as inducing multiannual or chaotic epidemics (London & Yorke, 1973; Schaffer, 1985; Earn et al., 2000b; Dalziel et al., 2016) or initiating ecological cascades (Jones et al., 1998; Glass et al., 2000; Luis et al., 2015). It is useful to distinguish between trends, predictable variability (such as seasonality), or non-predictable variability due to environmental and demographic stochasticity.

Some level of seasonality in transmission is very common in infectious disease dynamics and is usually reflected in seasonal cycles in incidence (Altizer et al., 2006); seasonality in incidence is the norm even for persistent infections for which prevalence may remain relatively stable. Influenza is the poster-child for seasonality in infection risk in the public eye (e.g., Bjørnstad & Viboud, 2016). Figure 6.1a shows the mean weekly influenza-related deaths in Pennsylvania between 1972 and 1998. The pronounced winter-peaked seasonality is linked to how climate conditions, such as temperature and absolute humidity affect rates of viral degradation in the environment (Shaman & Kohn, 2009; Dalziel et al., 2018). There is evidence of similar drivers of other airway viruses such as the respiratory syncytial virus (Pitzer et al., 2015).

We can illustrate various types of seasonality using four infectious diseases in Pennsylvania contained in the `paili`, `palymes`, `pagiard`, and `pameasle`

The chapter uses the following R packages: `deSolve` and `plotrix`.
A five minute epidemics MOOC on seasonality can be seen on youtube:
https://www.youtube.com/watch?v=TDuuM-wm6nw.

© The Author(s), under exclusive license to Springer Nature Switzerland AG 2023   105
O. N. Bjørnstad, *Epidemics*, Use R!, https://doi.org/10.1007/978-3-031-12056-5_6

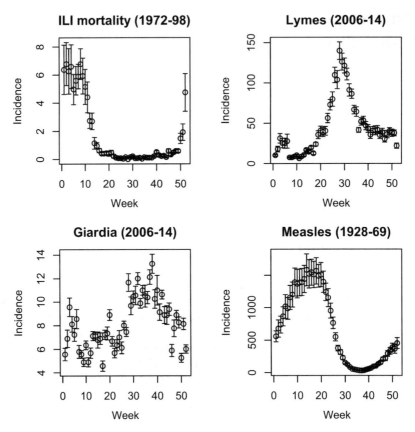

Fig. 6.1: Mean ($\pm$ 1 SD) weekly incidence of (**a**) deaths due to influenza like illness, (**b**) Lyme's disease, (**c**) giardiosis, and (**d**) pre-vaccination measles in Pennsylvania

datasets. The below is a simple function to extract and plot weekly average incidence (and standard errors) through the year from time series. Weekly incidence data occasionally has 53 reporting weeks (because years are 52.14 weeks, and leap years are 52.28 weeks). The function omits these extras.[1]

```
ppp = function(wk, x) {
    require(plotrix)
    x = x[wk < 53]
    wk = wk[wk < 53]
    ses = sapply(split(x, wk), mean, na.rm = TRUE)
    sesv = sapply(split(x, wk), sd, na.rm = TRUE)
    sesdv = sesv/sapply(split(x, wk), sd, na.rm = TRUE)
```

---

[1] `split` creates a `list` from a `vector` and `sapply` applies a function to a `list` to return a new `vector`.

```
    plotCI(x = c(1:52), y = ses, ui = ses + sesdv, li = ses -
        sesdv, xlab = "Week", ylab = "Incidence")
}
```

Figure 6.1 shows the seasonality in reported incidence of Lyme's disease, giardiosis, measles, and mortality from influenza-like illness (ILI) in Pennsylvania.

```
par(mfrow = c(2, 2))  #A four panel plot
ppp(paili[, "WEEK"], paili[, "PENNSYLVANIA"])
title("ILI mortality (1972-98)")
ppp(palymes[, "WEEK"], palymes[, "PENNSYLVANIA"])
title("Lymes (2006-14)")
ppp(pagiard[, "WEEK"], pagiard[, "PENNSYLVANIA"])
title("Giardia (2006-14)")
ppp(pameasle[, "WEEK"], pameasle[, "PENNSYLVANIA"])
title("Measles (1928-69)")
```

Seasonality arises from a variety of causes depending on the mode of transmission of the pathogen: air-borne (like influenza), vector-borne, or water-/food-borne. Lyme's disease, for example, is caused by tick-vectored bacteria in the genus *Borrelia*. Figure 6.1b shows the sharply seasonal incidence of human cases of Lyme's in Pennsylvania. The seasonality is the combined effect of seasonality in tick activity levels and human use of wilderness. Most mosquito-vectored pathogens also show strong seasonality because of the temperature- and precipitation-dependence of the vector life cycle. The seasonality of cholera infections, caused by the *Vibrio cholerae* bacterium, is among the most studied water-borne pathogens. The seasonality in southeast Asia is caused by rainfall variation associated with the monsoon season (Codeço, 2001; Ruiz-Moreno et al., 2007) (Fig. 1.3b). However, other water-borne diseases like giardiasis caused by protozoans in the genus *Giardia* also show marked seasonality (Fig. 6.1c). Host behavior can further cause seasonality in contact rates. Childhood disease dynamics, for example, are often shaped by "term-time" forcing: increased transmission when schools are open (e.g., Fine & Clarkson, 1982; Kucharski et al., 2015). Weekly average prevaccination incidence of measles in Pennsylvania, for instance, collapses as school closes for the summer only to resume robust circulation after the vacation ends (Fig. 6.1d). Additionally, seasonal urban–rural migration in Niger has been shown to generate strong seasonality in measles transmission (Ferrari et al., 2008). Seasonally varying birth rates can induce seasonality in susceptible recruitment in wildlife (Swinton et al., 1998; Peel et al., 2014) and humans (Martinez-Bakker et al., 2014).

6.2 The Seasonally Forced SEIR Model

To study the effect of seasonality in transmission, we modify the SEIR model (Eqs. (3.3)–(3.6)). We first consider the gradient functions for the undriven system. As in Sect. 4.4, we use with(as.list(...)) to evaluate the expression using the definitions in the parms vector.

```
seirmod = function(t, y, parms) {
    S = y[1]
    E = y[2]
    I = y[3]
    R = y[4]

    with(as.list(parms), {
        dS = mu * (N - S) - beta * S * I/N
        dE = beta * S * I/N - (mu + sigma) * E
        dI = sigma * E - (mu + gamma) * I
        dR = gamma * I - mu * R
        res = c(dS, dE, dI, dR)
        list(res)
    })
}
```

We can simulate 10 years of dynamics using the basic recipe introduced in Sect. 2.3. The seasonally forced SEIR model has been successfully applied to understand the dynamics of measles, such as those depicted in Fig. 1.4, and other immunizing childhood infections (e.g., Schwartz, 1985; Earn et al., 2000b; Bauch & Earn, 2003). To simulate a measles-like pathogen, assume a latent period of 8 days and an infectious period of 5 days. Assume the initial host population to be 0.1% infectious, 6% susceptibles, and the rest immune; the R_0 of measles is typically quoted in the 13–20 range, which means that the equilibrium fraction of susceptibles is somewhere around 5%. For simplicity, assume a host life span of 50 years and set $N = 1$ to model the fraction in each compartment.

```
require(deSolve)
times = seq(0, 10, by = 1/120)
paras = c(mu = 1/50, N = 1, beta = 1000, sigma = 365/8,
    gamma = 365/5)
start = c(S = 0.06, E = 0, I = 0.001, R = 0.939)
```

As discussed in Sect. 3.7, the R_0 for this system, assuming disease-induced mortality is negligible, is $\frac{\sigma}{\sigma+\mu}\frac{\beta}{\gamma+\mu}$.[2] We can verify that our choice of β places R_0 in the measles-like range. We use quote to define the equation for R_0.

```
R0 = quote(sigma/(sigma + mu) * beta/(gamma + mu))
with(as.list(paras), eval(R0))
```

```
## [1] 13.68888
```

The integrated ODEs plotted in time and in the phase plane reveal that, as is the case of the SIR model, the unforced SEIR model predicts dampened oscillations toward the endemic equilibrium when R_0 is above one (Fig. 6.2).

---

[2] If the infection has a case fatality ratio of, say, 30%, the additional *rate* of removal is $\alpha = -log(1 - 0.3)/ip$, where ip is the duration of infection and the appropriate calculation would be $R_0 = \sigma\beta/(\sigma+\mu)(\gamma+\mu+\alpha)$.

```
out = as.data.frame(ode(start, times, seirmod, paras))
par(mfrow = c(1, 2))   #Two plots side by side
plot(times, out$I, ylab = "Prevalence", xlab = "Time",
     type = "l")
plot(out$S, out$I, ylab = "Prevalence", xlab = "Susceptible",
     type = "l")
```

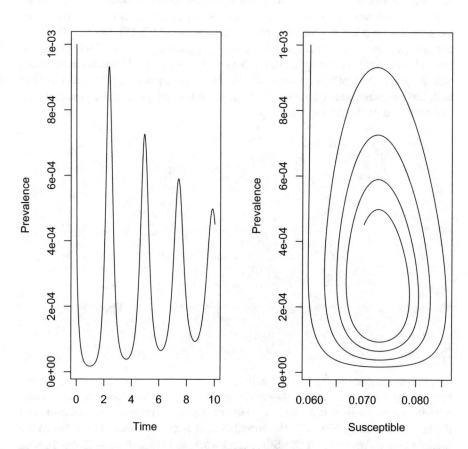

Fig. 6.2: Predicted prevalence from the SEIR model (**a**) in time, and (**b**) in the phase plane with $\mu = 1/50$, $N = 1$(to model fractions), $\beta = 1000$, $\sigma = 365/8$, and $\gamma = 365/5$. Ten years are not long enough for the simulation to settle on the endemic equilibrium, but the dampened cycles are apparent

6.3 Seasonality in β

The predicted dampened oscillations toward an equilibrium are at odds with the recurrent outbreaks seen in many immunizing infections (e.g., Fig. 1.4). Sustained oscillations require either additional predictable seasonal drivers—the topic of this chapter—or stochasticity (Sect. 8.2). An important driver in human childhood infections is seasonality in contact rates because of aggregation of children during the school term (Fine & Clarkson, 1982; Kucharski et al., 2015). For simplicity, we can analyze the consequences of seasonality by assuming sinusoidal forcing on the transmission rate[3] according to $\beta(t) = \beta_0(1 + \beta_1 cos(2\pi t))$. The mean transmission rate is β_0, but the realized transmission varies cyclically with a period of one time unit, and the magnitude of the seasonal variation is controlled by the parameter β_1. The modified gradient function is:

```
seirmod2 = function(t, y, parameters) {
    S = y[1]
    E = y[2]
    I = y[3]
    R = y[4]

    with(as.list(parameters), {
        dS = mu * (N - S) - beta0 * (1 + beta1 * cos(2 *
            pi * t)) * S * I/N
        dE = beta0 * (1 + beta1 * cos(2 * pi * t)) * S *
            I/N - (mu + sigma) * E
        dI = sigma * E - (mu + gamma) * I
        dR = gamma * I - mu * R
        res = c(dS, dE, dI, dR)
        list(res)
    })
}
```

With no seasonality, the model predicts dampened oscillation, and with moderate seasonality, the prediction is low-amplitude annual outbreaks. However, as seasonality increases (to $\beta_1 = 0.2$, say), we start seeing some surprising consequences of the seasonal forcing (Fig. 6.3): the appearance of harmonic resonance between the internal cyclic dynamics of the SEIR clockwork and the annual seasonal forcing function.

```
times  = seq(0, 100, by=1/120)
paras  = c(mu = 1/50, N = 1, beta0 = 1000, beta1 = 0.2,
    sigma = 365/8, gamma = 365/5)
start = c(S = 0.06, E = 0, I = 0.001, R = 0.939)
out = as.data.frame(ode(start, times, seirmod2, paras))
par(mfrow = c(1, 2)) #Side-by-side plot
plot(times, out$I, ylab="Infected", xlab="Time",
```

---

[3] It is possible to analyze more realistic patterns of seasonality, such as a more explicit term-time forcing; see Keeling et al. (2001) and Chap. 8. The qualitative (but not detailed) results appear to be robust to the exact shape of the forcing function.

```
        xlim = c(90, 100), ylim = c(0,
            max(out$I[11001:12000])), type = "l")
plot(out$S[11001:12000], out$I[11001:12000],
        ylab = "Infected", xlab = "Susceptible", type = "l")
```

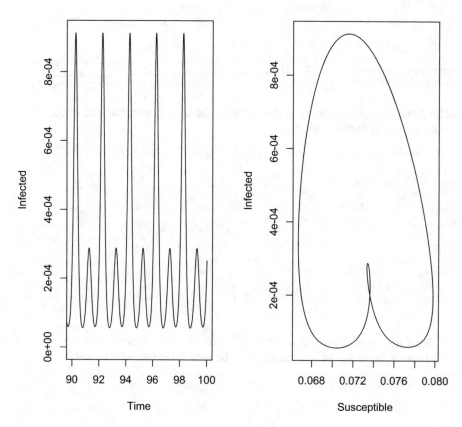

Fig. 6.3: The 10 last years of the forced SEIR model for $\beta_1 = 0.2$. (**a**) Predicted prevalence and (**b**) the S–I phase plane

The emergent pattern of recurrence in the forced SEIR model is the result of an interaction between the internal periodic clockwork (the damping period) of the SEIR flow and the externally imposed periodic forcing. The damping period is the focus of Chap. 10. However we can use the results previewed in Sect. 2.7: When working with a continuous-time ODE model which results in cyclic behavior like the SEIR model, the dominant eigenvalues of the <u>Jacobian matrix</u>—when evaluated at the equilibrium—are a conjugate pair of complex numbers $(a \pm bi)$ that determines the period according to $2\pi/b$.

The endemic equilibrium of the SEIR model is $S^* = 1/R_0$, $E^* = (\mu + \gamma)I^*/\sigma$ and $I^* = \mu(1 - 1/R_0)R_0/\beta$ (ignoring the absorbing compartment $R^* = 1 - S^* - E^* - I^*$):

```
mu = paras["mu"]
N = paras["N"]
beta0 = paras["beta0"]
beta1 = paras["beta1"]
sigma = paras["sigma"]
gamma = paras["gamma"]
R0 = sigma/(sigma + mu) * beta0/(gamma + mu)
# Equilibria
Sstar = 1/R0
Istar = mu * (1 - 1/R0) * R0/beta0
Estar = (mu + gamma) * Istar/sigma
eq = list(S = Sstar, E = Estar, I = Istar)
```

The D function can carry out symbolic differentiation to generate and evaluate the elements of the Jacobian matrix:

```
dS = quote(mu * (N  - S)  - beta0 * S * I / N)
dE = quote(beta0 * S * I / N - (mu + sigma) * E)
dI = quote(sigma*E - (mu + gamma) * I)
#Elements of Jacobian
j11 = D(dS, "S"); j12 = D(dS, "E"); j13 = D(dS, "I")
j21 = D(dE, "S"); j22 = D(dE, "E"); j23 = D(dE, "I")
j31 = D(dI, "S"); j32 = D(dI, "E"); j33 = D(dI, "I")
#Jacobian
J = with(eq,
matrix(c(eval(j11),eval(j12),eval(j13),
    eval(j21),eval(j22), eval(j23),
    eval(j31),eval(j32), eval(j33)),
    nrow=3, byrow=TRUE))
```

In this calculation, the dominant pair of complex conjugates is at the second and third places in the vector of eigenvalues. The associated resonant period is:

```
round(eigen(J)$values, 3)
```

```
  ## [1]  -118.725+0.000i   -0.107+2.667i    -0.107-2.667i
```

```
2 * pi/(Im(eigen(J)$values[2]))
```

```
  ## [1] 2.355891
```

So, the recurrent biennial epidemics are sustained because the internal epidemic clockwork cycles with a period of 2.3 years, but it is forced at an annual time scale, so as a compromise the epidemics are locked on to the annual clock, but with alternating major and minor epidemics such as seen, for example, in prevaccination measles in New York 1944–1958 (Fig. 1.4b) and London 1950–1965 (Fig. 1.4c). Section 6.8 introduces a general-purpose Jacobian calculator that makes these calculations less arduous.

6.4 Bifurcation Analysis

We can make a more comprehensive summary of the consequences of seasonality on the SEIR flow using a bifurcation analysis: A systematic search across a range of β_1 values. For annually forced models, this is best done by strobing the system once each year. To study the long-term (asymptotic) dynamics, we discard the initial transient part of the simulation. In the below, we hence use one data point per year for the last 42 years of simulation (which the `sel` variable flags) so that an annual cycle produces a single value (so will a fixed-point equilibrium), biannual cycles two values, etc. The resultant bifurcation plot shows when annual epidemics gives way to biannual cycles and finally chaotic dynamics as seasonality increases (Fig. 6.4). The irregular dynamics with strong seasonality comes about because there is no simple resonant compromise between the internal clock and the external forcing function. We may think of it as resonance giving place to dissonance in the dynamical system. That stronger seasonality pushes measles from regular to irregular epidemics has been predicted by the theoretical literature (e.g., Aron & Schwartz, 1984) and is supported by an empirical comparison of measles dynamics in prevaccination UK and USA by Dalziel et al. (2016) (see Sect. 11.2).

First define initial conditions and the sequence of parameter values to be considered for β_1 and then do the numerical integration for each of its values:

```
times = seq(0, 100, by = 1/120)
start = c(S = 0.06, E = 0, I = 0.001, R = 0.939)
beta1 = seq(0, 0.25, length = 101)
# Matrix to store infecteds
Imat = matrix(NA, ncol = 12001, nrow = 101)
# Loop over beta1's
for (i in 1:101) {
    paras = c(mu = 1/50, N = 1, beta0 = 1000, beta1 = beta1[i],
        sigma = 365/8, gamma = 365/5)
    out = as.data.frame(ode(start, times, seirmod2, paras))
    Imat[i, ] = out$I
}
```

For the visualization arbitrarily select the prevalence at the beginning of the 4th month each year of the simulations and plot the values against the associated β_1 values for the bifurcation plot (Fig. 6.4).

```
sel = seq(7001, 12000, by = 120)
plot(NA, xlim = range(beta1), ylim = c(1e-07, max(Imat[,
    sel])), log = "y", xlab = "beta1", ylab = "prevalence")
for (i in 1:101) {
    points(rep(beta1[i], length(sel)), Imat[i, sel], pch = 20)
}
```

Thus, with measles-like parameters, annual epidemics give way to biennial cycles at β_1 around 0.15 corresponding to a seasonal coefficient of variation (CV) in transmission of 10% and chaos for β_1 just over 0.2 corresponding to a CV of around 15%.

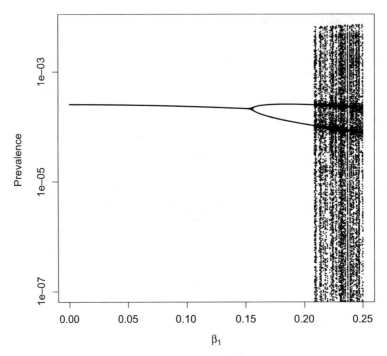

Fig. 6.4: The bifurcation plot of prevalence at the beginning of the 4th month of each year against seasonality for the forced SEIR model

6.5 Stroboscopic Section

Rand and Wilson (1991) studied the seasonally forced SEIR model with a set of parameters resulting in chaotic dynamics. It is interesting to integrate the model with these parameters for a very long time (in this case for 10,000 years) to better understand/visualize the meaning of quasi-periodic chaos. We will discuss this topic in greater detail in Sect. 11.2. Figure 6.5 shows a time series of prevalence and the dynamics in the S–I phase plane strobed at the annual time scale—the annual stroboscopic section of the S–I plane. The time series is erratic, but the paired S–I series trace out a very intricate pattern (Fig. 6.5b); the four-armed shape corresponds to the propensity of the chaotic pattern to adhere to a wobbly quasi-periodic 4-year recurrence. Chapter 11 will revisit on this attractor and its role in facilitating "chaotic stochasticity" and "stochastic resonance."

```
times = seq(0, 1e+05, by = 1/120)
start = c(S = 0.06, E = 0, I = 0.001, R = 0.939)
paras = c(mu = 1/50, N = 1, beta0 = 1800, beta1 = 0.28,
    sigma = 35.84, gamma = 100)
out = as.data.frame(ode(start, times, seirmod2, paras))
sel = seq(7001, 1.2e+07, by = 120)
```

```
par(mfrow = c(1, 2))
plot(out$time[7001:13001], out$I[7001:13001], type = "l",
     xlab = "Year", ylab = "Prevalence")
plot(out$S[sel], out$I[sel], type = "p", xlab = "S", ylab = "I",
     log = "y", pch = 20, cex = 0.25)
```

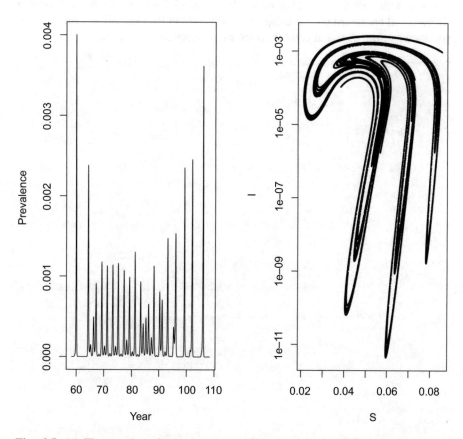

Fig. 6.5: (**a**) Time series of prevalence. (**b**) S–I phase plane of the annual strobo-scopic section of the quasi-periodic chaotic prevalence of a seasonally forced SEIR model ($\mu = 0.02$, $\beta_0 = 1800$, $\beta_1 = 0.28$, $\sigma = 35.84$, and $\gamma = 100$) (Rand & Wilson, 1991)

6.6 Susceptible Recruitment

The patterns of recurrent epidemics are also shaped by other characteristics of the host and pathogen. Earn et al. (2000b) studied how susceptible recruitment affects dynamics of the seasonally forced SEIR model by doing a bifurcation analysis over

μ (Fig. 6.6). As shown by Earn et al. (2000b), reduced susceptible recruitment in the seasonally forced SEIR model leads to a cascade from annual to biennial to coexisting annual and complex attractors.[4] To trace out the coexisting attractors, it is necessary to use multiple starting conditions because each attractor will have its own <u>basin of attraction</u>; that is, despite being a deterministic model, the dynamic behavior will change depending on the initial conditions. We do this by looping forward and backward over μ using the final values of the simulation with previous parameter values as initial conditions for the subsequent simulation.

```
times = seq(0, 100, by = 1/120)
start = c(S = 0.06, E = 0, I = 0.001, R = 0.939)
mu = seq(from = 0.005, to = 0.02, length = 101)
ImatF = ImatB = matrix(NA, ncol = 12001, nrow = 101)
#Forwards analysis
for(i in 1:101){
    paras  = c(mu = mu[i], N = 1, beta0 = 2500,
        beta1=0.12, sigma = 365/8, gamma = 365/5)
    out = as.data.frame(ode(start, times, seirmod2,
        paras))
    ImatF[i,] = out$I
    start = c(S = out$S[12001], E = out$E[12001],
        I = out$I[12001], R = out$R[12001])
}
#Backwards analysis
start = c(S = 0.06, E = 0, I = 0.001, R = 0.939)
for(i in 101:1){
    paras  = c(mu = mu[i], N = 1, beta0 = 2500,
        beta1 = 0.12, sigma = 365/8, gamma = 365/5)
    out = as.data.frame(ode(start, times, seirmod2,
        paras))
    ImatB[i,] = out$I
    start = c(S = out$S[12001], E = out$E[12001],
        I = out$I[12001], R = out$R[12001])
}
#Forward/backward bifurcation plot
sel = seq(7001, 12000, by = 120)
par(mfrow = c(1,1))
    plot(NA, xlim = range(mu),  ylim = range(ImatF[,sel]),
        log = "y", xlab = "mu", ylab = "prevalence")
for(i in 1:101){
    points(rep(mu[i], dim(ImatF)[2]), ImatF[i, ],
        pch = 20, cex = 0.25)
    points(rep(mu[i], dim(ImatB)[2]), ImatB[i, ],
        pch = 20, cex = 0.25, col = 2)
}
```

---

[4] We discuss coexisting attractors in further detail in Sect. 11.4.

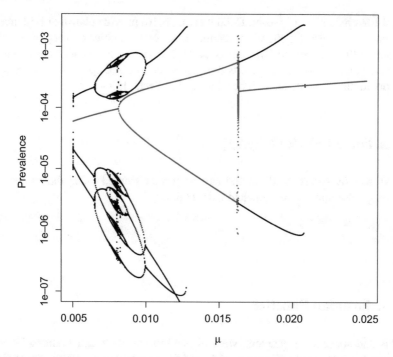

Fig. 6.6: The bifurcation plot of prevalence against birth rate μ for the forced SEIR model with intermediate (8.5% CV) seasonality. Black represents values from the forward analysis and red the backward analysis

In Fig. 6.6, the attractor from the forward analysis is shown in black and backward analysis in red. This color coding reveals the coexisting attractors for a range of parameter values. The predicted transition from biennial epidemics to annual when birth rates are above 25 per thousand per year is confirmed from changes in measles dynamics following the baby boom post-World War II in the UK (see Fig. 1.4c and Sect. 7.6). The complex dynamics at lower susceptible recruitment rates comes about for the same reasons as discussed in Sect. 6.4 because of dissonance between the external annual forcing and the internal periodic clock. With a per capita susceptible recruitment rate of 0.002/year which corresponds to 90% vaccination rate in the model parameterization, the dampening period is predicted to be 7.4 years (as calculated by changing parameter values in the code from Sect. 6.3; see also Chap. 10). Hence, Earn et al. (2000b) predicted that vaccination may, depending on seasonality, lead to chaotic epidemics. A complication in many real populations is that the troughs following major epidemics may be so deep that the chain of transmission will often break, leading to disease fade-out (Ferrari et al., 2008). In a mathematical study of rabies spread in European red fox, Mollison (1991) dubbed this the "atto-fox" of deterministic models; if the models predict that there is a 10^{-18}th of a rabid fox running around, deterministic predictions may not be very relevant to real-life epidemics. However, Dalziel et al. (2016) provide plausible evidence for sustained quasi-periodic chaotic epidemics in several US cities prevaccination. This evidence will be discussed further in Sect. 11.2. How non-persistent chaotic fluctuation may hamper eradication efforts through asynchronized epidemics and regional metapopulation persistence will be addressed in Sects. 15.6–15.8.

6.7 A Forced SEIR shinyApp

The seasonally forced SEIR model can be further studied using the seir.app shinyApp. The app can be launched from R through:

```
require(epimdr2)
runApp(seir.app)
```

6.8 A Jacobian Function

In this and subsequent chapters, we will need to construct and evaluate Jacobian matrices for a range of different models and for a variety of purposes. These topics include among other stability analysis, resonant periodicity calculation, and evaluation of transfer functions. Each case needs the Jacobian matrix evaluated with some parameters and at some point in the phase plane. R is not primarily design to do symbolic math, but a cobbled together general-purpose function is:[5]

```
jacobian = function(states, elist, parameters, pts) {
    paras = as.list(c(pts, parameters))
    k = 0
    jl = list(NULL)
    for (i in 1:length(states)) {
        assign(paste("jj", i , sep = "."), lapply(lapply(elist,
            deriv, states[i]), eval, paras))
    for (j in 1:length(states)) {
        k = k + 1
        jl[[k]] = attr(eval(as.name(paste("jj", i,
            sep="."))) [[j]], "gradient") [1, ]
        }
    }
    J = matrix(as.numeric(as.matrix(jl) [, 1]),
        ncol = length(states))
    return(J)
}
```

The function requires the following arguments:

---

[5] As for the nextgenR0 function introduced in Sect. 3.11, the internal syntax here involves quite a bit of acrobatics. Its construction involved a lot of trial and error on the authors part but it works.

- `states` is a vector naming all state variables.
- `elist` is a list that contains equations (as `quote`) for all state variables.
- `parameters` is a labeled vector of parameters.
- `pts` is a labeled vector of the point in the phase plane in which to evaluate the Jacobian (often the endemic or disease free equilibrium).

To illustrate its usage, consider the SIR model (Eqs. (2.1)–(2.3)). Because the R compartment is absorbing and does not influence the damping period, this class can be ignored.

```
#STEP 1: classes are $S$ and $I$
st = c("S", "I")
#STEP 2: Equations are:
el = c(dSdt = quote(mu * (N  - S)  - beta * S * I/N),
    dIdt = quote(beta * S * I/N - (mu + gamma) * I))
#STEP 3: Some arbitrary parameters are
parms  = c(mu = 1/(50 * 52), N = 1, beta =  2,
    gamma = 1/2)
#STEP 4: for this SIR the endemic equilibrium is
eeq = with(as.list(parms), c(I = (gamma + mu)/beta,
    S = mu * (beta/(gamma + mu) - 1)/beta))
#STEP 5: Invoke Jacobian  calculator:
JJ = jacobian(states = st, elist = el,
    parameters = parms, pts = eeq)
```

The endemic equilibrium is a stable focus with a resonant periodicity given by the imaginary coefficient of the dominant complex eigenvalues:

```
eigen(JJ)$value
```

```
## [1] -0.5000006+0.0240038i  -0.5000006-0.0240038i
```

```
# Resonant period
2 * pi/Im(eigen(JJ)$value[1])
```

```
## [1] 261.7575
```

Chapter 7
Time Series Analysis

7.1 Taxonomy of Methods

Analysis of epidemic time series is a large endeavor because of the richness of dynamical patterns and a plentitude of historical data (Rohani & King, 2010). A wide range of tools are used, some of which are borrowed from mainstream statistics and other of which are custom-made. The classic "mainstream" methods belong to two categories: the so-called time-domain and frequency-domain methods. The autocorrelation function and ARIMA models belong to the former class and spectral analysis, and the periodogram belongs to the latter. Hybrid time/frequency methods have become increasingly prominent in the form of wavelet analysis because it allows the study of changes in disease dynamics through time (Grenfell et al., 2001). This chapter discusses a variety of standard methods using a variety of time series data. Examples of more custom-made methods are mechanistically motivated models such as the time series SIR (TSIR) that is the focus of Chap. 9, semi-parametric models (Ellner et al., 1998), and nonparametric ("empirical dynamic") models. An example of the latter is discussed in Sect. 11.8.

7.2 Time Domain: ACF and ARMA

The autocorrelation function (ACF) and the autoregressive-moving-average (ARMA) model are classic tools for describing serial dependence in time series in the time domain. We first apply the ACF to the (weekly) time series of prevalence from the seasonally forced SEIR model. The ACF quantifies serial correlations at

---

This chapter uses the following R packages: `forecast`, `Rwave`, `imputeTS`, `nlts`, and `plotrix`.

Five minute epidemic MOOC videos on seasonality and patterns of endemicity can be watched on YouTube:
Seasonality https://www.youtube.com/watch?v=TDuuM-wm6nw
Patterns of endemicity https://www.youtube.com/watch?v=Mf_EZm5amxI.

O. N. Bjørnstad, *Epidemics*, Use R!, https://doi.org/10.1007/978-3-031-12056-5_7

different time lags; that is, for a given time series, it uses correlation analyses to consider statistical similarity of observations separated by each relevant time lag. Autocorrelation techniques are used in several context in the study of infectious disease dynamics. Chapter 13 discusses how *spatial* autocorrelation (how similarity in incidence depends on separating distance in space) can be used to study spatial and spatiotemporal disease dynamics. Chapter 18 shows how corrections for autocorrelation can be used to make valid inference in the face of interdependence of data points that would otherwise render standard methods that assume independence invalid.

As an illustration, consider the seasonally forced SEIR model introduced in Sect. 6.3 parameterized to the biennial regime with major epidemics in even years and minor epidemics in odd years. A simulated time series is constructed through integrating the ODEs numerically as in Chap. 6. Figure 7.1 shows the ACF for lags up to 3 years (=156 weeks) as calculated using the `acf` function.

```
require(deSolve)
times = seq(0, 100, by = 1/52)
paras = c(mu = 1/50, N = 1, beta0 = 1000, beta1 = 0.2,
    sigma = 365/8, gamma = 365/5)
xstart = c(S = 0.06, E = 0, I = 0.001, R = 0.939)
out = as.data.frame(ode(xstart, times, seirmod2, paras))

par(mfrow = c(1, 2))
plot(times, out$I, ylab = "Infected", xlab = "Time", xlim = c(90,
    100), type = "l")
acf(out$I, lag.max = 156, main = "")
```

The major peak in autocorrelation at 104 week lag represents the dominant 2 year periodicity in the simulation, the minor peak at 52 week lag reflects the subdominant annual periodicity, and the nadirs at 26 and 78 weeks reflect, respectively, how 2 year lags align dynamics perfectly, 1 year lags align major and minor peaks (and major and minor troughs), and half year and one-and-a-half year reflect the opposition between epidemic peaks and troughs.

For noncyclic time series, the ACF is an important tool for characterizing the duration of serial dependence in time series. The ACF will drop to zero at the horizon where influence of past values is lost.

7.3 ARMA

Autoregressive-moving-average models have been used to forecast disease dynamics for respiratory (e.g., Choi & Thacker, 1981), water-borne (e.g., Baker-Austin et al., 2013), and vector-borne diseases (e.g., Linthicum et al., 1999). The ARMA(p,q) model assumes that the future incidence (Y_t) can be predicted according to $Y_t = a_1 Y_{t-1} + \ldots + a_p Y_{t-p} + \varepsilon_t - b_1 \varepsilon_{t-1} - \ldots - b_q \varepsilon_{t-q}$, where the ε's rep-

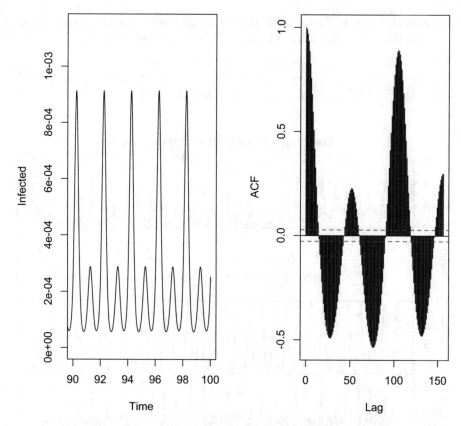

Fig. 7.1: The ACF of prevalence from the seasonally forced SEIR model with $\mu = 0.02$, $\beta_0 = 1000$, $\beta_1 = 0.2$, $\sigma = 45$, and $\gamma = 73$ and all rates are 1/year. (a) Time series. (b) ACF

resent stochasticity and the echo of past stochasticity.[1] The ARMA model applied to the monthly influenza-like illness reported from Iceland can be done using the forecast package:

```
require(forecast)
data(icelandflu)
```

For the analysis, convert the data frame into a time series ts object and do a seasonal decomposition (Fig. 7.2). Because the epidemics are very peaky, it is useful to

---

[1] The ARMA model is usually considered a purely statistical model (i.e., not containing biological mechanism), though it can be shown that for example the linearized discrete-time SIR model with stochastic transmission can be approximately mapped onto an ARMA(2,1) model (see Sect. 10.9). Bjørnstad et al. (2001) and Bjørnstad et al. (2004) provide additional examples of how ARMA processes arise from a variety of ecological interactions.

square-root transform the numbers. There is a slight trend through the data, but as expected the winter seasonality is the dominant feature of the time series.

```
ilits = ts(sqrt(icelandflu$ili), start = c(1980, 1), end = c(2009,
    12), frequency = 12)
plot(decompose(ilits))
```

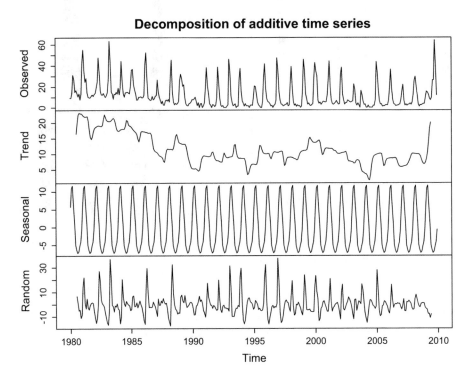

Fig. 7.2: A decomposition of the Iceland ILI time series

As an example of statistical forecasting, the seasonal ARMA(2,1) model can be trained on the data from 1990 through 2000 to predict the following 24 months (Fig. 7.3):

```
wts = window(ilits, start = c(1990, 6), end = c(2000,
    5))
fit = arima(sqrt(wts), order = c(2, 0, 1), list(order = c(1,
    0, 0), period = 12))
coef(fit)

##         ar1         ar2         ma1        sar1   intercept
##   1.4460827  -0.7323795  -0.7819940   0.2026528   2.4823415

fore = predict(fit, n.ahead = 24)
```

```
# Calculate approximate upper (U) and lower (L)
# prediction intervals
U = fore$pred + 2 * fore$se
L = fore$pred - 2 * fore$se
# plot observed and predicted values
ts.plot(sqrt(wts), fore$pred, U, L, col = c(1, 2, 4, 4),
    lty = c(1, 1, 2, 2), ylab = "Sqrt(cases)")
legend("bottomleft", c("ILI", "Forecast", "95% Error Bounds"),
    col = c(1, 2, 4), lty = c(1, 1, 2))
```

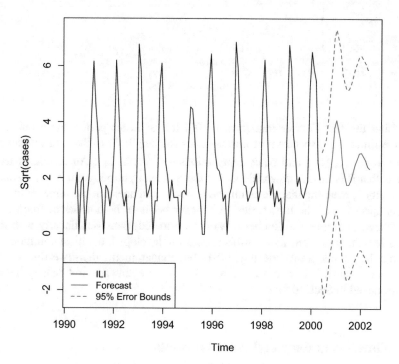

Fig. 7.3: Forecast of square-root transformed ILI incidence in Iceland for the 2001 and 2002 seasons using a seasonal ARMA(2,1) model

While ARMA forecasting is useful in many disciplines and is an important part of the broad statistical toolbox, it suffers from lacking mechanism and can therefore not answer questions like "how are dynamics likely to change if we vaccinate 50% of susceptible children?" It furthermore assumes that time series are stationary, essentially meaning that dynamical patterns do not change radically over time. As is frequently seen in infectious diseases, this is not a good assumption. Chapter 8 discusses how time series methods that incorporate more biological mechanisms (like the time series SIR model) are better able to capture and predict dynamic transitions.

7.4 Frequency Domain

The Schuster periodogram is a direct way of estimating and testing for significant periodicity. The periodogram decomposes a time series into cycles of different frequencies (where frequency = 1/period). The importance of each frequency is measured by the spectral amplitude. As an illustration, the spectrum function calculates the periodogram for the time series from the seasonally forced SEIR model. The analysis clearly identifies the two superimposed periods (Fig. 7.4).

```
my.spec = spectrum(out$I)
par(mfrow = c(1, 2))
#default plot (less default lables)
plot(my.spec, xlab = "Frequency", ylab = "Log-amplitude",
    main = "", sub = "")
#plot with period (rather than frequency)
plot(1/my.spec$freq/52, my.spec$spec, type = "b",
    xlab = "Period (year)", ylab = "Amplitude", xlim = c(0, 5))
```

Using the fast Fourier transform (FFT), the Schuster periodogram automatically estimates the spectrum of a time series (of length T) at the $T/2$ frequencies $f = \{\frac{1}{T}, \frac{2}{T}, \ldots, \frac{T/2}{T}\}$ and equivalent periods $\{T, \frac{T}{2}, \ldots, 2\}$). An upside of using FFT is that it is fast. A downside is that the Schuster periodogram is not a *consistent* method, meaning that the estimated periodogram does not converge on the true power spectrum as the time series gets longer because the number of frequencies considered (and thus the number of values estimated) increases linearly with time series length. Numerous fixes of this have been developed, the most common is to smooth the periodogram (Priestley, 1981), but nonparametric density estimation has also been proposed. Kooperberg et al.'s (1995) log-spline spectral density method is introduced in Sect. 10.8.

7.5 Time/Frequency Hybrids: Wavelets

The wavelet spectrum is an extension of spectral analysis that allows an additional time axis and therefore allows the study of changes in dynamics over time (Torrence & Compo, 1998; Grenfell et al., 2001). Unlike the periodogram, wavelets do not have canonical periods for decomposition so these have to be user specified. Using the Morlet wavelet (which is provided by for example the cwt function in the Rwave package), the periods are given via the number of octaves, no, and voices, nv. With 8 octaves, the main periods will be $\{2^1, 2^2, \ldots, 2^8\} = \{2, 4, \ldots, 256\}$. The number of voices specifies how many subdivisions to estimate within each octave. With four voices, the resultant periods will be $\{2^1, 2^{1.25}, 2^{1.5}, 2^{1.75}, 2^2, 2^{2.25}, \ldots\}$. Consider first the simulated time series of prevalence for the unforced SEIR model (Fig. 7.5).

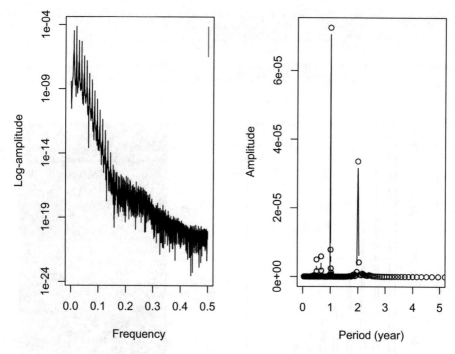

Fig. 7.4: The power spectrum of prevalence for the seasonally forced SEIR model. (**a**) Default plot of log-amplitude against frequency and (**b**) amplitude against period (in years)

```
# Simulate and plot time series
times = seq(0, 25, by = 1/52)
paras = c(mu = 1/50, N = 1, beta = 1000, sigma = 365/8,
    gamma = 365/5)
xstart = c(S = 0.06, E = 0, I = 0.001, R = 0.939)
out2 = as.data.frame(ode(xstart, times, seirmod, paras))
par(mfrow = c(1, 2)) #Side-by-side plots
plot(times, out2$I, type = "l", xlab = "Time", ylab = "Infected")
```

The wavelet decomposition is

```
#Wavelet analysis
require(Rwave)
#Set the number of "octaves" and "voices"
no = 8; nv = 32
#Calculate periods
a = 2^seq(1, no + 1 - 1/nv, by = 1/nv)
#Do the continous wavelet decomposition
wfit = cwt(out2$I, no, nv, plot = FALSE)
#Calculate the wavelet spectrum
wspec = Mod(wfit)
```

```
#Wavelet plot with contours
image(x = times, wspec, col = gray((12:32)/32),
      y = a/52,  ylim = c(0, 4), xlab = "Time", ylab = "Period")
contour(x = times, wspec, y = a/52, ylim = c(0, 4),
        zlim = c(mean(wspec), max(wspec)), add = TRUE)
```

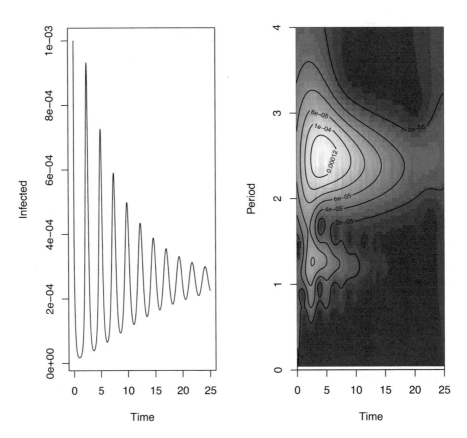

Fig. 7.5: Prevalence against time for the unforced SEIR model ($\mu = 1/50$, $N = 1$, $\beta = 1000$, $\sigma = 365/8$, $\gamma = 365/5$) with associated wavelet spectrum

The initial inter-epidemic period at around 2.5 years is strong (recall that the dampening period of the SEIR with these parameters is 2.3 years; Sect. 6.3) but then wanes as the system converges toward the stable endemic equilibrium. We see this clearly illustrated if we compare the wavelet spectrum at, for example, the beginning of year 2 and the beginning of year 10 (Fig. 7.6).

```
plot(a/52, wspec[104, ], type = "l", ylab = "Amplitude",
     xlab = "Period")
lines(a/52, wspec[1040, ], type = "l", lty = 2, col = "red")
```

```
legend("topright", legend = c("Year 2", "Year 10"), lty = c(1,
    2), col = c("black", "red"))
```

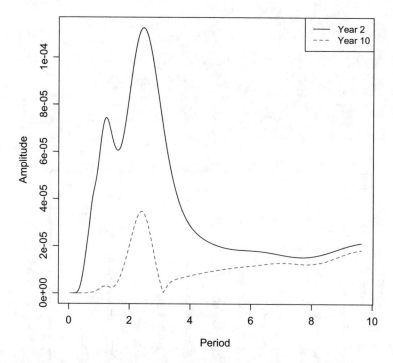

Fig. 7.6: The estimated wavelet spectrum at the first week of year 2 and year 10 for the unforced SEIR model

7.6 Measles in London

The prevaccination incidence of measles shows interesting nonstationarities that have been traced back to changing susceptible recruitment due to the post-World War II baby boom (Grenfell et al., 2002; Becker et al., 2019, Fig. 7.7). The meas dataset contains the biweekly incidence and births from 1944 to 1965.

```
data(meas)
head(meas)
```

```
##    year week      time London    B
## 1    44    2 44.00000    180 1725
## 2    44    4 44.03846    271 1725
## 3    44    6 44.07692    423 1725
```

```
## 4    44    8 44.11538    465 1725
## 5    44   10 44.15385    523 1725
## 6    44   12 44.19231    649 1725
```

```r
par(mar = c(5, 5, 2, 5))  #Make room for two axes
plot(meas$time, meas$London, type = "b", xlab = "Week",
    ylab = "Incidence", ylim = c(0, 8000))
par(new = T)  #Superimposed births plot
plot(meas$time, meas$B, type = "l", col = "red", axes = FALSE,
    xlab = NA, ylab = NA, ylim = c(1000, 2700))
axis(side = 4)
mtext(side = 4, line = 3, "Births")
legend("topright", legend = c("Cases", "Births"), lty = c(1,
    1), col = c("black", "red"))
```

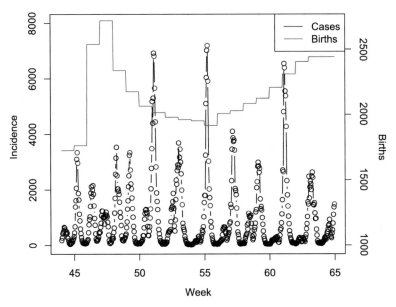

Fig. 7.7: Biweekly incidence of measles in London between 1944 and 1965 with susceptible recruitment (births) superimposed

In addition to providing a continuous wavelet transform, the Rwave package has a crazy climber algorithm to highlight ridges in the wavelet spectrum (implemented with the crc and cfamily functions). When applied to the London measles data, the crazy climber reveals the background annual rhythm and the punctuated appearance of the biennial cycle in the early 1950s (Fig. 7.8).

```r
# Set octaves, voices and associated periods
no = 8
nv = 32
a = 2^seq(1, no + 1 - 1/nv, by = 1/nv)
# Continous  wavelet  decomposition
```

```
wfit = cwt(meas$London, no, nv, plot = FALSE)
wspec = Mod(wfit)
# Crazy climber
crcinc = crc(wspec, nbclimb = 10, bstep = 100)
fcrcinc = cfamily(crcinc, ptile = 0.5, nbchain = 1000,
    bstep = 10)

  ## There are 2 chains.

ridges = fcrcinc[[1]]
ridges[which(ridges == 0)] <- NA
# Wavelet plot with crazy-climber and contours
image(x = meas$time, wspec, col = gray((12:32)/32), y = a/26,
    ylim = c(0.1, 3), ylab = "Period", xlab = "Year")
contour(x = meas$time, wspec, y = a/26, ylim = c(0, 3),
    nlevels = 6, zlim = c(mean(wspec), max(wspec)), add = TRUE)
image(x = meas$time, y = a/26, z = ridges, add = TRUE,
    col = gray(0))
```

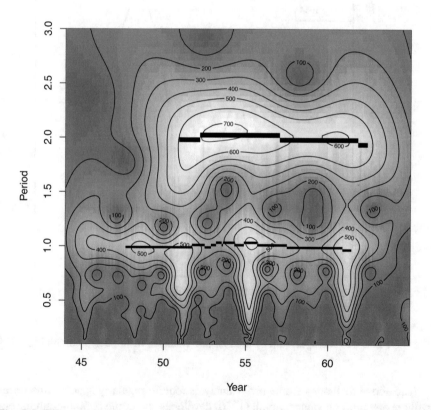

Fig. 7.8: The wavelet spectrum of the London measles incidence with crazy climber ridges. The appearance of a significant biennial rhythm in the 1950s is conspicuous

Figure 7.9 contrasts the spectrum of the first biweek of January 1945 and the first biweek of January 1954. The transition from a dominance of annual to biennial epidemics is conspicuous. Two-year cycles are pronounced when birth rates are around 20 per thousand per year; annual epidemics are associated with higher birth rates. This transition due to the post-World War II baby boom is as predicted by the seasonally forced SEIR model with dropping birth rates (Earn et al., 2000b, Fig. 6.6) and will be discussed further in Chap. 8.

```
plot(a/26, wspec[261, ], type = "l",xlim = c(0, 3),
     xlab = "period (years)", ylab = "amplitude")
lines(a/26, wspec[27, ], type = "l",  lty = 2,
     col = "red")
legend("topleft", legend = c("1945", "1954"),
     lty = c(2, 1), col = c("red", "black"))
```

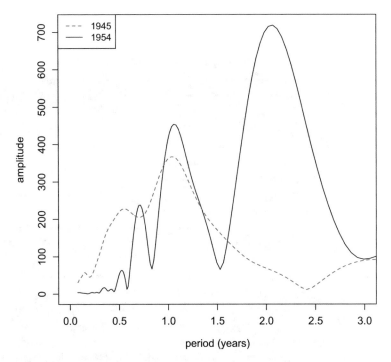

Fig. 7.9: The wavelet spectrum of the London measles in Jan 1945 versus Jan 1954

The above methods of time series analysis require regularly spaced time series without any missing values. Lomb (1976) developed the Lomb periodogram for un-equally spaced data. Furthermore, the classic spectral methods are poorly adapted to quantify rhythms in nonmetric data such as the presence/absence of infection. Legendre et al. (1981) developed the contingency periodogram for such situations. The nlts package has the `spec.lomb` and `contingency.periodogram` functions to carry out such analyses. The `mvcwt` package has functions that do wavelet analyses of time series with missing data or unequally spaced data.

7.7 Project Tycho

Project Tycho (http://www.tycho.pitt.edu) is a great resource for time series on historical disease incidence. The data used in Sect. 6.1 were downloaded from this database. Weekly data of whooping cough (1925–1947), diphtheria (1914–1947), and measles (1914–1947) in the city of Philadelphia are from Project Tycho and are saved in the `tywhooping`, `tydiphtheria`, and `tymeasles` datasets. These were all important causes of childhood mortality in the early twentieth century and were therefore "reportable infections" in the USA. Whooping cough is caused by bacterial colonization of the lower respiratory tract by congeneric species in the genus *Bordetella*, most notably *B. pertussis*, and causes violent coughing, vomiting, and pneumonia. Diphtheria is caused by infection by *Corynebacterium diphtheriae* whose toxin caused a range of health complications before a vaccine was available.[2] Measles is a severely immuno-compromising paramyxovirus that still kills more than fifty thousand children each year (Dixon et al., 2021). These time series are helpful to illustrate some additional aspects of disease dynamics and time series methods.

```
data(tywhooping)
tywhooping$TIME = tywhooping$YEAR + tywhooping$WEEK/52
tywhooping$TM = 1:length(tywhooping$YEAR)
data(tydiphtheria)
data(tymeasles)
tydiphtheria$TIME = tymeasles$TIME = tymeasles$YEAR +
    tymeasles$WEEK/52
```

These time series have occasional weeks of missing data that have to be interpolated using the `imputeTS` package for ease of analyses. But first we can use the whooping cough data to illustrate the use of the Lomb periodogram for spectral analysis of unevenly spaced data.

7.8 Lomb Periodogram: Whooping Cough

There are 14 missing weeks in the `tywhooping` data set. For frequency-domain analyses of this data, we either have to interpolate the missing weeks or use the Lomb periodogram. Compare the two approaches:

---

[2] The first smallpox vaccines are dated to China in the fifteenth century (Plotkin, 2011). Thereafter, the diphteria toxoid vaccine developed in the 1920s was among the very first to be broadly administered (Relyveld, 2011).

```
data(tywhooping)
whp = na.omit(tywhooping)

#data with missing values interpolated
require(imputeTS)
sum(is.na(tywhooping$PHILADELPHIA))

  ## [1] 14

tywhooping$PHILADELPHIA=
    na_interpolation(ts(tywhooping$PHILADELPHIA))

#Classic periodogram
my.spec = spectrum(sqrt(tywhooping$PHILADELPHIA))
#Lomb periodogram
require(nlts)
my.lomb = spec.lomb(x = whp$TM,
    y = sqrt(whp$PHILADELPHIA))

plot(1/my.spec$freq/52, my.spec$spec, type = "b",
    xlab = "Period (year)", ylab = "Amplitude")
par(new = TRUE)
plot(1/my.lomb$freq/52, my.lomb$spec, axes = FALSE,
    type = "b", col = 2, xlab = "", ylab = "")
legend("topright", legend = c("Classic", "Lomb"),
    lty = c(1, 1), pch = c(1, 1), col = c("black", "red"))
```

With only 14 missing values in a 1000+ week long time series, the shape of the
Schuster periodogram (on interpolated data) and the Lomb periodogram are almost
identical (Fig. 7.10). With a higher fraction of a time series missing, interpolation
will introduce biased or spurious patterns in the analysis so the Lomb method will
be essential.

7.9 Triennial Cycles: Philadelphia Measles

Like in London, prevaccination measles dynamics in Philadelphia exhibit interesting
nonstationarities that are highlighted by a wavelet analysis. There are 24 missing
weeks to interpolate to ease the wavelet analysis:

```
data(tymeasles)
sum(is.na(tymeasles$PHILADELPHIA))

  ## [1] 24

tymeasles$PHILADELPHIA =
    na_interpolation(ts(tymeasles$PHILADELPHIA))
```

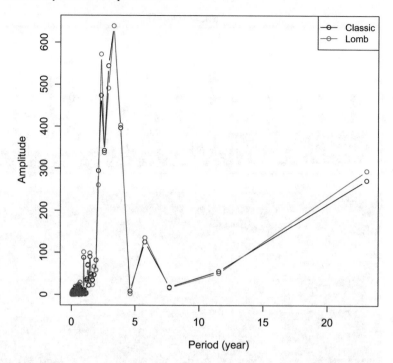

Fig. 7.10: The Lomb periodogram and the classic periodogram (on interpolated data) of the Philadelphia whooping cough time series

We can twiddle with the graphics margins and layout using the par and layout functions to make a prettier compound graphic (Fig. 7.11).

```
par(mfrow = c(2, 1), mar = c(2, 4, 2, 1))
layout(matrix(c(1, 1, 2, 2, 2), ncol = 1))
plot(tymeasles$TIME, sqrt(tymeasles$PHILADELPHIA), type = "b",
    ylab = "Sqrt(incidence)")
title("Measles 1914-47")

no = 8
nv = 16
a = 2^seq(1, no + 1 - 1/nv, by = 1/nv)
wfit = cwt(sqrt(tymeasles$PHILADELPHIA), no, nv, plot = FALSE)
wspec = Mod(wfit)
par(mar = c(1, 4, 0.25, 1))
image(z = wspec, y = a/52, ylim = c(0, 4), ylab = "Period(year)",
    col = gray((12:32)/32), xaxt = "n")
contour(z = wspec, y = a/52, ylim = c(0, 4), nlevels = 6,
    zlim = c(mean(wspec), max(wspec)), add = TRUE)
```

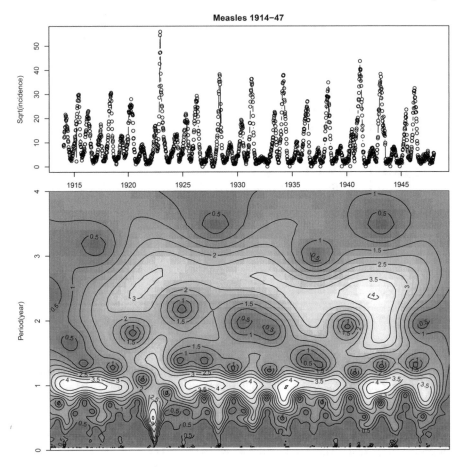

Fig. 7.11: Wavelet spectrum of measles in Philadelphia

The early annual epidemics give way to irregular triennial epidemic cycles from
1920 onward (Fig. 7.12). The triennial cycles are the hallmarks of chaotic epidemics
(Li & Yorke, 2004; Dalziel et al., 2016). This will be discussed further in Sect. 11.2.

```
plot(a/52,wspec[54,], type = "l", xlim = c(0, 4),
     xlab = "Period (years)", ylab = "Amplitude",
     col = "red", lty = 2)
lines(a/52, wspec[1357,], type = "l", xlim = c(0, 4))
legend("topleft", legend= c("1915", "1940"),
     lty = c(2, 1), col = c("red","black"))
```

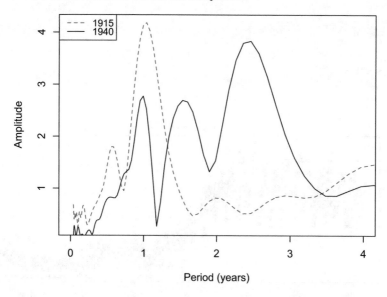

Fig. 7.12: The Jan 1915 versus Jan 1940 New York measles wavelet spectrum. Annual epidemics gave way to triennial cycles

7.10 Wavelet Reconstruction and Wavelet Filter: Diphtheria

Diphtheria exhibited conspicuous annual cycles during the beginning of the twentieth century until the addition of an adjuvant to the toxoid vaccine in 1926 led to a strong secular downward trend and effectively the elimination of the disease (Fig. 7.13). The wavelet allows the study of how the reduction in incidence is associated with a loss of periodicity and increase in high-frequency variability ("noise") (Fig. 7.13). There are 18 missing values to interpolate prior to the analysis.

```
data(tydiphtheria)
sum(is.na(tydiphtheria$PHILADELPHIA))

  ## [1] 18

tydiphtheria$PHILADELPHIA =
    na_interpolation(ts(tydiphtheria$PHILADELPHIA))

par(mfrow = c(2, 1), mar = c(2, 4, 2, 1))
layout(matrix(c(1, 1, 2, 2, 2), ncol = 1))
plot(tydiphtheria$TIME, sqrt(tydiphtheria$PHILADELPHIA),
    type = "b", ylab = "Sqrt(incidence)")
title("Diphteria 1914-47")

no = 8; nv = 16; a = 2^seq(1,no+1-1/nv, by = 1/nv)
wfit = cwt(sqrt(tydiphtheria$PHILADELPHIA),
    no, nv, plot = FALSE)
wspec = Mod(wfit)
```

```
par(mar = c(1, 4, 0.25, 1))
image(z = wspec, y = a/52, ylim = c(0, 3),
    ylab = "Period(year)", col = gray((12:32)/32), xaxt = "n")
contour(z = wspec, y = a/52, ylim = c(0, 3), nlevels = 6,
    zlim = c(mean(wspec), max(wspec)), add = TRUE)
```

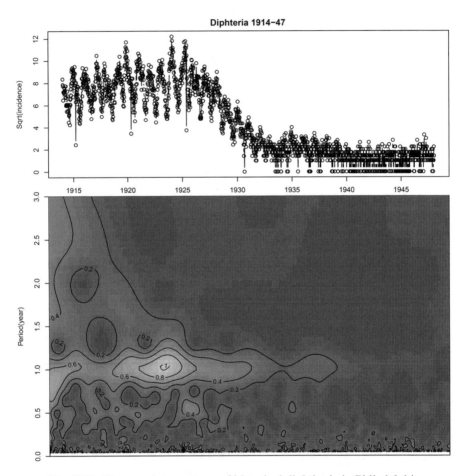

Fig. 7.13: The wavelet spectrum of historical diphtheria in Philadelphia

It is sometimes of interest to use the wavelet as a signal filter. We may for example want to quantitate how the strength of the annual cycle of diphtheria (in the
45–60 week range, say) changes over time. To do this, we use wavelet reconstruction around the relevant time scales (Fig. 7.14). For the Morlet wavelet, the formula
for reconstruction using the j'th through $j + s$'th scales is provided by Torrence and
Compo (1998). The mid-pass filter clearly illustrates the loss of annual signal over
time (Fig. 7.14).

```
#midpass filter
sel = a > 45 & a < 60
rec = 0.6 * apply(Re(wfit[ ,sel])/sqrt(a[sel]), 1,
    sum)/(0.776 * (pi^(-1/4)))
data = pi * scale(sqrt(tydiphtheria$PHILADELPHIA))/2
plot(tydiphtheria$TIME, data, type = "b", xlab = "Year",
    ylab = "Scaled cases")
lines(tydiphtheria$TIME, rec, type = "l", col = 2, lwd = 3)
legend("topright", legend = c("Scaled cases",
    "Annual reconstruction"), pch=c(1, NA), lty = c(1, 1),
    lwd = c(1, 3), col = c("black", "red"))
```

7.11 Advanced: FFT and Reconstruction

One-hundred-and-twenty years ago, Arthur Schuster proposed the bold idea that any discrete-time series can be decomposed and exactly reconstructed from a sum of trigonometric functions. Given its nonstationary transition from annual to biennial epidemics, the prevaccination 1944–1964 London measles time series (in the meas dataset) offers a nice testbed for this assertion.

The below code generates an animated visualization of the reconstruction. Section 12.7 discusses making in-line and permanent animations in more detail. A web-optimized animated gif can be found at https://tinyurl.com/4yb6ta2f.

If z is the fast Fourier transform of the time series, then the trigonometric "signal" of the k'th frequency is $\frac{1}{T}(\sum_f (Re(z)\cos(2\pi(k-1)f)) - Im(z)\sin(2\pi(k-1)f))$, where $Re()$ and $Im()$ represent the real and imaginary parts. We first piece together relevant bits for the formula and then do the reconstruction in the rec2 object where the contribution of each frequency is weighed by its amplitude:

```
# fft
x = meas$London
p = length(x)
z = fft(x)
f = seq(from = 0, length = p, by = 1/p)
a = Re(z)
b = Im(z)
# reconstruction
rec2 = matrix(NA, ncol = p, nrow = p)
for (k in 1:p) {
    rec2[, k] = (a * cos(2 * pi * (k - 1) * f) - b * sin(2 *
        pi * (k - 1) * f))/p
}
```

The below code provides a sequential reconstruction of the time series from the Schuster periodogram.

```
# fft
x = meas$London
```

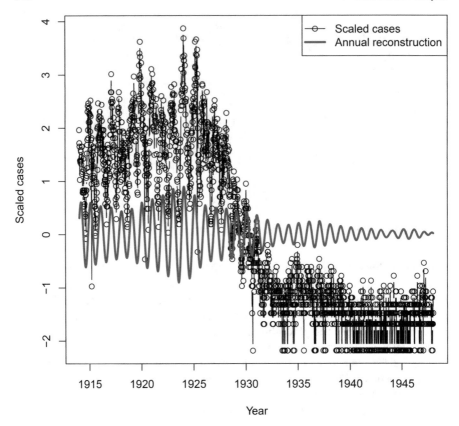

Fig. 7.14: Wavelet reconstructed variability in the 45–60 week range of diphtheria in Philadelphia during the first half of the twentieth century

```
p = length(x)
z = fft(x)
f = seq(from = 0, length = p, by = 1/p)
a = Re(z)
b = Im(z)
# reconstruction
rec2 = matrix(NA, ncol = p, nrow = p)
for (k in 1:p) {
    rec2[, k] <- (a * cos(2 * pi * (k - 1) * f) - b *
        sin(2 * pi * (k - 1) * f))/p
}
```

Finally, we can visualize the convergence on the original signal using the sequence of frequencies order by amplitude (highest to lowest importance). In the animation, the upper right inset shows the *log*-amplitude associated with each trigonometric function.

```r
sim = rep(0, p)
n = 0
samp = order(a^2 + b^2, decreasing = TRUE)
for(g in samp){
n = n+1
par(mfrow = c(1, 2))
plot(x, ylim = c(0, 11000), ylab = "Incidence",
    xlab = "Biweek")
title(paste("nfreq = ", n))
sim = sim + rec2[g,]
lines(sim, col = 2)
par(new = TRUE)
sc = scale((cos(2 * pi * (0:(p - 1)) * f[g]) -
    sin(2 * pi * (0:(p - 1)) * f[g]))/p)
plot(sc * (a^2 + b^2)[g]/max(a^2 + b^2), type = "l",
    col = gray(0.5), ylim = c(-8, 2), axes = FALSE,
    xlab = "", ylab = "")
plot(x, sim, ylab = "Reconstructed", xlab = "Observed",
    ylim = c(0, 8000))
#Sys.sleep() makes R wait a bit for visalisation
Sys.sleep(.2)
}
```

Chapter 8
TSIR

8.1 Estimating Parameters in Dynamic Models

There are many strategies for estimating the parameters of dynamic models from time series data. They differ conceptually in the way they handle demographic and environmental stochasticity (sometimes referred to jointly as "process error"), observation error, and partial (missing) observation. The strategies also often vary by whether the underlying dynamics is thought to be best approximated in continuous time (differential models) or discrete time (difference models).

In reality, disease dynamics is always affected by some level of demographic and environmental stochasticity, and observation error comes in the form of both inaccuracies in observation and missing information. The exposed (latent) class of an SEIR-like system, for example, is very rarely monitored (tuberculosis perhaps being an exception). Furthermore, while disease dynamics very rarely play out in discrete generation (in-host dynamics of *Eimeria* and sometimes *Plasmodium* being exceptions; Mideo et al., 2013), they also never rarely follow the exponential waiting-time distributions implicit in ODE models (Fig. 2.6). As discussed in Sect. 2.9, various types of distributed-delay models or renewal equations can cover the continuum between fixed (discrete) and exponential distributions—the original SIR formulation by Kermack and McKendrick (1927) is an early example of how to embrace such biological detail—but these come at a prize of mathematical/computational overhead.

The previous implementation of Ferrari et al.'s (2005) removal method (Sect. 3.4) for fitting the chain-binomial model for a simple epidemic is an example of a model that assumes that all process error is due to demographic stochasticity (according to the chain binomial) and that observation error is sufficiently insignificant to be ignored. The method finds parameters (S_0 and β) that predict an epidemic curve that most closely (in a likelihood sense) resembles the data. This is an example of the strategy of trajectory matching; choose parameters that produce a predicted

---

This chapter uses the following R packages: imputeTS and plotrix.

O. N. Bjørnstad, *Epidemics*, Use R!, https://doi.org/10.1007/978-3-031-12056-5_8

trajectory that comes most close to the observed. It is also common to use trajectory matching for a continuous-time SIR model of simple epidemics, but instead assume that all process error is sufficiently insignificant to be ignored. In this case, we find parameters that predict prevalence curves that most closely resemble the data assuming an underlying deterministic epidemic clockwork cloaked only by observation error (see Chap. 9). A variety of approaches have been proposed to fit dynamical models to ecological and epidemiological time series models including:

- Trajectory matching: Assume no/negligible stochasticity in transmission dynamics and find parameters that make a model trajectory best line up with observations (see Sect. 9.3).
- Gradient matching: Fitting ODEs in the presence of significant process noise (Ellner et al., 2002). The idea is to estimate derivatives dx/dt along the time series (for example by fitting a spline and calculating its derivatives) and then relate them to relevant state variables.
- Probe matching was introduced by Kendall et al. (1999), and its statistical properties were later formalized in Wood's (2010) synthetic likelihood. The idea is to choose parameters that make the model most closely reproduce what are deemed to be the critical dynamical features of the system.
- Hierarchical models using MCMC (e.g., Clark & Bjørnstad, 2004) that has been much refined as partially observed Markov processes in the pomp package (King et al., 2015b). See Sect. 11.5 for some usage.
- One of the simpler methods that tries to balance the need for both observational errors and stochasticity is the time series SIR model (Finkenstädt & Grenfell, 2000; Bjørnstad et al., 2002a; Grenfell et al., 2002) to which this chapter is devoted.

8.2 Stochastic Variability

Much environmental forcing is non-predictable environmental stochasticity. In such cases, stochastic simulation can be very useful.[1] One can use stochastic analogues of the continuous-time deterministic compartmental models using event-based simulations (see Sect. 9.2) or consider extensions of the chain-binomial model we introduced in Sects. 3.4 and 3.5. This chapter is focused on a variant of the chain-binomial model dubbed the time series SIR (TSIR) model (Bjørnstad et al., 2002a; Finkenstädt et al., 2002; Grenfell et al., 2002).

The TSIR model is as follows: If we use a discrete time step equal to the serial interval of the pathogen (about 2 weeks in the case of infections such as measles, diphtheria, scarlet fever, and chicken pox), we can write the model (subsuming a latent period) as

---

[1] It is also possible to use more powerful mathematical approaches in such cases with signal theory and transfer functions; see Sect. 10.8.

$$S_{t+1} = S_t + B_t - I_t, \tag{8.1}$$

$$\lambda_{t+1} = \beta_u \frac{S_t}{N_t} I_t^\alpha, \tag{8.2}$$

where S_t and I_t are the numbers of susceptibles and infecteds in pathogen generation t, B_t is the number of susceptible recruits (births) during the time interval, N
is the population size, and β_u is the seasonally forced transmission rate. The α is
an exponent (normally just under 1) that accounts for discretizing the underlying
continuous process (Glass et al., 2003).[2] The final variable λ_{t+1} represents the expectation for the new number of infecteds in generation $t+1$. The actual number of
infecteds that will appear in generation $t+1$ will follow some stochastic distribution
around λ_{t+1}. For example, $I_{t+1} \sim Po(\lambda_{t+1})$ or $I_{t+1} \sim NegBin(\lambda, I_t)$ depending on
the exact assumptions regarding the variability in the underlying process (Bjørnstad
et al., 2002a). The negative binomial that is employed here arises from assuming an
epidemic birth-and-death process in which case the offspring distribution from each
infected follows a geometric distribution (Kendall, 1949), and the sum of I_t identical
geometrics is a negative binomial with clumping parameter I_t. The link to the chain
binomial comes about because $1 - exp(-\phi) \simeq \phi$, when ϕ is small, and the binomial
process—for which we need to know the susceptible denominator (which is usually
unknown)—can be approximated with a Poisson or negative binomial distribution
neither of which require known denominators (Bjørnstad et al., 2002a).

Stochasticity may further enter through variable numbers of births or random
variation in the transmission rates. The `tsirSim` function does stochastic simulation akin to the chain-binomial simulator of Sect. 3.5 but with the possibility of
having stochastic variation in β (controlled by the `sdbeta` argument in the below
code):

```
tsirSim = function(alpha = 0.97, B = 2300, beta = 25,
    sdbeta = 0, S0 = 0.06, I0 = 180, IT = 520, N = 3300000) {
    # Set up simulation
    lambda = rep(NA, IT)
    I = rep(NA, IT)
    S = rep(NA, IT)
    # Add initial conditions
    I[1] = I0
    lambda[1] = I0
    S[1] = S0 * N

    # Run simulation
    for (i in 2:IT) {
        lambda[i] = rnorm(1, mean = beta, sd = sdbeta) *
            I[i - 1]^alpha * S[i - 1]/N
        if (lambda[i] < 0) {
            lambda[i] = 0
```

---

[2] The logic behind this tweak is that the model predicts the number of cases several days into the
future, which means that for highly contagious pathogens, it will somewhat overpredict during epidemic peaks because the time discreteness does not account for the continuous and rapid depletion
of susceptibles at such times.

```
        }
        I[i] = rpois(1, lambda[i])
        S[i] = S[i - 1] + B - I[i]
    }
    # Return result
    list(I = I, S = S)
}
```

In the function, IT is the length of the time series to be simulated. S0 and I0 are the initial conditions, and B is the susceptible recruitment number during each serial interval. The parameters in the model are provided with default values. These values correspond roughly to estimates from the measles time series for London for the period 1944–1965 (see Sect. 8.5), a city with 3.3 million inhabitants at the time. The trajectories in time and in the phase plane are (Fig. 8.1)

```
out = tsirSim()
par(mfrow = c(1, 2))
plot(out$I, ylab = "Infected", xlab = "Time", type = "l")
plot(out$S, out$I, ylab = "Infected", xlab = "Susceptible",
    type = "l")
```

8.3 Estimation Using the TSIR

Estimation using the TSIR came out of a pragmatic attempt at dealing with the complexities of disease dynamics and incidence data using basic statistical tools. In its original form, it assumes that process noise is due to demographic stochasticity, and observation error is in the form of time-invariant'ish underreporting that in large populations can be adequately corrected for in a deterministic fashion.

Consider the biweekly incidence (number of cases for each 2-week period) of measles from London between 1944 and 1965 (Fig. 7.8) introduced in Sect. 7.6:

```
data(meas)
head(meas)

##    year week     time London    B
## 1    44    2 44.00000    180 1725
## 2    44    4 44.03846    271 1725
## 3    44    6 44.07692    423 1725
## 4    44    8 44.11538    465 1725
## 5    44   10 44.15385    523 1725
## 6    44   12 44.19231    649 1725
```

The incidence is accessed as meas$London. In addition, the dataset contains columns reporting meas$year and meas$week that combine into meas$time, and biweekly number of births (meas$B). Birth numbers are annual, so in the dataset, this number is evenly distributed across the 26 biweeks of each year. We

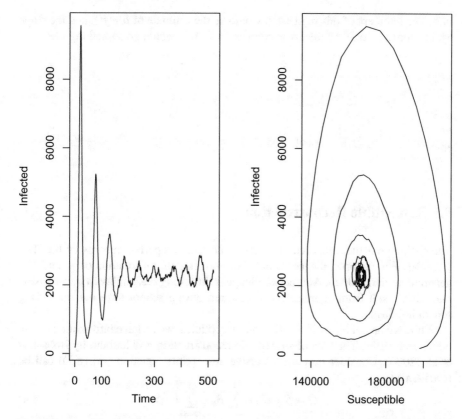

Fig. 8.1: A stochastic realization from the TSIR model with demographic stochasticity and parameters corresponding roughly to measles during prevaccination conditions in London. (**a**) Incidence in time. (**b**) The phase plane

should be able to use this data to estimate key epidemiological parameters. However, we somehow have to reconstruct the susceptible time series (and correct for underreporting)...

8.4 Inference (Hypothetical)

Given Eqs. (8.1)–(8.2) and time series of I and S, the candidate for estimation is obvious:

$$log(I_{t+1}) = log(\beta) + \alpha log(I_t) + log(S_t) - log(N). \qquad (8.3)$$

Estimate the unknown parameters β and α by a regression of $log(I_{t+1})$ on $log(I_t)$ with $log(S_t)$ and $-log(N)$ as *offsets* (i.e., the slope for the $log(S)$, and the $-log(N)$ variables are fixed at unity) or the equivalent generalized linear model with a log link. The intercept of this regression would be the estimate of $log(\beta)$, and the slope against $log(I_t)$ would be the estimate of α. In R, this would go something like:

```
# Align time series
IT = length(meas$London)
Inow = log(meas$London[2:IT])
Ilag = log(meas$London[1:(IT - 1)])
Slag = log(S[1:(IT - 1)])   #This does not yet exist
# now the regression
glm(Inow ~ Ilag + offset(Slag) + offset(-N))
```

8.5 Susceptible Reconstruction

The challenge is that most real datasets do not contain perfect records on the state variables. For example, the `meas` data does not contain information on `S`, and `I` is generally underreported. Another challenge is the strong seasonality in transmission rates that result from aggregation of children during school term but not during school holidays.

While we do not have observation on susceptibles, we do have information on the number of births. The idea of susceptible reconstruction was laid out by Bobashev et al. (2000). Consider how the recursive susceptible equation (Eq. (8.1)) can be rewritten as

$$S_t = \bar{S} + D_0 + \sum_{k=0}^{t} B_k - \sum_{k=0}^{t} I_k/\rho, \tag{8.4}$$

where $\bar{S}$ is the mean number of susceptibles, D_0 is the unknown deviations around the mean at time 0, and ρ is the (known or unknown) reporting rate. We can reconstruct the time series D_t of how the susceptible numbers deviate from the mean value, $D_t = S_t - \bar{S}$, by rewriting (8.4) as

$$\sum_{k=0}^{t} B_k = \bar{S} + D_0 + 1/\rho \sum_{k=0}^{t} I_k + D_t, \tag{8.5}$$

from which it is clear that D_t is the residual from the regression of the cumulative number of births on the cumulative number of cases. Note that this reconstruction still works when the reporting rate ρ is unknown because underreporting can be accounted for by the slope of the cumulative–cumulative regression.

As it turns out, reporting rates sometimes vary subtly through time so it is good to use a slightly more flexible model than linear regression (Finkenstädt et al., 2002), for example, a smoothing spline with 5 degrees of freedom (Fig. 8.2).

```
cum.reg = smooth.spline(cumsum(meas$B), cumsum(meas$London),
     df = 5)
D = -resid(cum.reg)   #The residuals
plot(cumsum(meas$B), cumsum(meas$London), type = "l",
```

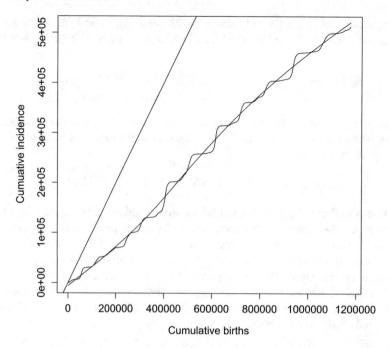

Fig. 8.2: Cumulative incidence versus cumulative births. The straight line is the 1-to-1 reference line

```
    xlab = "Cumulative births", ylab = "Cumuative incidence")
lines(cum.reg)
abline(a = 0, b = 1)
```

The 1-to-1 line generated by the `abline` command shows that the cumulative number of reported cases is less than the cumulative number of births (Fig. 8.2). The discrepancy is informative because we know from serology that almost all children were infected with the common childhood infections before the age of 20 in the pre-vaccine era; Black's (1959) data, for example, has seroprevalence >95% by age 15 in prevaccination Connecticut (Sect. 5.2). The slope of the cumulative regression, therefore, is an estimate of the reporting rate. We can get the estimated reporting rates for each time step from the slope of the fitted spline:

```
rr = predict(cum.reg, deriv = 1)$y
summary(rr)

##    Min. 1st Qu.  Median    Mean 3rd Qu.    Max.
##  0.3485  0.3841  0.4424  0.4522  0.5214  0.5635
```

The reporting rate is fairly steady across the 20 years at around 45%. We can create time series corrected for reporting of both incidence, `Ic`, and susceptible deviation, `Dc`:

```
Ic = meas$London/rr
Dc = D/rr
```

To estimate parameters, rewrite the model (Eq. (8.3)) in terms of the data and unknown parameters on a log-scale (recall that λ_{t+1} is the expected number of cases in serial interval $t+1$):

$$log(\lambda_{t+1}) = log(\beta_u) - log(N) + log(D_t + \overline{S}) + \alpha log(I_t).$$

This is almost (but not quite) a linear regression with unknown parameters β_u, α, and $\overline{S}$. Before ready to estimate the parameters, however, it is neccesary to consider the fact that β_u varies seasonally (because of the school year), thus the subscript u. The most flexible model is to assume that each of the 26 biweeks of the year has its own transmission rate. Under that assumption, there are 28 parameters to estimate (26 βs, α, and $\overline{S}$). So define a vector that flags the periodic βs across the 21 years, and create the three vectors of logged current (`lInew`) and lagged infecteds (`lIold`) and lagged "residual susceptibles" (`Dold`):

```
seas = rep(1:26, 21)[1:545]
lInew = log(Ic[2:546])
lIold = log(Ic[1:545])
Dold = Dc[1:545]
```

Given a value for $\overline{S}$, the models fall neatly within the linear regression framework.[3] We can therefore use `glm` to find a profile likelihood estimate of $\overline{S}$. It is known from serology that the average proportion of susceptibles in measles is somewhere in the 2%–20% range, and given the size of London at the time (3.3M), postulate a reasonable range of candidate values:

```
N = 3300000
Smean = seq(0.02, 0.2, by = 0.001) * N
offsetN = rep(-log(N), 545)
```

The following sets up a vector to store the log-likelihood values corresponding to each candidate and loop over the candidate values to generate a likelihood profile for $\overline{S}$ (Fig. 8.3).

```
llik = rep(NA, length(Smean))
for (i in 1:length(Smean)) {
    lSold = log(Smean[i] + Dold)
    glmfit = glm(lInew ~ -1 + as.factor(seas) + lIold +
        offset(lSold + offsetN))
    llik[i] = glmfit$deviance/2
```

---

[3] Though had it not, we could write out the likelihood and use `optim` or `mle2` to find maximum likelihood estimates as in Chap. 3.

```
}
par(mfrow = c(1, 1))
plot(Smean/3300000, llik, ylim = c(min(llik), 25), xlab = "Sbar",
    ylab = "Neg log-lik")
```

The `-1` in the regression formula removes the intercept, so that `as.factor(seas)` becomes the estimates of the log-βs. Note further that `glmfit$deviance` holds -2*log-likelihood, so the negative log-likelihood is ½ the deviance.[4] The London estimate for the measles TSIR model is

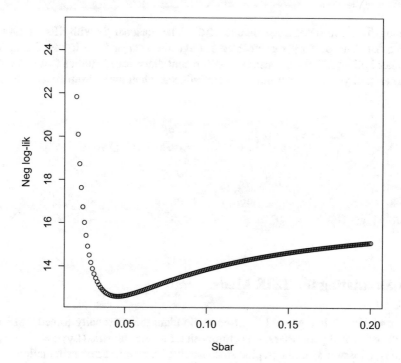

Fig. 8.3: The likelihood profile for $\bar{S}$ from the TSIR applied to the London measles time series

```
lSold = log(Smean[which(llik == min(llik))] + Dold)
glmfit = glm(lInew ~ -1 + as.factor(seas) + lIold +
    offset(lSold + offsetN))
```

---

[4] An alternative to the Gaussian likelihood is to use a counting likelihood such as the Poisson quasi-likelihood with a `log` link. For this, the code would be
```
lnew = Ic[2:546]
glmfit = glm(lnew ~ -1 +as.factor(seas) + lIold + offset(lSold +
offsetN), family = quasipoisson(link = "log")).
```

That is, $\overline{S}$ is

```
Smean[which.min(llik)]/3300000
```

```
## [1] 0.045
```

and α is

```
glmfit$coef[27]
```

```
##       lIold
## 0.9636908
```

The log-βs are in `glmfit$coef[1:26]`. The seasonal βs with SEs are plotted in Fig. 8.4. The βs vary significantly through the year and are lowest during the summer holidays. This is consistent with recent diary-based studies that show that children and youth contact numbers are reduced when away from school (Eames et al., 2011).

```
require(plotrix)
beta = exp(glmfit$coef[1:26])
ubeta = exp(glmfit$coef[1:26] + summary(glmfit)$coef[1:26,
    2])
lbeta = exp(glmfit$coef[1:26] - summary(glmfit)$coef[1:26,
    2])
plotCI(x = c(1:26), y = beta, ui = ubeta, li = lbeta,
    xlab = "Biweek", ylab = expression(beta))
```

8.6 Simulating the TSIR Model

The `tsirSim2` is a general function to simulate the seasonally forced TSIR using the estimated parameters. It performs either a deterministic (`type="det"`) or stochastic (assuming demographic stochasticity, `type="stoc"`) simulation.

```
tsirSim2 = function(beta, alpha, B, N, inits = list(Snull = 0,
    Inull = 0), type = "det") {
    type = charmatch(type, c("det", "stoc"), nomatch = NA)
    if (is.na(type))
        stop("method should be \"det\", \"stoc\"")
    IT = length(B)
    s = length(beta)
    lambda = rep(NA, IT)
    I = rep(NA, IT)
    S = rep(NA, IT)

    I[1] = inits$Inull
    lambda[1] = inits$Inull
    S[1] = inits$Snull
```

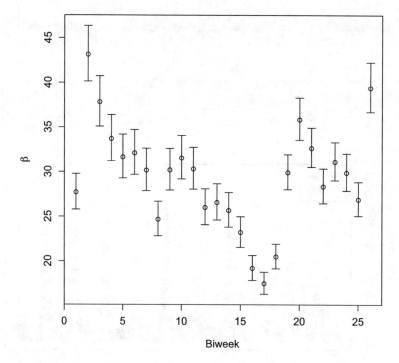

Fig. 8.4: The estimated seasonal βs with SEs from the London measles time series

```
for (i in 2:IT) {
    lambda[i] = beta[((i - 2)%%s) + 1] * S[i - 1] *
        (I[i - 1]^alpha)/N
    if (type == 2) {
        I[i] = rpois(1, lambda[i])
    }
    if (type == 1) {
        I[i] = lambda[i]
    }
    S[i] = S[i - 1] + B[i] - I[i]
}
return(list(I = I, S = S))
}
```

Simulated dynamics is sensitive to the value of α, and there is evidence that the TSIR regression is biased with respect to this parameter.[5] A simulation using the estimated parameters (with a small correction in α) is shown in Fig. 8.5. While not perfect, the model nicely captures the transition from annual to biennial epidemics as birth rates fall following the post-World War II baby boom.

---

[5] Metcalf et al. (2011a) proposed to use a "Whittle estimator" of α to re-estimate this variable by matching simulated and observed power spectra.

```
sim = tsirSim2(beta = exp(glmfit$coef[1:26]), alpha = 0.966,
    B = meas$B, N = N, inits = list(Snull = Dc[1] +
    Smean[which(llik == min(llik))], Inull = Ic[1]))
plot(sim$I, type = "b", ylim = c(0, max(Ic)),
    ylab = "Incidence", xlab = "Biweek")
lines(exp(lInew), col = "red")
legend("topleft", legend = c("sim", "Ic"), lty = c(1, 1),
    pch = c(1, NA), col = c("black", "red"))
```

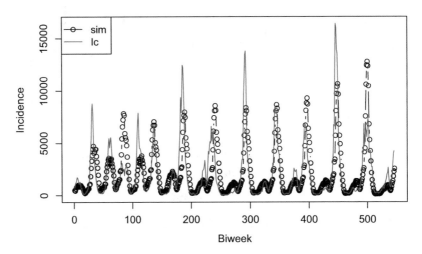

Fig. 8.5: Observed and TSIR simulated dynamics for measles in London 1944–1965

A more comprehensive TSIR analysis across almost 100 years of data is provided by Becker et al. (2019). This study also introduces a dedicated tsiR package for R (Becker & Grenfell, 2017).

8.7 Emergent Simplicity

Chapters 4 and 5 focused on the importance of age-structure and age-structured mixing in shaping real-world disease dynamics. The TSIR model generally attains a very good fit for long-term measles dynamics (e.g., Fig. 8.5; Grenfell et al., 2002; Becker et al., 2019) despite seemingly ignoring such age-structured complexities altogether... There is however a mathematical framework to understand this because when an age-structured S–I system is on the trajectory governed by the underlying attractor of Eqs. (4.1)–(4.5) introduced in Chap. 4, the aggregate system $\bar{S}$ and $\bar{I}$ will follow the "dynamic homogeneity" model proposed by Earn et al. (2000b) and further discussed by Mahmud (2017). The so-called unity calculations for the SIR are

$$\frac{d\bar{S}}{dt} = \mu N - \hat{\beta}(t)\bar{S}\bar{I} - \mu\bar{S} \tag{8.6}$$

$$\frac{d\bar{I}}{dt} = \hat{\beta}(t)\bar{S}\bar{I} - \gamma\bar{I} - \mu\bar{I} \tag{8.7}$$

$$\hat{\beta}(t) = \frac{1}{\bar{S}\bar{I}} \sum_{i=1}^{A} \sum_{j=1}^{A} \beta_{ij}(t)S_i I_j, \tag{8.8}$$

where $\beta_{ij}(t)$ corresponds to seasonal age-specific variation in transmission as laid out in the intersection between Sects. 4.4 and 6.3, and $\hat{\beta}(t)$ is the time-varying susceptible/prevalence-by-age weighted effective transmission rate. There are two important insights from this. The first is that when demographies and contact patterns are level, the full age-structured transmission can be captured by less elaborate models. Grenfell et al. (2006) termed this "emergent simplicity." The second is that while the school schedule represents an on/off switch with respect to term-time forcing, the overall FoI and thus effective transmission rate will vary in a more subtle fashion (as evidenced in Fig. 8.4) because of the differential removal of individuals of higher risk of exposure and onward transmission versus lower risk individuals. Demographers have long discussed such modulations of population-level averaged rates as "frailty effects" or "heterogeneities ruses" (Keyfitz & Littman, 1979; Vaupel et al., 1979; Vaupel & Yashin, 1985). Emergent simplicity appears to capture broad dynamic patterns of highly transmissible infections. Bansal et al. (2007) discuss situations where more elaborate network models are important for providing further insights. Chapter 14 will visit on this.

8.8 Project Tycho

Bjørnstad et al. (2002a) and Grenfell et al. (2002) expanded on the above TSIR analysis of measles in London to 60 cities and villages in prevaccination England and Wales to better understand dynamics and how it scales with community size. They found that R_0 was independent of population size, suggesting that even if transmission is density dependent, the social clique size does not differ between large cities and small towns. They speculated that this is because school classes are relatively similar in size across population numbers. Ferrari et al. (2011) discussed this within a social network context.

The TSIR has also been used to study the dynamics of rubella (Metcalf et al., 2011a), hand-foot-and-mouth disease caused by various enteroviruses (Takahashi et al., 2016), a variety of other childhood diseases (e.g., Metcalf et al., 2009; Mahmud et al., 2017) and the in-host dynamics of malaria (see Sect. 8.9).

Dalziel et al. (2016) compiled measles and demographic data consistent with the level-2 measles data in Project Tycho for 40 cities in the USA (1906–1948) and 40 cities in the UK (1944–1964). The full dataset is available from datadryad.org. The US portion of the data is in the `dalziel` dataset.

```
data(dalziel)
```

`dalziel$pop` contains interpolated population sizes from the 10-year census surveys, and `dalziel$rec` contains the reconstructed number of births. The data are
biweekly to roughly match that the serial interval can use this data to fit the TSIR
to other diseases with a two-week'ish serial interval. The Philadelphia scarlet fever
data is weekly from Jan 1915 to Dec 1947. The disease is caused by streptococcus A
bacterial infection. Before antibiotics, it was an important cause of death in children.
To prepare it for TSIR modeling, delete the occasional 53rd week and aggregate in
two-week intervals:

```
data(tyscarlet)
tyscarlet = tyscarlet[tyscarlet$WEEK < 53, ]
tyscarlet = tyscarlet[tyscarlet$YEAR > 1914, ]
ag = rep(1:(dim(tyscarlet)[1]/2), each = 2)
scarlet2 = sapply(split(tyscarlet$PHILADELPHIA, ag), sum)
```

Then merge it with the appropriate part of the `dalziel` dataset (and impute a
dozen missing values):

```
require(imputeTS)
philly = dalziel[dalziel$loc == "PHILADELPHIA", ]
philly = philly[philly$year > 1914 & philly$year < 1948,]
philly$cases = na_interpolation(ts(scarlet2))
```

The susceptible reconstruction is:

```
cum.reg = smooth.spline(cumsum(philly$rec), cumsum(philly$cases),
    df = 10)
D = -resid(cum.reg)  #The residuals
rr = predict(cum.reg, deriv = 1)$y
summary(rr)

  ##    Min. 1st Qu.  Median    Mean 3rd Qu.    Max.
  ## 0.03348 0.09533 0.10971 0.10995 0.13719 0.16678
```

The reporting rate is around 10% so it is necessary to create a time series corrected
for underreporting of both incidence, `Ic`, and susceptible deviation, `Dc`:

```
Ic = philly$cases/rr
Dc = D/rr
seas = rep(1:26, 21)[1:597]
lInew = log(Ic[2:598])
lIold = log(Ic[1:597])
Dold = Dc[1:597]
N = median(philly$pop)
offsetN = rep(-log(N), 597)
```

The vector for the profile likelihood on $\bar{S}$ and loop over all candidates is:

```
Smean = seq(0.02, 0.6, by = 0.001) * N
llik = rep(NA, length(Smean))
for (i in 1:length(Smean)) {
    lSold = log(Smean[i] + Dold)
    glmfit = glm(lInew ~ -1 + as.factor(seas) + lIold +
        offset(lSold + offsetN))
    llik[i] = glmfit$deviance
}
Smean[which(llik == min(llik))]/N
```

```
## [1] 0.206
```

Recalling the basic result from Chap. 3 that the fraction of susceptibles is regulated around $s^* = 1/R_0$, the estimate suggests an R_0 of around 5. The best estimates of α are:

```
lSold = log(Smean[which.min(llik)] + Dold)
glmfit = glm(lInew ~ -1 + as.factor(seas) + lIold + offset(lSold +
    offsetN))
# alpha
glmfit$coef[27]
```

```
##      lIold
## 0.8336856
```

The log-βs with SEs are shown in Fig. 8.6. The lower transmission during the summer holiday is conspicuous.

```
beta = exp(glmfit$coef[1:26])
ubeta = exp(glmfit$coef[1:26] + summary(glmfit)$coef[1:26, 2])
lbeta = exp(glmfit$coef[1:26] - summary(glmfit)$coef[1:26, 2])
plotCI(x = c(1:26), y = beta, ui = ubeta, li = lbeta,
    xlab = "Biweek", ylab = expression(beta))
```

8.9 In-Host Malaria Dynamics

When *Plasmodium* parasites enter the blood phase of its mammalian host to cause malaria, it usually causes a period of acute anemia with subsequent rebound from erythropoiesis (production of red blood cells). The rebound may in part be due to host immunity or a delayed response to decline in the parasite population because of depletion of susceptible host cells. Metcalf et al. (2011b, 2012) noted the analogies between the TSIR-like dynamics of immunizing human pathogens and the within-host dynamics of malaria-causing parasites. During the blood stage of infection, infected red blood cells (RBC) burst open in synchrony every 24, 48, or 72h depending on species to release 6–30 merozoites (depending on species).[6] Merozoites

---

[6] The harmonic and subharmonics of the Plasmodium circadian rhythm are still an unresolved mystery (Mideo et al., 2013; Greischar et al., 2014).

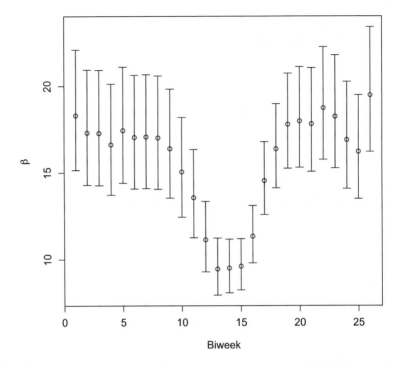

Fig. 8.6: The estimated seasonal βs with SEs for scarlet fever in Philadelphia between 1914 and 1948

then have a narrow time window to find and invade susceptible cells to start the next replication cycle. The malaria TSIR model assumes that the number of infected cells at generation t+1 is captured by $I_{t+1} = P_{E,t}I_tS_t$, where in this *in-host* model I_t and S_t are the number of infected and uninfected RBCs and $P_{E,t}$ is the time-varying effective propagation number (analogous to the βs of the previous sections). This quantity can be thought of as the product of merozoite burst size, evasion of host immunity, contact rates between merozoites and uninfected RBCs, and invasion probability given that a contact has occurred.

We will consider data for the 24h replicating *Plasmodium chabaudi* mouse parasite and use daily data from day three to 21 of 10 laboratory mice infected with the AQ strain as collected by Sylvie Huijben (we will revisit on these data in Sects. 17.7 and 18.4). The chabaudi data is in long format (each measurement on separate lines). The reshape function can convert this into matrices with the time series of infected (paras) and uninfected (RBCs) red blood cells for each mouse as lines (wide format). Some basic further data formatting are:

```
data(chabaudi)
#subset RBC data
chabaudirbc = chabaudi[ ,-c(1, 3, 4, 7, 8, 10, 11)]
#Bump up RBC to microliter
chabaudirbc[ ,4] = chabaudirbc[,4] * 10^6
#subset parasitemia data
chabaudipara = chabaudi[ ,-c(1, 3, 4, 7, 8, 9, 10)]

#reshape to wide
chabaudirbcw = reshape(chabaudirbc, idvar = "Ind2",
     direction = "wide", timevar = "Day")
chabaudipw = reshape(chabaudipara, idvar = "Ind2",
     direction = "wide", timevar = "Day")
#delete duplicate columns
chabaudirbcw = chabaudirbcw[ ,-seq(4, 50, by = 2)]
names(chabaudirbcw)[2] = "Treatment"
chabaudipw = chabaudipw[, -seq(4, 50, by = 2)]
names(chabaudipw)[2] = "Treatment"

#drop last columns of data not counted every day
chabaudipw = chabaudipw[, -c(22:27)]
chabaudirbcw = chabaudirbcw[, -c(22:27)]
#Pull out AQ mice
paras = chabaudipw[1:10, -c(1:2)]
chabaudirbcw = as.matrix(chabaudirbcw[1:10, -c(1:2)])
#Uninfected are total RBCs less infected
RBCs = as.matrix(chabaudirbcw-paras)
```

The time series of infected and susceptible RBCs are shown in Fig. 8.7. The acute anemia is very strong.

```
par(mfrow = c(1, 2), bty = "l")
matplot(t(log(RBCs)), type = "l",xlab = "Day",
     ylab = "Uninfected logRBC")
matplot(t(log(paras)),type = "l", xlab = "Days",
     ylab = "Infected logRBC")
```

Finally, the in-host TSIR model can be fit after log-transforming and lagging as needed:

```
Tmax = length(paras[1, ])  ##max number of days
Nind = length(paras[, 1])  ##number of individuals
day = matrix(rep(1:(Tmax - 1), each = Nind), Nind, Tmax -
    1)
day = c(day)

# Log infected cells
log.para = log(paras[, 2:Tmax])
log.para.lag = log(paras[, 1:(Tmax - 1)])
log.para = unlist(c(log.para))
log.para.lag = unlist(c(log.para.lag))

# Log uninfected cells
```

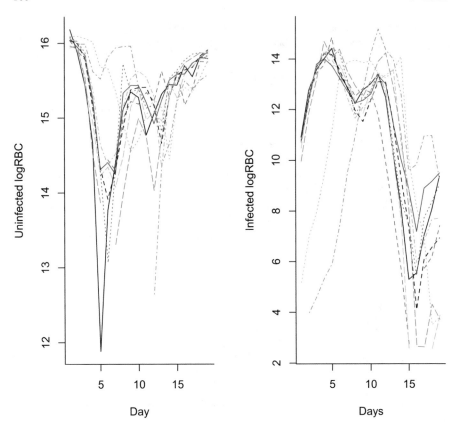

Fig. 8.7: The numbers of infected and susceptible red blood cells in mice infected by the *P.chabaudi* AQ strain in 10 different mice

```
log.rbcs.lag = log(RBCs[, 1:(Tmax - 1)])
log.rbcs.lag = unlist(c(log.rbcs.lag))
```

Occasionally, the parasite count is below the detection limit. These zeros (leading to $-\infty$ log values) are best replaced with the minimum observed non-zero values:

```
log.para[!is.finite(log.para)] =
    min(log.para[is.finite(log.para)] , na.rm = TRUE)
log.para.lag[!is.finite(log.para.lag)] =
    min(log.para[is.finite(log.para)] , na.rm = TRUE)
```

The model fitting algorithm is similar to that done for measles, except that *Plasmodium* replication occurs in discrete, synchronous cycles (Mideo et al., 2013) so the model does not need the α exponent introduced in Sect. 8.2 that corrects for non-discreteness of generations.

```
data = data.frame(log.para = log.para, day = day,
  log.para.lag = log.para.lag,
  log.rbcs.lag = log.rbcs.lag)
fit = glm(log.para ~ -1 + as.factor(day) +
  offset(log.para.lag + log.rbcs.lag), data = data)
```

Figure 8.8 shows the estimated daily propagation numbers and associated in-host effective reproductive numbers ($R_{E,t} = P_{E,t}S_t$). The $R_{E,t}$s are initially around six, which is close to (but a little smaller than) the burst size of *P. chabaudi* merozites. This drops to around one after a week. Metcalf et al. (2011b) discuss how the drop in R_E reflects a combination of depletion of red blood cells in the early phase and the action of innate and acquired immunity. The acquired immunity kicks in after about 2 weeks.

```
par(mfrow = c(1, 2))
require(plotrix)
ses = summary(fit)$coeff[, 2]
beta = exp(fit$coef)
ubeta = exp(fit$coef + ses)
lbeta = exp(fit$coef - ses)
plotCI(x = c(3:20), y = beta, ui = ubeta, li = lbeta,
    xlab = "Day", ylab = expression(P[E]))
points(x = c(3:20), exp(fit$coeff), type = "b", pch = 19)
plotCI(x = c(3:20), y = beta * colMeans(RBCs)[-19], ui = ubeta *
    colMeans(RBCs)[-19], li = lbeta * colMeans(RBCs)[-19],
    xlab = "Day", ylab = expression(R[E]))
points(x = c(3:20), beta * colMeans(RBCs)[-19], type = "b",
    pch = 19)
abline(h = 1, lty = 3)
```

8.10 A TSIR shinyApp

The tsir.app explores the nonseasonal TSIR model. It can be launched from R through:

```
require(epimdr2)
runApp(tsir.app)
```

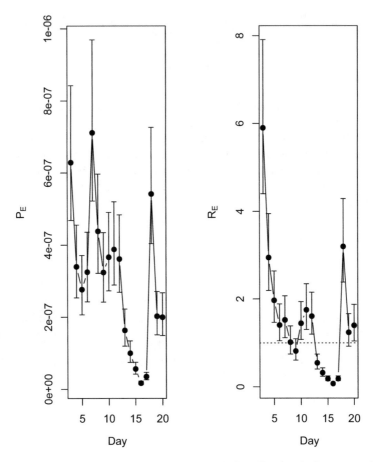

Fig. 8.8: Estimated (**a**) propagation numbers and (**b**) effective in-host reproductive numbers of *P. chabaudi* in mice infected with the AQ strain

8.11 Malapropos: A Ross–Macdonald Malaria Model

This monograph is primarily devoted to computations regarding directly transmitted infectious diseases, but it is pertinent to highlight that the conceptual principles discussed herein also apply to vector-borne diseases. The Ross–Macdonald framework for example is a large literature on modeling malaria dynamics (Smith et al., 2012). A version of this model was proposed by Aron and May (1982) as an ODE system tracking the fraction of infected humans (x) and infected mosquitos (y).

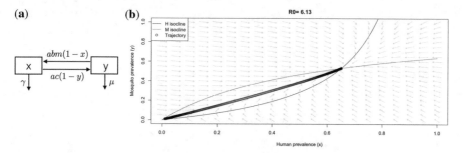

Fig. 8.9: **(a)** Flow diagram of the Aron–May version of Ross–Macdonald malaria transmission model. **(b)** Isoclines in phase plane with parameter values $\gamma = 0.14/\text{day}$, $a = 0.25/\text{day}$, $b = 0.1$, $c = 1$, $\mu = 0.14/\text{day}$, and $m = 20$

The basic equations due to Aron and May (1982) are (Fig. 8.9a)

$$dx/dt = (abY/X)y(1-x) - \gamma x \tag{8.9}$$
$$dy/dt = acx(1-y) - \mu y, \tag{8.10}$$

where $Y/X = m$ is the mosquito-to-human ratio, γ is the human recovery rate (so $1/\gamma$ is the human infectious period), $1/\mu$ is the adult mosquito life expectancy, a is the biting rate (1 / gonotrophic cycle duration), b is the human probability of getting infected by infected mosquito, and c is the probability of mosquito infection from an infected human. We can apply similar logic as in Sect. 3.7 to derive the reproduction number for this system: During the $1/\gamma$ infectious period of the host transmission to mosquitos happens at a rate ac, infected mosquitos are infectious for their lifespan $1/\mu$ and transmit back at a rate abm. Thus $R_0 = \frac{ac}{\gamma} \frac{abm}{\mu} = \frac{a^2 cbm}{\gamma \mu}$.

The isoclines in this system are given by the solution to the equations $dx/dt = 0$ and $dy/dt = 0$ and partition the phase plane into regions where x and y are increasing and decreasing according to (Fig. 8.9b)

$$y = \frac{\gamma x}{(abm)(1-x)} \tag{8.11}$$

$$y = \frac{cx}{acx + \mu}, \tag{8.12}$$

respectively. The endemic equilibrium is

$$x^* = (R_0 - 1)/(R_0 + ac/\mu) \tag{8.13}$$

$$y^* = \frac{R_0 - 1}{R_0} \frac{ac/\mu}{1 + ac/\mu}. \tag{8.14}$$

While the model is simplistic in terms of not considering acquired immunity from lifetime exposure, it is nevertheless useful for considering the fundamental kinetics of vector-borne infections. The `ross.app` can be launched via

```
require(epimdr2)
runApp(ross.app)
```

Chapter 9
Stochastics

9.1 Preamble: Prevalence versus Incidence

When fitting mechanistic models to data, we have to consider carefully the relation-ship between the nature of the data versus the nature of the model state variables. For example, when working with continuous-time S(E)IR models, it is important to keep in mind that incidence is not prevalence. The results from integrating the com-partmental models represent prevalence over time (i.e., the number or fraction of a population that is infected). Most public health data, in contrast, tracks incidence—the number of new cases in any given time interval. We thus need to do something more than trying to match simulated prevalence with observed incidence. We there-fore start with a toy example in which the simulated data actually represents preva-lence.

When/if one can assume that dynamics is largely unaffected by process noise (demographic and environmental stochasticity), models can be fit from data using trajectory matching (e.g., Bhattacharyya et al., 2015). The assumption is that dis-crepancies between the observations and the predictions from the dynamic model are due to observational errors. The upside of trajectory matching is that we can easily fit continuous-time models to variably spaced observations on any/all state variable, and the downside is that these assumptions are restrictive; though highly transmissible, seasonally forced, immunizing pathogens in large populations may effectively erase long-term signatures of stochasticity (Grenfell et al., 2002).[1] The purpose of this chapter is three-fold: To introduce methods for parameter estima-tion using trajectory matching; before then to introduce algorithms for event-based stochastic simulation to explore plausible real-world outcomes; and finally to dis-cuss how these estimations have important bearings on decisions regarding outbreak response vaccination.

This chapter uses the following R package: deSolve.

[1] Yao and Tong (1998; 2000) proposed general statistical time series methods to test for operational determinism in stochastic dynamic systems.

O. N. Bjørnstad, *Epidemics*, Use R!, https://doi.org/10.1007/978-3-031-12056-5_9

9.2 Event-Based Stochastic Simulation

To begin, we consider how to stochastically simulate the continuous-time SIR model (Eqs. (2.1)–(2.3)). Previously, we considered stochastic simulation using the discrete-time chain-binomial framework (Sect. 3.4) for plausible epidemic trajectories. An alternative is to do continuous-time stochastic simulation using an event-based approach via the Gillespie exact algorithm (Gillespie, 1977) and the associated τ-leap approximation (Gillespie, 2001). As discussed in Sect. 2.9, the S(E)IR model (and all compartmental ODEs) implies exponentially distributed waiting times between individual transitions to other compartments. The Gillespie exact algorithm takes advantage of this idea. If we for example consider how the states of the SIR flows (Eqs. (2.1)–(2.3)) should change over time, we expect the following six possible changes:

- $S \to S+1$ at rate μN from births
- $S \to S-1$ at rate μS from deaths
- $S \to S-1$ and $I \to I+1$ at rate $\beta SI/N$ from infection
- $I \to I-1$ at rate μI from deaths
- $I \to I-1$ and $R \to R+1$ at rate γI from recovery
- $R \to R-1$ at rate μR from deaths

Thus, the system is expected to change by an overall summed rate of $r = \mu N + \mu S + \beta SI/N + \mu I + \gamma I + \mu R$. We can therefore draw a random exponential waiting time with mean r to update a continuous-time clock, then draw a random event from a multinomial distribution with probabilities given by the relative rates, update the state variables accordingly, and repeat. . .

Because of the many versions of compartmental models used in studying disease dynamics, it is useful to write a general-purpose stochastic simulator that can be applied to any set of rate equations. To this end, we first define a `rlist` list of equations corresponding to the rates for the six transitions of the SIR flows. The `quote` formalism allows us to set up the list such that all equations can be evaluated in a single `sapply` call as the simulation progress.

```
rlist = c(quote(mu * (S + I + R)), #Births
quote(mu * S), #Sucseptible deaths
quote(beta * S * I /(S + I + R)), #Infection
quote(mu * I), #Infected death
quote(gamma * I), #Recovery
quote(mu * R)) #Recovered death
```

The transition matrix associated with each SIR event has three columns that correspond to changes in S, I, and R, respectively; the rows correspond to the six possible events.

```
emat = matrix(c(1, 0, 0,
    -1, 0, 0,
    -1, 1, 0,
     0, -1, 0,
```

```
    0, -1, 1,
    0, 0, -1),
    ncol = 3, byrow = TRUE)
```

A general-purpose simulator using the Gillespie exact algorithm is provided by the `gillespie` function. The idea is to write a function that is sufficiently robust and general that it can be applied to event-based stochastic simulation of any model that fits within a compartmental framework. The function takes five arguments to accomplish this:

- `rateqs` A list of rate equations corresponding to each of the possible events using the `quote` formalism
- `eventmatrix` A matrix of changes to each of the state variables associated with each event
- `parameters` A vector of parameter values
- `initialvals` A vector of initial values for the states
- `numevents` The number of events to be simulated

```
gillespie = function(rateqs, eventmatrix, parameters,
    initialvals, numevents) {
    res = data.frame(matrix(NA, ncol = length(initialvals) +
        1, nrow = numevents + 1))
    names(res) = c("time", names(inits))
    res[1, ] = c(0, inits)
    for (i in 1:numevents) {
        # evaluate rates
        rat = sapply(rateqs, eval, as.list(c(parameters,
            res[i, ])))
        # update clock
        res[i + 1, 1] = res[i, 1] + rexp(1, sum(rat))
        # draw event
        whichevent = sample(1:nrow(eventmatrix), 1, prob = rat)
        # updat states
        res[i + 1, -1] = res[i, -1] + eventmatrix[whichevent,
            ]
    }
    return(res)
}
```

For the SIR model, an exact Gillespie stochastic simulation assuming an infectious period of 20 days, $R_0 = 26$, and a per capita birth/death rate of one per year (recalling that $\beta = R_0 * (\mu + \gamma) = 500.5$ for the basic SIR model) is shown in Fig. 9.1:

```
paras = c(mu = 1, beta = 26 * (1 + 365/20), gamma = 365/20)
inits = c(S = 100, I = 2, R = 0)
sim = gillespie(rlist, emat, paras, inits, 1000)
matplot(sim[, 1], sim[, 2:4], type = "l", ylab = "Numbers",
    xlab = "Time", log = "y")
legend("topright", c("S", "I", "R"), lty = c(1, 1, 1),
    col = c(1, 2, 3))
```

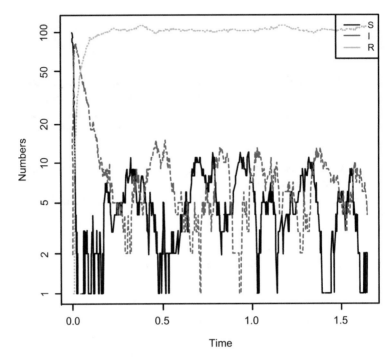

Fig. 9.1: A Gillespie exact simulation of the stochastic SIR model with $\mu = 1$, $\gamma = 365/20$, and $R_0 = 26$, giving a β of 500.5

The Gillespie algorithm provides an "exact" stochastic simulation in the sense that the time evolution of the system is changing exactly according to a random realization of the stochastic differential system. It is, however, computationally expensive as every event is recorded separately. Gillespie's τ-leap method uses the Poisson approximation corresponding to the discussion of Sect. 8.2. If we assume that the interval, Δt, is sufficiently short that any change in the rates is negligible, the number of events should be Poisson distributed with summed rates multiplied by Δt and multinomially divided among the events according to their relative rates.[2]

The below tau function is a general τ-leap simulator for the SEIR model or any other compartmental models such as, for example, Li et al.'s (2017) application to the Ebola SEIHFR model discussed in Sect. 3.9. The SEIR model has eight possible events:

- $S \to S + 1$ at rate μN from births
- $S \to S - 1$ at rate μS from deaths

---

[2] Mathematically speaking, the τ-leap implementation of a stochastic SIR model is related to the chain-binomial model (Eqs. (3.1)–(3.2)) discussed in Sect. 3.4 because Binomial$(S, 1 - \exp^{-\beta I \Delta t/N}) \to$ Poisson$(\beta S I \Delta t/N)$ as $S \to \infty$ if $\beta I \Delta t/N$ is small, where the latter expression is the force of infection.

- $S \rightarrow S - 1$ and $E \rightarrow E + 1$ at rate $\beta SI/N$ from infection
- $E \rightarrow E - 1$ at rate μE from deaths
- $E \rightarrow E - 1$ and $I \rightarrow I + 1$ at rate σE from becoming infectious
- $I \rightarrow I - 1$ at rate μI from deaths
- $I \rightarrow I - 1$ and $R \rightarrow R + 1$ at rate γI from recovery
- $R \rightarrow R - 1$ at rate μR from deaths

We thus have the following four column event matrices:

```
emat2 = matrix(c(1, 0, 0, 0,
    -1, 0, 0, 0,
    -1, 1, 0, 0,
    0, -1, 0, 0,
    0, -1, 1, 0,
    0, 0, -1, 0,
    0, 0, -1, 1,
    0, 0, 0, -1),
  ncol = 4, byrow = TRUE)
```

The SEIR equations associated with each event are:

```
rlist2 = c(quote(mu * (S + E + I + R)),
    quote(mu * S),
    quote(beta * S * I/(S + E + I + R)),
    quote(mu * E),
    quote(sigma * E),
    quote(mu * I),
    quote(gamma * I),
    quote(mu * R))
```

A general-purpose τ-leap simulator is:

```
tau = function(rateqs, eventmatrix, parameters, initialvals,
    deltaT, endT) {
    time = seq(0, endT, by = deltaT)
    res = data.frame(matrix(NA, ncol = length(initialvals) +
        1, nrow = length(time)))
    res[, 1] = time
    names(res) = c("time", names(inits))
    res[1, ] = c(0, inits)
    for (i in 1:(length(time) - 1)) {
        # calculate overall rates
        rat = sapply(rateqs, eval, as.list(c(parameters,
            res[i, ])))
        evts = rpois(1, sum(rat) * deltaT)
        if (evts > 0) {
            # draw events
            whichevent = sample(1:nrow(eventmatrix), evts,
                prob = rat, replace = TRUE)
            mt = rbind(eventmatrix[whichevent, ], t(matrix(res[i,
                -1])))
            mt = matrix(as.numeric(mt), ncol = ncol(mt))
            # update states
```

```
                    res[i + 1, -1] = apply(mt, 2, sum)
                    res[i + 1, ][res[i + 1, ] < 0] = 0
            } else {
                    # if no events in deltaT
                    res[i + 1, -1] = res[i, -1]
            }
    }
    return(res)
}
```

With an initial population comprised of 1000 individuals and 1 initial infected, a stochastically simulated daily incidence for 2 years with measles-like parameters is:[3]

```
paras = c(mu = 1, beta = 1000, sigma = 365/8, gamma = 365/5)
inits = c(S = 999, E = 0, I = 1, R = 0)
sim2 = tau(rlist2, emat2, paras, inits, 1/365, 2)
matplot(sim2[, 1], sim2[, 2:5], type = "l", log = "y",
    ylab = "Numbers", xlab = "Time")
legend("bottomright", c("S", "E", "I", "R"), lty = c(1,
    1, 1, 1), col = c(1, 2, 3, 4))
```

Following the virgin epidemic, the inherent birth/death stochasticity leads to low-amplitude oscillations (Fig. 9.2) according to the resonant periodicity of the SEIR model (see details in Chap. 10).

9.3 Trajectory Matching

Trajectory matching assumes that the discrepancies between models and data are due to error of observation. The event-based, stochastic simulation breaks with this assumption as model discrepancies are due to demographic stochasticity. Let us nevertheless see if we can fit the SEIR model to the event-based simulation. We first recall the gradient function for the system:

```
require(deSolve)
seirmod = function(t, y, parms) {
    S = y[1]
    E = y[2]
    I = y[3]
    R = y[4]

    with(as.list(parms), {
        dS = mu * (N - S) - beta * S * I/N
        dE = beta * S * I/N - (mu + sigma) * E
        dI = sigma * E - (mu + gamma) * I
        dR = gamma * I - mu * R
```

---

[3] Recalling that for the SEIR model $R_0 = \frac{\sigma}{\sigma+\mu} \frac{\beta}{\gamma+\mu}$, these parameters yield an R_0 of around 21.

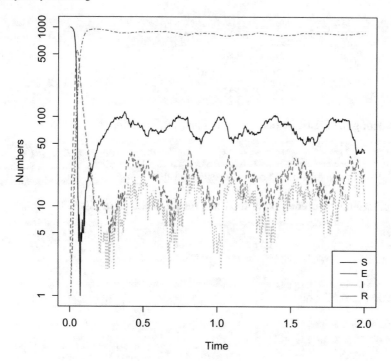

Fig. 9.2: A τ-leap simulation of the SEIR model using a daily time step for 2 years assuming $\mu = 1$, $\beta = 1000$, an infectious period of 8 days, a latent period of 5 days, and an initial population comprised of 1000 individuals one of which is infected

```
        res = c(dS, dE, dI, dR)
        list(res)
    })
}
```

Using the ideas introduced in Sect. 3.4, define a likelihood function to estimate parameters. The Gaussian negative log-likelihood is $\frac{n}{2}\log(\text{RSS}) + \text{const}$, where n is the length of the time series, RSS is the residual sum-of-squares, and the constant is $n(\log(n) - \log(2\pi) - 1)/2$ (Aitkin et al., 2005).[4] The function to calculate this is thus

```
lfn = function(p) {
    times = seq(0, 2, by = 1/365)
    start = c(S = 999, E = 0, I = 1, R = 0)
    paras = exp(c(mu = p[1], N = p[2], beta = p[3], sigma = p[4],
        gamma = p[5]))
    out = as.data.frame(ode(start, times = times, seirmod,
```

---

[4] If in a hurry we can ignore the constant and minimize $\frac{n}{2}\log(RSS)$ because it is the relative likelihood that matters.

```
        paras))
    n = length(sim2$I)
    rss = sum((sim2$I - out$I)^2)
    return(log(rss) * (n/2) - n * (log(n) - log(2 * pi) -
        1)/2)
}
```

Calculating the MLEs involves, as previously, minimizing the function:

```
# initial values for mu, N, beta, sigma, gamma
paras0 = log(c(2, 500, 500, 365/7, 365/7))
fit = optim(paras0, lfn, hessian = TRUE)
```

The deterministic prediction of the fitted model is shown in Fig. 9.3.

```
times = seq(0, 2, by = 1/365)
paras = exp(c(mu = fit$par[1], N = fit$par[2], beta = fit$par[3],
    sigma = fit$par[4], gamma = fit$par[5]))
start = c(S = 999, E = 0, I = 1, R = 0)
out = as.data.frame(ode(start, times, seirmod, paras))
plot(out$time, out$I, xlab = "Time", ylab = "Prevalence",
    type = "l")
lines(sim2$time, sim2$I, col = 2, type = "l")
legend("topright", c("Gillespie simulation", "SEIR fit"),
    lty = c(1, 1), col = c(2, 1))
```

The trajectory-matched fit predicts the virgin epidemic and the next dampened epidemic well, but not the subsequent stochastically excited low-amplitude cycles (Fig. 9.3). In addition to finding parameter estimates, we are usually interested in uncertainty and trade-offs among parameters in producing a fit to the data...

9.4 Likelihood Theory 101

Maximum likelihood principles were used in several previous analyses of, for example, the chain binomial (Sect. 3.4), the catalytic (Sect. 5.3), and the TSIR (Chap. 8) models. However, it is useful to discuss likelihood theory in a more formal fashion.[5] For this purpose, it is useful to summarize the key results with respect to inference from elementary likelihood theory with maximum brevity (see, for example, appendix A of McCullagh & Nelder, 1989):

- Let $L(\theta|D)$ be the function that calculates the likelihood for a set of data, D; i.e., the probability of observing the data given some values for the parameters, θ. The values that maximize this probability are the maximum likelihood estimates (MLEs) of the parameters, $\hat{\theta}$.

---

[5] Bolker (2008) is an excellent broad discussion on estimation for ecologically realistic models using a variety of methods.

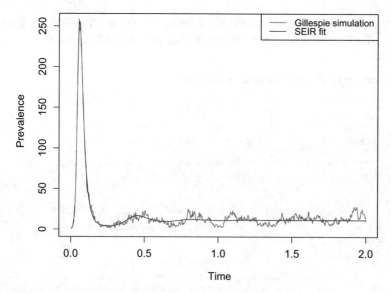

Fig. 9.3: SEIR fitted predicted trajectory superimposed on the τ-leap simulation of the SEIR model

- The negative log-likelihood $(-\log L = \ell(\theta|D))$ shows what $\hat{\theta}$ are the values that minimize $\ell(\theta)$. If data points are independent, then the joint log-likelihood is simply the sum of the log-likelihoods over the data points.
- The MLE is a minimum of ℓ, so the *score function* $U(\theta) = \partial\ell/\partial\theta$ is zero at the MLE.
- The likelihood profile graphs how $\ell(\theta)$ changes with θ. The 95% confidence interval is the set of values of θ for which $\ell(\theta)$ is within $\chi^2(0.95,p)/2$ of the minimum, where p is the number of parameters. The quantity $2\ell(\theta)$ is referred to as the *deviance*, so if we work with the deviance we would use $\chi^2(0.95,p)$ as the cut-off.
- The second derivative of $\ell(\theta)$ with respect to θ is called the *Fisher informa-tion*, $\iota(\theta) = \partial^2\ell/\partial\theta^2$. The inverted information matrix is an approximation of the variance–covariance matrix of the parameters, so we can obtain approximate standard errors as the square-root of the diagonal of the inverted information matrix. The approximate correlation matrix is the standardized inverted information matrix.
- A matrix of second derivatives is generally referred to as a <u>Hessian matrix</u>. If we call optim(..., hessian=TRUE), R will numerically estimate the hessian at the minimum, so if the function to be minimized is the negative log-likelihood, we can obtain approximate SEs and the approximate correlation matrix from this Hessian.
- If we have two alternative models that are *nested*—meaning that the more com-plex model contains all the parameters of the simpler—then we can test for

significant model improvement; the difference in the log-likelihood is $\chi^2(df = \Delta p)/2$-distributed, where Δp is the number of extra parameters in the complex model.[6]

We can apply these ideas to the model fit:

```
# MLEs
round(exp(fit$par), 4)

  ## [1]    1.5165 642.3009 563.3407   50.3001   69.6786

# Approximate SEs
round(exp(sqrt(diag(solve(fit$hessian)))), 4)

  ## [1] 1.2744 1.2441 1.2561 1.0224 1.0240

# Correlation matrix (Normalized inverted Hessian)
round(cov2cor(solve(fit$hessian)), 4)

  ##             [,1]     [,2]     [,3]     [,4]     [,5]
  ## [1,]   1.0000 -0.9976 -0.9972  0.6107 -0.9546
  ## [2,]  -0.9976  1.0000  0.9974 -0.5872  0.9649
  ## [3,]  -0.9972  0.9974  1.0000 -0.6421  0.9543
  ## [4,]   0.6107 -0.5872 -0.6421  1.0000 -0.4653
  ## [5,]  -0.9546  0.9649  0.9543 -0.4653  1.0000
```

The true parameter values used in the simulation were $\mu = 1$, $N = 1000$, $\beta = 1000$, $\sigma = 45.6$, and $\gamma = 73$. So while the model prediction gives a decent fit, the parameter estimates are not particularly accurate. This is where it is useful to apply the likelihood theory more extensively. From the normalized inverted hessian, we see that several of the parameters are highly (positively or negatively) correlated, and several with correlations more extreme than ± 0.9. That means that a different parameter combination may provide a very similar fit to the data. This is an illustration of identifiability problems because of multicollinearites; with observations only on the infectious stage, for instance, a relatively short infectious period and high transmission rate will predict a similar trajectory to a relatively short latent period and a lower transmission rate. Furthermore, a smaller population size and higher birth rate can result in an identical susceptible recruitment rate of a larger population with lower birth rate. For inference, it is therefore normally best to inform the analysis with any known biological quantities; for example, if the latent and infectious periods are known from household or clinical studies, it may be best not to attempt to infer these from the time series alone (though, as King et al. 2008 point out for cholera dynamics, conventional wisdom may not always be consistent with dynamical patterns). Moreover, if there are strong correlations, the individual standard errors (and confidence intervals derived there from) may be a poor representation of parametric uncertainty. It may then be better to look at pairwise confidence ellipses (e.g., Bolker, 2008).

---

[6] If the models are non-nested, formal tests are not available but information theoretical rankings of models using AIC, BIC, AIC weights, etc., are useful (Burnham & Anderson, 2003).

9.5 SEIR with Error

We can use the `ode` function from the `deSolve` package to integrate the SEIR gradient function (`seirmod`) introduced in Sect. 6.2 to which we can add noise to generate a dataset that adheres to the assumption that the dynamics is only affected by observational noise. A 10 year simulation of weekly data assuming measles'ish parameters and 6% of initial susceptibles is

```
times = seq(0, 10, by = 1/52)
paras = c(mu = 1/50, N = 1, beta = 1000, sigma = 365/8,
    gamma = 365/5)
start = c(S = 0.06, E = 0, I = 0.001, R = 0.939)
out = as.data.frame(ode(start, times, seirmod, paras))
```

The `jitter` function can be used to add some noise to the data (Fig. 9.4),

```
datay = jitter(out$I, amount = 1e-04)
plot(times, datay, ylab = "Infected", xlab = "Time")
lines(times, out$I, col = 2)
```

Then define a Gaussian likelihood function,

```
lfn = function(p, data) {
    times = seq(0, 10, by = 1/52)
    start = c(S = 0.06, E = 0, I = 0.001, R = 0.939)
    paras = c(mu = p[1], N = p[2], beta = p[3], sigma = p[4],
        gamma = p[5])
    out = as.data.frame(ode(start, times = times, seirmod,
        paras))
    n = length(data)
    rss = sum((data - out$I)^2)
    return(log(rss) * (n/2) - n * (log(n) - log(2 * pi) -
        1)/2)
}
```

and estimate parameters using the jittered observations:

```
paras0 = c(mu = 1/30, N = 1, beta = 1500, sigma = 365/4,
    gamma = 365/10)
fit = optim(paras0, lfn, data = datay, hessian = TRUE)
```

The estimates are

```
# MLEs:
round(fit$par, 3)

  ## [1]     0.036    1.031 2179.946    71.197   138.851

# Approximate SEs:
round(sqrt(diag(solve(fit$hessian))), 3)

  ## [1]     0.003    0.066 200.261     7.584     8.718
```

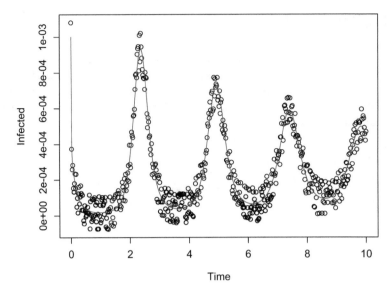

Fig. 9.4: Fraction infectious and jittered data from the SEIR model assuming $\mu = 0.02$, $\beta = 1000$, $\sigma = 45.6$, and $\gamma = 73$/year

```
# Correlation matrix:
round(cov2cor(solve(fit$hessian)), 3)

##          [,1]   [,2]   [,3]   [,4]   [,5]
## [1,]   1.000 -0.743 -0.330 -0.407  0.374
## [2,]  -0.743  1.000  0.820 -0.258  0.204
## [3,]  -0.330  0.820  1.000 -0.658  0.714
## [4,]  -0.407 -0.258 -0.658  1.000 -0.821
## [5,]   0.374  0.204  0.714 -0.821  1.000
```

The likelihood framework, again, reveals important multicolinearities among parameters that highlight uncertainties that will require additional epidemiological data or clinical measurements in order to be resolved.

Uncertainties regarding appropriate model formulations and parameterizations are canonical in the face of emerging diseases, and the inverted hessian allows a quantitation of where parametric uncertainties are strongest. However, from a decision and policy-making point of view Shea et al. (2014) discuss how some uncertainties are more critical to resolve than others using the value-of-information protocol. With respect to identifying the critical uncertainties with respect to the 2014 West African Ebola outbreak, Li et al. (2017) used the event-based stochastic framework introduced in Sect. 9.2 for an expected-value-of-perfect-information (EVPI) analysis to help prioritize fact-finding among the various unknowns. Shea et al. (2020) provide a succinct introduction to this type of decision-theory analysis with an associated shinyApp for further exploration.

9.6 Boarding School Flu Data

The boarding school flu dataset introduced in Sect. 3.6 has an approximate match between *observation* and *prevalence* because the data represents the number of children confined to bed each day, and while the average stay in bed (3–7 days) is maybe a bit different than the infectious period, the durations are comparable.

```
data(flu)
```

Recalling the `sirmod` gradient functions from Sect. 2.3, the likelihood function assuming normally distributed errors is

```
lfn2 = function(pp, II, mu = 0, N = 726) {
    times = seq(1, 14, by = 1)
    start = c(S = N, I = 1, R = 0)
    paras = c(mu = mu, N = N, beta = pp[1], gamma = pp[2])
    out = as.data.frame(ode(y = start, times = times,
        sirmod, paras))
    n = length(II)
    rss = sum((II - out$I)^2)
    return(log(rss) * (n/2) - n * (log(n) - log(2 * pi) -
        1)/2)
}
```

There are two parameters to estimate: β and γ. The time scale is daily so plausible parameter guesses to be optimized are $\beta = 2$ and $\gamma = 0.5$.

```
# beta, gamma
paras0 = c(2, 1/2)
flufit = optim(paras0, lfn2, II = flu$cases, hessian = TRUE)
```

The estimated parameters and basic reproduction number are

```
# parameters
flufit$par

    ## [1] 1.9427860 0.4482372

# R0:
flufit$par[1]/flufit$par[2]

    ## [1] 4.334281
```

The R_0 estimate is comparable to the estimate made in Chap. 3. The observed and predicted outbreaks are seemingly a good match (Fig. 9.5):

```
times = seq(1, 20, by = 0.1)
start = c(S = 762, I = 1, R = 0)
paras = c(beta = flufit$par[1], gamma = flufit$par[2],
    N = 763)
out = as.data.frame(ode(start, times = times, sirmod,
    paras))
```

```
plot(out$time, out$I, ylab = "Prevalence", xlab = "Day",
    type = "l")
points(flu$day, flu$cases)
```

As discussed in Sect. 3.6, the reproduction number is higher than broadly seen for influenza presumably due to the high contact rates among pupils within a boarding school setting.

9.7 Measles

Consider, again, the measles incidence data collected by Doctors Without Borders (MSF) during the 2003–2004 outbreak in Niamey, Niger (Fig. 9.6; Sect. 3.4) but using data at a daily resolution. The compiled daily *incidence* vector y is

```
y = as.vector(table(niamey_daily))
```

The challenge for model fitting is to make the SEIR formulation relevant to the data. The complication is that I represents prevalence (i.e., the current number of infected individuals), while incidence y represents appearance of new cases (i.e., flux) into the infected class. If recasting the SEIR model to also keep track of cumulative incidence (*K*), the differenced K time series (using the diff function) is a pre-

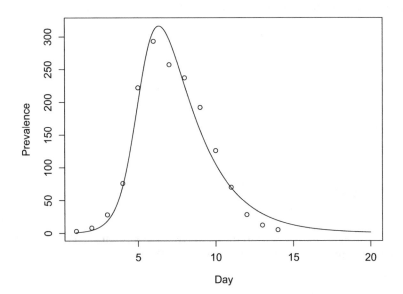

Fig. 9.5: Predicted and observed influenza prevalence for the 1978 boarding school data

diction of incidence (y). The SEIRK model (assuming known latent and infectious periods of 8 and 5 days, respectively) thus provides a vehicle to link model and data quantities.

```
times = unique(niamey_daily$day)
paras = c(mu = 0, N = 1, beta = 5, sigma = 1/8, gamma = 1/5)
start = c(S = 0.999, E = 0, I = 0.001, R = 0, K = 0)
```

The resultant gradient function is

```
seirkmod = function(t, x, params) {
    S = x[1]
    E = x[2]
    I = x[3]
    R = x[4]
    K = x[5]

    with(as.list(params), {
        dS = mu * (N - S) - beta * S * I/N
        dE = beta * S * I/N - (mu + sigma) * E
        dI = sigma * E - (mu + gamma) * I
        dR = gamma * I - mu * R
        dK = sigma * E
        res = c(dS, dE, dI, dR, dK)
        list(res)
    })
}
```

The likelihood function (assuming Poisson distributed counting errors) for the unknown transmission rate, β, and initial susceptible number, N, are as per above protocols. According to the MSF outbreak response protocol, an outbreak is declared once five cases have been confirmed. The unknown initial infectious fraction is thus $5/N$.

```
lfn4 = function(p, I) {
    times = unique(niamey_daily$day)
    xstart = c(S = (p[1] - 5)/p[1], E = 0, I = 5/p[1],
        R = 0, K = 0)
    paras = c(mu = 0, N = p[1], beta = p[2], sigma = 1/8,
        gamma = 1/5)
    out = as.data.frame(ode(xstart, times = times, seirkmod,
        paras))
    predinci = c(xstart["I"], diff(out$K)) * p[1]
    ll = -sum(dpois(I, predinci, log = TRUE))
    return(ll)
}
```

For starting values assuming initial susceptible numbers $N = 11,000$ and $\beta = 5$, the optimization is

```
# N, beta
paras0 = c(11000, 5)
measfit = optim(paras0, lfn4, I = y, hessian = TRUE)
day = 1:230
xstart = c(S = (measfit$par[1] - 5)/measfit$par[1], E = 0,
```

```
    I = 5/measfit$par[1], R = 0, K = 0)
paras = c(mu = 0, N = measfit$par[1], beta = measfit$par[2],
    sigma = 1/8, gamma = 1/5)
out = as.data.frame(ode(xstart, times = day, seirkmod,
    paras))
plot(table(niamey_daily), xlab = "Day", ylab = "Incidence")
lines(out$time, c(xstart["I"], diff(out$K)) * measfit$par[1],
    col = 2, lwd = 2)
```

The estimated effective reproduction number, R_E, at the beginning of the outbreak
is comparable to the estimates based on biweekly data using the chain-binomial
framework of Sect. 3.4:

```
with(as.list(paras), sigma/(sigma + mu) * 1/(gamma + mu) *
    beta/N)
```

```
## [1] 1.761133
```

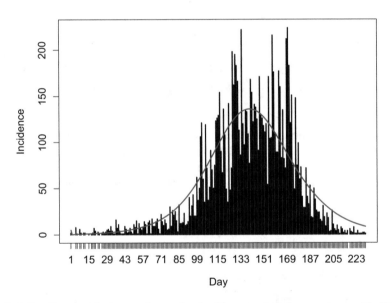

Fig. 9.6: Predicted and observed measles incidence using the maximum likelihood
estimates from the Poisson likelihood

9.8 Outbreak Response Vaccination

Grais et al.'s (2008) objective in fitting a model to the Niamey outbreak data was
to evaluate the effectiveness of outbreak response vaccination (ORV) in reducing
the burden of disease during an ongoing outbreak. For vaccine preventable diseases,

there are four broad categories of intervention. Routine vaccination is immunizations administered during routine pediatric visits. For measles , this typically entails a first dose at 9–12 months of age, followed by one or two more doses before the age of five. Because some children may not have full access to routine medical attention, so-called supplementary immunization activities (SIA) are undertaken intermittently in many (often low or mid income) countries. These typically happen every five to 10 years and have a broader age target group such as 1–15 year olds. The objective of SIAs is to prop up vaccine-induced herd immunity in the face of slow buildup of susceptibles from incomplete vaccine cover. Manifestations of such are for example the resurgence of measles in 1996–1997 in São Paulo, Brazil (Fonnesbeck et al., 2018), and in 2010 in Malawi (Kundrick et al., 2018) both areas have had control of measles prior to these significant flare-ups. Cocoon vaccination discussed in Sect. 5.5 is the strategy to attempt to socially isolate children too young for immunization from exposure (Lavine et al., 2011; Althouse & Scarpino, 2015). The fourth deployment strategy is ORV that is the attempt to aggressively use vaccination to stem an ongoing outbreak such as the 2003–2004 epidemic of measles in Niamey, Niger. At the time, the WHO guidelines were to prioritize palliative care of measles cases (Grais et al., 2008). The goal of the computational exercise was to ask the extent to which ORV can help mitigate the burden of disease during accelerating epidemics of highly transmissible infections.

In the case of the Niamey 2003–2004 outbreak, the Médicine Sans Frontiers ORV campaign began on day 161 after the beginning of the epidemic with a goal of vaccinating 50% of all children of ages between 9 months and 5 years. After 10 days, almost 85,000 (57%) of this at-risk group was vaccinated (without knowledge of previous disease or vaccination status). Assuming that vaccination was at random with respect to immune status, we can write a modified SEIR function incorporating a punctuated ORV to study the problem; the vaccine cover is a fraction—effectively a *probability*—so this needs to be translated into a rate using the relation discussed in Sect. 3.2: $r = -\log(1-p)/D$, where D is now the length of the campaign. We can define two functions to carry out the efficacy calculations. The `sirvmod` function integrates the SIR that includes outbreak response vaccination, and the `retrospec` function compares predicted epidemic trajectories with and without the ORV.

```
sirvmod = function(t, x, parms) {
    S = x[1]
    E = x[2]
    I = x[3]
    R = x[4]
    K = x[5]
    with(as.list(parms), {
        Q = ifelse(t < T | t > T + Dt, 0, (-log(1 - P)/Dt))
        dS = -B * S * I - q * Q * S
        dE = B * S * I - r * E
        dI = r * E - g * I
        dR = g * I + q * Q * S
        dK = r * E
        res = c(dS, dE, dI, dR, dK)
        list(res)
    })
}
```

```
retrospec = function(R, day, vaccine_efficacy, target_vaccination,
    intervention_length, mtime, LP = 7, IP = 7, N = 10000) {
    steps = 1:mtime
    out = matrix(NA, nrow = mtime, ncol = 3)
    # starting values
    xstrt = c(S = 1 - 1/N, E = 0, I = 1/N, R = 0, K = 0)
    beta = R/IP   #transmission rate
    # Without ORV
    par = c(B = beta, r = 1/LP, g = 1/IP, q = vaccine_efficacy,
        P = 0, Dt = 0, T = Inf, R = R)
    outv = as.data.frame(ode(xstrt, steps, sirvmod, par))
    fsv = max(outv$K)
    # With ORV
    par = c(B = beta, r = 1/LP, g = 1/IP, q = vaccine_efficacy,
        P = target_vaccination, Dt = intervention_length,
        T = day)
    outi = as.data.frame(ode(xstrt, steps, sirvmod, par))
    fsi = max(outi$K)
    res = list(redn = fsi/fsv, out = outv, orv = outi,
        B = par["B"], r = par["r"], g = par["g"], q = par["q"],
        P = par["P"], Dt = par["Dt"], T = par["T"], R = R)
    class(res) = "retro"
    return(res)
}
```

Section 14.2 will discuss S3 class programming more formally; however, as a preview, we define a plot.retro function for objects of class retro returned by the retrospec function:

```
plot.retro = function(x) {
    plot(x$out[, 1], x$out[, "I"], type = "l", ylim = c(0,
        max(x$out[, "I"])), xlab = "Day", ylab = "Prevalence")
    polygon(c(x$T, x$T, x$T + x$Dt,
        x$T + x$Dt), c(-0.1, 1, 1, -0.1), col = "gray")
    lines(x$out[, 1], x$out[, "I"])
    lines(x$orv[, 1], x$orv[, "I"], col = "red")
    title(paste("Final size: ", round(100 * (x$redn), 1),
        "% (R=", x$R,", target=", 100*x$P, "%)", sep=""))
    legend(x = "topleft", legend = c("Natural epidemic",
        "With ORV"), col = c("black", "red"), lty = c(1, 1))
    text(x = x$T + x$Dt, y = 0, pos = 4,
        labels = paste(x$intervention_length,
        "ORV from ", x$T))
}
```

Assuming the model is correct and that the vaccine either elicits instantaneous protection or after two or four weeks for the B and T cell response to mature (Sect. 5.1), the ORV is predicted to have reduced the epidemic by 25%, 15%, or 8%, respectively:

```
red1 = retrospec(R = 1.8, 161, vaccine_efficacy = 0.85,
    target_vaccination = 0.5, intervention_length = 10,
    mtime = 250, LP = 8, IP = 5, N = 16000)
red2 = retrospec(R = 1.8, 161 + 14, vaccine_efficacy = 0.85,
    target_vaccination = 0.5, intervention_length = 10,
    mtime = 250, LP = 8, IP = 5, N = 16000)
```

```
red3 = retrospec(R = 1.8, 161 + 28, vaccine_efficacy = 0.85,
    target_vaccination = 0.5, intervention_length = 10,
    mtime = 250, LP = 8, IP = 5, N = 16000)
1 - red1$redn  #protection from 1st day (161) of ORV

  ## [1] 0.2612989

1 - red2$redn  #1st day + 14 of ORV

  ## [1] 0.1509867

1 - red3$redn  #1st day + 28 of ORV

  ## [1] 0.07827277
```

Figure 9.7 depicts the predicted epidemic curve with and without outbreak response vaccination assuming instantaneous protection from vaccine. The key insight is that for ORVs to work they need to be implemented early (Grais et al., 2008).

```
plot(red1)
```

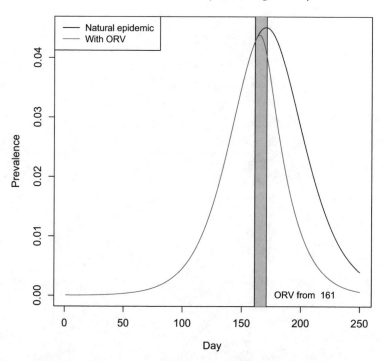

Fig. 9.7: Epidemic curve with and without outbreak response vaccination starting on day 161 with instantaneous protection, a target of 50%, a vaccine efficacy of 85%, a campaign duration of 10 days, and an effective reproduction number of 1.8

9.9 An ORV shinyApp

The `epimdr2` package contains the `orv.app` with more detailed sensitivity analyses of outbreak response vaccine scenarios. The shinyApp can be launched from R through:

```
require(epimdr2)
runApp(orv.app)
```

Chapter 10
Stability and Resonant Periodicity

10.1 Preamble: Rabies

The rabies virus infects a wide range of mammalian carnivores across the world with spillovers to non-competent hosts[1] including humans. While not always classified as rabies, there are a wide range of related lyssaviruses of bats that can also spill over to humans. These viruses are transmitted from saliva during aggressive encounters involving biting. The incubation period is relatively long 3–7 weeks depending on species as the virus slowly migrates through the peripheral and central nervous system to the brain. In humans, the typical incubation period is 2–3 months, which is why, as an unusual case, the vaccine is effective after infection. Rabies is an interesting case where the incubation period determines the effective latent period;[2] in competent hosts, virus can present in saliva a week earlier, but it is only after behavioral changes following the onset of symptomatic disease that onward transmission begins.

Rabies usually invades a naive host range in spatial waves (spatial aspect of which will be discussed in Sect. 15.4). This has been documented in great detail for fox rabies in continental Europe and raccoon rabies in Eastern USA. Raccoon rabies appeared in Virginia/West Virginia in 1977, before which the area was rabies free, following some translocation event from Florida/Georgia that at the time was raccoon rabies endemic.

The `rabies` dataset collected by CDC is the monthly number of rabid raccoons by state. The time column starts from first month of invasion for each state (Childs et al., 2000). The incidence patterns follow the characteristic pattern of major virgin epidemics followed by a fuzzy but distinct periodic recurrence intervals of around 4 years (Fig. 10.1). Theory should allow us to predict such recurrence intervals.

This chapter uses the following R packages: `nleqslv` and `polspline`.

[1] In this context, non-competent means host species that has no onward transmission; Sect. 15.1 will discuss interspecific spillover in more detail.

[2] Recall the incubation period is the time to onset of symptoms, while the latent period is the time to new pathogen presentation such as to be ready for onward transmission.

O. N. Bjørnstad, *Epidemics*, Use R!, https://doi.org/10.1007/978-3-031-12056-5_10

```
data(rabies)
matplot(rabies[, 2:7], ylab = "Cases", xlab = "Month")
legend("topright", c("CT", "DE", "MD", "MA", "NJ", "NY"),
    pch = as.character(1:6), col = 1:6)
```

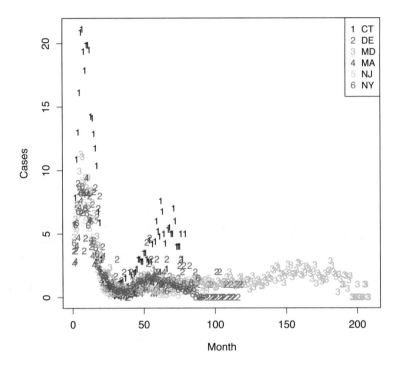

Fig. 10.1: Incidence of raccoon rabies by state since first appearance in Virginia/West Virginia in 1977 (Childs et al., 2000)

10.2 Linear Stability Analysis

As briefly introduced in Sect. 2.7, linear stability analysis is very useful for two reasons: classification of types of equilibria and the calculation of resonant periodicities (i.e., recurrence intervals) in the case of stable or unstable foci.

If we work with continuous-time models (ODEs such as the SEIR), equilibria are stable if all the real parts of eigenvalues of the Jacobian matrix—when evaluated at the equilibrium—are smaller than 0. An equilibrium is: (i) a *node* (i.e., all trajectories move monotonically toward/away from the equilibrium) if the largest eigenvalue has only real parts and (ii) a *focus* (i.e., trajectories spiral toward or away from the equilibrium) if the largest eigenvalues are a conjugate pair of complex numbers $(a \pm bi)$. The resonant period of a focus is $2\pi/b$.[3]

If we work with discrete-time models such as the TSIR discussed in Chap. 8 or the Nicholson–Bailey parasitoid–host model (see Chap. 16), equilibria are stable if the absolute value of all the eigenvalues of the Jacobian—when evaluated at the equilibrium—are smaller than 1. Conditions for nodes versus foci are as for continuous-time models, but the resonant period for such difference equations is $2\pi/\arctan(b/a)$.

10.3 Finding Equilibria

To carry out such calculations, we need to construct the Jacobian and gather the values corresponding to the equilibrium of interest. An equilibrium is where the state variables do not change. So in the case of ODEs, we may consider three strategies of decreasing desirability: (i) solve analytically for when all gradient functions are zero, (ii) solve numerically for when all gradient functions are zero, or (iii) simulate the ODEs a long time and record the state of the system at the end. The latter is the worst because it will not find any unstable solutions, and (ii) is less good than (i) because it is less exact, but (i) may be difficult if you are a biologist working with complex models.

Consider the SIR model (Eqs. (2.1)–(2.3)). The equilibria occur when dS/dt, dI/dt, and dR/dt all equal zero.

Strategy 1: Setting N to 1 (i.e., modeling fractions rather than numbers), the disease free equilibrium (dfe) is $\{S^* = 1, I^* = 0, R^* = 0\}$. The endemic equilibrium is as follows: The I equation of the SIR implies that $S^* = (\gamma + \mu)/\beta = 1/R_0$, which when substituted into the S equation gives $I^* = \mu(R_0 - 1)/\beta$, and finally, $R^* = N - I^* - S^*$. Thus the evaluation for a given set of parameters is

```
parms = c(mu = 1/(50 * 52), N = 1, beta = 2.5, gamma = 1/2)
N = parms["N"]
gamma = parms["gamma"]
beta = parms["beta"]
mu = parms["mu"]
Istar = as.numeric(mu * (beta/(gamma + mu) - 1)/beta)
Sstar = as.numeric((gamma + mu)/beta)
Sstar
```

```
## [1] 0.2001538
```

```
Istar
```

```
## [1] 0.0006147934
```

---

[3] And a "center" that produces amplitude-neutral oscillations like that seen in the Lotka–Volterra predator–prey model if it has only imaginary parts.

Strategy 2: For a numerical solution, the `nleqslv` package solves coupled equations by any desired level of accuracy. Note, now, that the state variables, x, are the unknown quantities to solve so the below `rootfn` function provides the set of equations that needs to be solved for the value of all zeros.

```
require(nleqslv)
rootfn = function(x, params) {
    r = with(as.list(params), c(mu * (N - x[1]) - beta *
        x[1] * x[2]/N, beta * x[1] * x[2]/N - (mu + gamma) *
        x[2], gamma * x[2] - mu * x[3]))
    r
}
parms = c(mu = 1/(50 * 52), N = 1, beta = 2.5, gamma = 1/2)
ans = nleqslv(c(0.1, 0.5, 0.4), fn = rootfn, params = parms)
ans$x

  ## [1] 0.2001523463 0.0006147945 0.7992328592
```

The numerical solution is accurate to the fifth decimal place for the endemic equilibrium. The unstable disease free equilibrium $\{S^* = 1, I^* = 0, R^* = 0\}$ also appears numerically when using this protocol to explore across a wide range of initial guesses.

```
ans = grid = expand.grid(seq(0, 1, by = 0.25), seq(0,
    1, by = 0.25), seq(0, 1, by = 0.25))
ans[, ] = NA
for (i in 1:nrow(ans)) {
    ans[i, ] = nleqslv(as.numeric(grid[i, ]), fn = rootfn,
        params = parms)$x
}
ans2 = round(ans, 4)
ans2[!duplicated(ans2), ]

  ##      Var1   Var2    Var3
  ## 1 1.0000 0e+00 0.0000
  ## 6 0.2002 6e-04 0.7992
```

The two equilibria show up.

Strategy 3: This probably should not be used for final analyses because numerically integrating differential equations is much more fraught than numerically solving nonlinear equations. However, as a shortcut if there already is a gradient function defined, one can integrate the equations for the time required to reach equilibrium and then use those final values.[4]

```
sirmod = function(t, y, parameters) {
    S = y[1]
    I = y[2]
```

---

[4] NB: Unstable equilibria will not be found with this protocol, and if there are more than one steady state (as discussed further in Chap. 11), only one will show up depending on chosen initial conditions.

```
    R = y[3]
    with(as.list(parameters), {
        dS = mu * (N - S) - beta * S * I/N
        dI = beta * S * I/N - (mu + gamma) * I
        dR = gamma * I - mu * R
        res = c(dS, dI, dR)
        list(res)
    })
}

paras = c(mu = 1/(50 * 52), N = 1, beta = 2.5, gamma = 1/2)
equil = ode(y = c(S = 1 - 1e-04, I = 1e-04, R = 0), times = seq(0,
    1e+05, by = 1), func = sirmod, parms = paras)
round(tail(equil[, -1], 1), 5)

##              S       I       R
## [100001,] 0.20015 0.00061 0.79923
```

10.4 Evaluating the Jacobian

If we work on fractions of individuals in each compartment ($N = S + I + R = 1$), the R compartment of the SIR model does not affect dynamics. So for analysis, one only needs to consider the coupled S–I system. The calculations are easily done using the general-purpose jacobian function introduced in Sect. 6.3.

STEP 1: classes are S and I

```
states = c("S", "I")
```

STEP 2: The list of equations is

```
elist=c(dS = quote(mu * (N - S) - beta * S * I / N),
    dI = quote(beta * S * I / N - (mu + gamma) * I))
```

STEP 3: Parameters are

```
parms = c(mu = 1/(50 * 52), N = 1, beta = 2, gamma = 1/2)
```

STEP 4: For this model, the endemic equilibrium is $\{S^* = \beta/(\gamma + \mu), I^* = \mu(\beta/(\gamma + \mu) - 1)/\beta\}$, and the disease free equilibrium is $\{S^* = 1, I^* = 0\}$.

```
eeq = with(as.list(parms), c(S = (gamma + mu)/beta, I = mu *
    (beta/(gamma + mu) - 1)/beta))
deq = list(S = 1, I = 0, R = 0)
```

STEP 5: Invoke the Jacobian calculator and calculate eigenvalues:

```
JJ = jacobian(states = states, elist = elist, parameters = parms,
    pts = eeq)
# Eigen values are:
eigen(JJ)$value
```

```
## [1] -0.00076864+0.02400384i -0.00076864-0.02400384i
```

The solution is a pair of complex conjugates with negative real parts. So the endemic equilibrium is a stable focus. The resonant periodicity is

```
2 * pi/Im(eigen(JJ)$value[1])
```

```
## [1] 261.7575
```

So just over 5 years. Next consider the disease free equilibrium:

```
deq = list(S = 1, I = 0, R = 0)
JJ = jacobian(states = states, elist = elist, parameters = parms,
    pts = deq)
# Eigen values are:
eigen(JJ)$values
```

```
## [1]   1.4996153846 -0.0003846154
```

The leading eigenvalue is real-only and > 0; the disease free equilibrium is an unstable node (because $R_0 > 1$). What if the transmission rate is 0.3?

```
parms = list(mu = 1/(50 * 52), N = 1, beta = 0.3, gamma = 1/2,
    S = 1, I = 0)
JJ = jacobian(states = states, elist = elist, parameters = parms,
    pts = deq)
# Eigen values are:
eigen(JJ)$values
```

```
## [1] -0.2003846154 -0.0003846154
```

```
# R0
with(parms, beta/(mu + gamma))
```

```
## [1] 0.5995388
```

The leading eigenvalue is real-only and less than zero; the disease free equilibrium is a stable node (because $R_0 \simeq 0.6$ is smaller than one). So this system would be resistant to disease invasion and establishment as previously discussed in Sect. 3.1.

10.5 Influenza

The mystery of the annual epidemics of influenza that peak in the Northern hemisphere in the Northern winter and in the Southern hemisphere in the Southern winter (Hope-Simpson, 1981) has been discussed as an exemplar par excellence in resonant periodicities in epidemiology (Dushoff et al., 2004; Bjørnstad & Viboud, 2016). Seasonal influenza epidemics are caused by subtypes B, A/H3N2, and A/H1N1 in various mixtures in any given year. At the aggregate level, the flu can be modeled as a susceptible–infected–recovered–(re)susceptible (SIRS) system (Axelsen et al., 2014) with transient immune protection upon recovery lasting around 4–6 years due to epochal evolution (Koelle et al., 2006). The SIRS model is

$$\frac{dS}{dt} = \underbrace{\mu N}_{\text{birth}} - \underbrace{\beta I \frac{S}{N}}_{\text{infection}} + \underbrace{\omega R}_{\text{resusceptible}} - \underbrace{\mu S}_{\text{death}} \tag{10.1}$$

$$\frac{dI}{dt} = \underbrace{\beta I \frac{S}{N}}_{\text{infection}} - \underbrace{\gamma I}_{\text{recovery}} - \underbrace{\mu I}_{\text{death}} \tag{10.2}$$

$$\frac{dR}{dt} = \underbrace{\gamma I}_{\text{recovery}} - \underbrace{\omega R}_{\text{lost immmunity}} - \underbrace{\mu R}_{\text{death}}, \tag{10.3}$$

where ω is the rate of loss of immunity (~ 0.25 year^{-1}). Carrat et al. (2008) suggest an infectious period ($1/\gamma$) of 3.8 days, and Axelsen et al. (2014) suggest an R_0 of 2.9. Modeling fractions ($N = 1$) of the weekly SIRS flu-appropriate parameters are

```
N = 1
gamma = 7/3.8
omega = 1/(52 * 4)
mu = 1/(52 * 70)
R0 = 2.9
```

STEP 3: The call for back-calculating β to get the right R_0 and gathering parameters is

```
# R0 = beta / (gamma + mu)
beta = R0 * (gamma + mu)
paras = c(beta = beta, gamma = gamma, mu = mu, omega = omega)
```

STEP 4: The endemic equilibrium of the SIRS model is $S^* = 1/R_0$, $I^* = \frac{\mu(1-1/R_0)}{\gamma+\mu-\frac{\omega\gamma}{\omega+\mu}}$, and $R^* = \gamma I^*/(\omega+\mu)$:

```
Sstar = 1/R0
Istar = mu * (1 - 1/R0)/(gamma + mu - (omega * gamma)/(omega +
    mu))
Rstar = gamma * Istar/(omega + mu)
eq = list(S = Sstar, I = Istar, R = Rstar)
eq
```

```
## $S
## [1] 0.3448276
##
## $I
## [1] 0.001802665
##
## $R
## [1] 0.6533697
```

STEP 1-2: Defining states and equations and applying the `jacobian` function to the endemic equilibrium are

```
#states
states=c("S", "I", "R")

#equations
elist=c(
dS = quote(mu * (1-S)  - beta * S * I / N +
    omega * R),
dI = quote(beta * S * I / N - (mu + gamma) * I),
dR = expression(gamma * I - (mu +omega) * R))

JJ = jacobian(states = states, elist = elist,
    parameters = paras, pts = eq)
```

Finally, the eigenvalues and resonant frequency from the dominant conjugate pair predict a stable focus (real parts are negative) with a resonant period of 47 weeks:

```
round(eigen(JJ)$values, 4)
```

```
   ## [1] -0.0074+0.1332i  -0.0074-0.1332i  -0.0003+0.0000i
```

```
2 * pi/Im(eigen(JJ)$values)[1]
```

```
   ## [1] 47.17804
```

For the SIRS model, there is an approximate equation for the resonant period (Keeling & Rohani, 2008): $T = 4\pi/\sqrt{(4(R_0 - 1)/(G_I G_R) - ((1/G_R) - (1/A))^2)}$, where A is the mean age of infection $(= \frac{\omega+\mu+\gamma}{(\omega+\mu)(\beta-\gamma-\mu)})$, G_I is the infectious period $(= 1/(\gamma+\mu))$, and G_R is the average duration of immunity $(= 1/(\omega+\mu))$. We can check the accuracy of the approximation against the resonant frequency of the linearized system.

```
A = (omega + mu + gamma)/((omega + mu) * (beta - gamma -
    mu))
GI = 1/(gamma + mu)
GR = 1/(omega + mu)
T = 4 * pi/sqrt(4 * (R0 - 1)/(GI * GR) - ((1/GR) - (1/A))^2)
T
```

```
   ## [1] 47.11307
```

The approximate equation is in very good agreement with the Jacobian-calculated period.

10.6 Raccoon Rabies

Coyne et al. (1989) developed a compartmental model for rabies in raccoons (Fig. 10.2). The flow is from susceptible (S), infected but not yet infectious hosts that eventually become rabid (E_1), infected hosts that recover with immunity (E_2), rabid raccoons (I), immune raccoons (R), and vaccinated raccoons (V). The total number of raccoons (N) is the sum of these. The model is

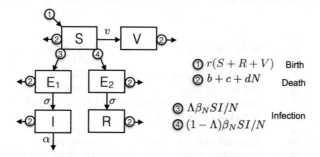

Fig. 10.2: The flow diagram for the raccoon rabies model of Coyne et al. (1989). The compartments are susceptible (S), vaccinated (V), exposed on path to disease (E_1), exposed on path to recovery (E_2), rabid (I), and immune (R). Death rates are assumed density-dependent as numbers approach the carrying capacity with additional mortality from rabies

The equations are Eqs. (10.4)–(10.10) with parameters as defined in Table 10.1.[5]

$$\frac{dS}{dt} = \underbrace{a(S+R+V)}_{\text{birth}} - \underbrace{\beta_N SI/N}_{\text{infection}} - \underbrace{(b+c+dN)S}_{\text{density-dependent death}} - \underbrace{vS}_{\text{vaccination}} \qquad (10.4)$$

$$\frac{dE_1}{dt} = \underbrace{\Lambda \beta_N SI/N}_{\text{to } I} - \underbrace{(b+c+dN)E_1}_{\text{density-dependent death}} - \underbrace{\sigma E_1}_{\text{to } I} \qquad (10.5)$$

$$\frac{dE_2}{dt} = \underbrace{(1-\Lambda)\beta_N SI/N}_{\text{to } I} - \underbrace{(b+c+dN)E_2}_{\text{density-dependent death}} - \underbrace{\sigma E_2}_{\text{to } R} \qquad (10.6)$$

---

[5] The notation has been changed from the original publication to conform to conventions in the current text.

$$\frac{dI}{dt} = \underbrace{\sigma E_1}_{\text{from } E_1} - \underbrace{(b+c+dN)I}_{\text{density-dependent death}} - \underbrace{\alpha I}_{\text{disease death}} \tag{10.7}$$

$$\frac{dR}{dt} = \underbrace{\sigma E_2}_{\text{from } E_2} - \underbrace{(b+c+dN)R}_{\text{density-dependent death}} \tag{10.8}$$

$$\frac{dV}{dt} = \underbrace{vS}_{\text{vaccination}} - \underbrace{(b+c+dN)V}_{\text{density-dependent death}} \tag{10.9}$$

$$N = S + E_1 + E_2 + I + R + V. \tag{10.10}$$

In this model, transmission is assumed to scale in a density-dependent fashion ($\beta_N = \beta N$) (see Sect. 4.1) so the overall transmission term cancels to βSI in the below code.

a	Intrinsic birth rate	1.34/year
b	Intrinsic death rate	0.836/year
r	Intrinsic rate of increase ($= a - b$)	0.504
K	Carrying capacity	12.69/km^2
d	Index of density dependence (=r/K)	0.0397 km^2/year
$(1 - \Lambda)$	Probability of recovery	0.20
σ	Rate of transition from latents	7.5/year
α	Disease-induced mortality	66.36/year
β_N	Transmission rate	33.25N/year
v	Vaccination rate	Variable
c	Culling rate	Variable

Table 10.1: Parameters and values for the Coyne et al.'s (1989) raccoon   rabies model. Transmission related parameters are represented with symbols and host related parameters by letters

Considering a slightly simplified system without vaccination (so without the V class and v parameter). The deSolve package can integrate the model using the "log-trick" introduced in Sect. 2.9 to solve the system in log-coordinates.[6]

```
coyne2 = function(t, logx, parms) {
    x = exp(logx)
    S  = x[1]
    E1 = x[2]
    E2 = x[3]
```

---

[6] Note again how initial values are log-transformed in start, the first line in the function is x = exp(logx), and the last line returns dS/S, etc., in place of dS that comes from the chain-rule of differentiation and the fact that $D(\log x) = 1/x$.

```
    I = x[4]
    R = x[5]
    N = sum(x)
    with(as.list(parms), {
        dS = a * (S + R) - beta * S * I - (b + c + d *
            N) * S
        dE1 = lambda * beta * S * I - (b + c + d * N) *
            E1 - sigma * E1
        dE2 = (1 - lambda) * beta * S * I - (b + c + d *
            N) * E2 - sigma * E2
        dI = sigma * E1 - (b + c + d * N) * I - alpha *
            I
        dR = sigma * E2 - (b + d + c * N) * R
        res = c(dS/S, dE1/E1, dE2/E2, dI/I, dR/R)
        list(res)
    })
}
```

The integrated system is

```
times = seq(0, 100, by = 1/520)
paras = c(d = 0.0397, b = 0.836, a = 1.34, sigma = 7.5,
    alpha = 66.36, beta = 33.25, c = 0, lambda = 0.8)
start = log(c(S = 12.69/2, E1 = 0.1, E2 = 0.1, I = 0.1,
    R = 0.1))
out = as.data.frame(ode(start, times, coyne2, paras))
```

Figure 10.3 is a plot of the predicted prevalence time series and the dynamics in the S–I phase plane (anti-logging the log-coordinate variables to convert them to abundances). The model predicts transient cycles toward the endemic equilibrium.

```
par(mfrow = c(1, 2))
plot(times, exp(out$I), ylab = "Infected", xlab = "Time",
    type = "l")
plot(exp(out$S), exp(out$I), ylab = "Infected",
    xlab = "Susceptible", type = "l")
```

Childs et al. (2000) used this model to study how the predicted inter-epidemic period compares to the data (Fig. 10.1). We can repeat this analysis by calculating the resonant frequency of the system. This calculation needs the 5×5 Jacobian matrix and values for the endemic equilibrium.

```
#states
states=c("S", "E1", "E2", "I", "R")

#equations
elist = c(dS = quote(a * (S + R) - beta * S * I -
    d * (S + E1 + E2 + I + R) * S  - (b + c) * S),
dE1= quote(lambda * beta * S * I -
    d * (S + E1 + E2 + I + R) * E1  - (b + sigma + c) * E1),
dE2 = quote((1-lambda) * beta * S * I -
    d * (S + E1 + E2 + I + R) * E2  - (b + sigma + c) * E2),
```

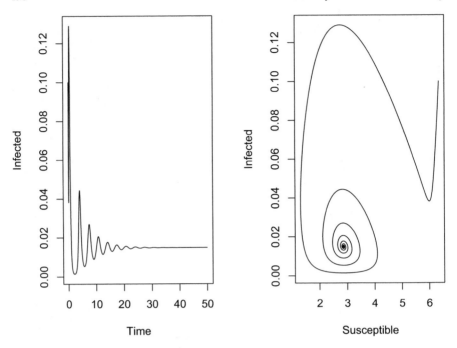

Fig. 10.3: Rabies dynamics predicted by the model of Coyne et al. (1989) (**a**) in time and (**b**) in the phase plane using the parameters defined in Table 10.1

```
dI = quote(sigma * E1  - d * (S + E1 +
     E2 + I + R) * I  - (b.+ alpha + c) * I),
dR = quote(sigma * E2 - d * (S + E1 +
     E2 + I + R) * R  - (b + c) * R))
```

The already defined `coyne2` gradient function can be used to identify the steady state, so we can use the lazy option (strategy 3):

```
equil = exp(tail(out[, -1], n = 1))
```

The Jacobian at the endemic equilibrium and the dominant eigenvalues are

```
# Evaluate  Jacobian  elements
JJ = jacobian(states = states, elist = elist, parameters = paras,
    pts = equil)
# Eigen decomposition
wh = which.max(Re(eigen(JJ, only.values = TRUE)$values))
round(eigen(JJ)$values, 4)

  ## [1]  -75.8478+0.0000i  -8.4686+0.0000i  -0.2008+1.9235i
  ## [4]   -0.2008-1.9235i   -0.7870+0.0000i
```

The dominant eigenvalues are the conjugate pair with a real part of -0.20. The endemic equilibrium is thus a stable focus with a resonant period of

```
2 * pi/Im(eigen(JJ)$values[wh])
```

```
## [1] 3.266555
```

Hence, the model predicts recurrent outbreaks with a mean period of 3.3 years during the rabies invasion that is 9 months shorter than that observed in the data. Childs et al. (2000) varied the ρ parameter (the fraction of exposed raccoons escaping infection with immunity) to find a model that more closely matched the data (around 48 months) if recovery is higher than conventional wisdom from the literature. However, it appears that alternatively a lower carrying capacity closer to that reported by Rosatte et al. (2007) also produces patterns in good agreement with the empirical data:

```
paras["lambda"] = 0.95
paras["d"] = 0.1
out = as.data.frame(ode(start, times, coyne2, paras))
equil = exp(tail(out[, -1], n = 1))
JJ = jacobian(states = states, elist = elist, parameters = paras,
     pts = equil)
wh = which.max(Re(eigen(JJ, only.values = TRUE)$values))
2 * pi/Im(eigen(JJ)$values[wh])
```

```
## [1] 4.472992
```

10.7 Critical Host Density

Section 3.1 introduced the notion that for many directly transmitted wildlife diseases, there may be a critical host density below which contact rates are insufficient to initiate a robust chain of transmission. Anderson et al. (1981) derived an explicit equation for the critical host density for fox rabies of $K = (\sigma + a)(\alpha + a)/\beta\sigma$, where α is the rate of disease-induced mortality (so 1/average time to death of rabid foxes), a is the birth rate, β is the transmission rate , and $1/\sigma$ is the latent period (see also Murray et al., 1986). For the slightly more elaborate raccoon rabies model of Coyne et al. (1989), we can apply the next-generation tools from Sect. 3.11 to explore this notion further. In the rabies model, the carrying capacity of the host is $K = r/d$. By varying d, we can change host density and study resultant changes in R_0. First make the appropriate setup for the next-generation calculations. Next define the `Istates`, the vector naming all infected classes, the `Flist` that contains equations (as `quotes`) for completely new infections entering each infected compartment, the `Vlist` that contains the equations for losses out of each infected compartment minus the equations for all gains into each infected compartment that

does not represent new infections but transfers among infected classes with model
parameters and the value of all states at the disease free equilibrium (recall Sect. 3.11
for details).

```
#STEP 1: Infected classes
istates = c("E1", "E2", "I")

#STEP 2: All new infections
flist=c(dE1=quote(lambda * beta * S * I),
   dE2=quote((1-lambda) * beta * S * I),
   dIdt=quote(0))

#STEP 3--5:
#Losses from E1, E2, I
Vm1 = quote(d * (S + E1 + E2 + I + R) * E1   + (b + c) * E1)
Vm2 = quote(d * (S + E1 + E2 + I + R) * E2   +
   (b + sigma + c) * E2)
Vm3 = quote(d * (S + E1 + E2 + I + R) * I   + (b + alpha + c) * I)

#Gained transfers
Vp1 = 0
Vp2 = 0
Vp3 = quote(sigma * E1)

#To Make Vlist, subtract Vp from Vm
V1 = substitute(a - b, list(a = Vm1, b = Vp1))
V2 = substitute(a - b, list(a = Vm2, b = Vp2))
V3 = substitute(a - b, list(a = Vm3, b = Vp3))
vlist = c(V1, V2, V3)

#STEP 7:
#Define parameters
paras = c(d = 0.0397, b = 0.836, a = 1.34, sigma = 7.5,
   alpha = 66.36, beta = 33.25, c = 0, lambda = 0.8)

#Specify the disease free equilibrium
df = list(S = 1, E1 = 0, E2=0, I = 0, R = 0)

#STEP 6 and 8:
#Invoke R0 calculator
nextgenR0(Istates = istates, Flist = flist, Vlist = vlist,
   parameters = paras, dfe = df)

## [1] 4.230338
```

So with Coyne et al.'s (1989) default parameters and a carrying capacity of 12.7/km
R_0 is around 4.2. Exploring a range of carrying capacities by changing the value of
d indicates a relatively unchanging R_0 in the 3–4.5 range that drops rapidly with a
carrying capacity below 5/km^2. Nevertheless, the critical host density is predicted as

low as $0.3/\text{km}^2$ (Fig. 10.4)—a quarter that predicted by Anderson et al. (1981) for fox rabies—so invasion should be robust across most raccoon populations according to this model.

```
d = seq(0.02, 3, by = 0.01)
K = (paras["a"] - paras["b"])/d
R0 = rep(NA, length(d))
for (i in 1:length(d)) {
    paras["d"] = d[i]
    R0[i] = nextgenR0(Istates = istates, Flist = flist,
        Vlist = vlist, parameters = paras, dfe = df)
}
plot(K, R0, type = "l", lwd = 2, ylab = expression(R[0]))
abline(h = 1)
K[which(R0 < 1)[1]]

    ## [1] 0.2458537
```

10.8 Advanced: Transfer Functions

We can predict the entire power spectrum of a linearized stochastic system using transfer functions (Priestley, 1981; Nisbet & Gurney, 1982; Bjørnstad et al., 2004). In matrix form, the transfer function for a coupled continuous-time system is

$$\mathbf{T}(\boldsymbol{\varpi}) = (\mathbf{I}\boldsymbol{\varpi}\imath - \mathbf{J})^{-1}\mathbf{A}(\boldsymbol{\varpi}), \qquad (10.11)$$

where $\mathbf{I}$ is the identity matrix, $\boldsymbol{\varpi}$ is the *angular* frequency (between 0 and π; so $\boldsymbol{\varpi}/(2*\pi)$ and $2*\pi/\boldsymbol{\varpi}$ correspond to the frequencies (f) and periods discussed in Sect. 7.4), $\mathbf{J}$ is the Jacobian matrix (evaluated at the equilibrium), $\mathbf{A}$ is the matrix of gradients differentiated with respect to the stochastic term(s), and $^{-1}$ denotes the matrix inverse.[7] If the stochasticity is uncorrelated white noise, the power spectrum is predicted by the modulus of the transfer function.

Example 1: Let us consider the SIR model from Sect. 2.7 and assume that variability enters through stochasticity in β. We first need the equilibrium values for the linearization:

---

[7] This equation stems from the result that if $\tilde{\mathbf{X}}(\boldsymbol{\varpi})$ denotes the Fourier transform of the vector of state variables, the transform of $\frac{d\mathbf{X}}{dt}$ will be $\tilde{\mathbf{X}}(\boldsymbol{\varpi})\imath\boldsymbol{\varpi}$; rearranging in matrix form yields $\tilde{\mathbf{X}}(\boldsymbol{\varpi}) = \tilde{\mathbf{T}}(\boldsymbol{\varpi})\tilde{\mathbf{A}}(\boldsymbol{\varpi})$. For discrete-time systems, the transfer function is $\tilde{\mathbf{T}}(\boldsymbol{\varpi}) = (\tilde{\mathbf{I}} - e^{-\imath\boldsymbol{\varpi}}\tilde{\mathbf{J}})^{-1}\mathbf{A}(\tilde{\boldsymbol{\varpi}})$ because the Fourier transform of X_{t-1} is $\tilde{\mathbf{X}}(\boldsymbol{\varpi})e^{-\imath\boldsymbol{\varpi}}$ (see example 2 below).

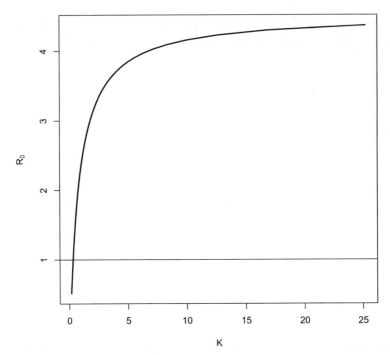

Fig. 10.4: R_0 as a function of carrying capacity for the raccoon rabies model

```
paras = c(mu = 1/(50 * 52), N = 1, beta = 2.5, gamma = 1/2)
eq = with(as.list(paras), c(S = (gamma + mu)/beta, I = mu *
    (beta/(gamma + mu) - 1)/beta))
```

Next the Jacobian matrix evaluated at the equilibrium is

```
#states
states=c("S", "I")

#equations
elist = c(dS = quote(mu * (N  - S)   - beta * S * I / N),
    dI = quote(beta * S * I / N - (mu + gamma) * I))

JJ = jacobian(states = states, elist = elist,
    parameters = paras, pts = eq)
```

The **A** matrix is the linearization with respect to the stochastic term. Assuming stochasticity in β, the last pieces needed for the transfer function are

```
a1 = D(elist$dS, "beta")
a2 = D(elist$dI, "beta")
```

```
A = with(as.list(c(paras, eq)), matrix(c(eval(a1), eval(a2)),
    ncol = 1))
Id = diag(2)
```

Finally, evaluate the transfer function (across 500 frequencies between 0 and π):

```
wseq = seq(0, pi, length = 500)
Fr = vector("list", 500)   #set up empty list of matrices
# Loop to fill matrices for each frequency
for (i in 1:500) {
    # Solve gives matrix inverse
    Fr[[i]] = matrix(solve(Id * (0+1i) * wseq[i] - JJ) %*%
        A, ncol = 1)
}
```

and calculate the theoretical power spectrum from the modulus of the transfer function:

```
PS = matrix(NA, ncol = 2, nrow = 500,
    dimnames = list(1:500, c("S","I")))
#Power spectra from real and imaginary
# parts of the Fourier transform
for(i in 1:500){
    PS[i, ] = sqrt(Re(Fr[[i]])^2 + Im(Fr[[i]])^2)
}
plot(wseq, PS[,2], type = "l", log = "x",
    xlab = "Frequency (in radians)", ylab = "Amplitude")
#The dominant period in weeks
2 * pi/wseq[which.max(PS[, 2])]

  ## [1] 249.5
```

So the stochastic system with variability in β is predicted to oscillate with a period of around 250 weeks (just shy of 5 years) (Fig. 10.5). Thus the stochastically excited cycles have a period that is comparable but slightly longer than the resonant frequency of the deterministic system (Sect. 2.7).

Example 2: Section 8.2 discussed how to do simulation using the TSIR model with a stochastic transmission term. We can apply the transfer function theory to this model. The TSIR model is a discrete-time model, so the transfer function is $\tilde{\mathbf{T}}(\varpi) = (\tilde{\mathbf{I}} - e^{-\iota\varpi}\tilde{\mathbf{J}})^{-1}\tilde{\mathbf{A}}$. The equilibrium for the TSIR model is $S^* = \frac{B^{1-\alpha}N}{\beta}$ and $I^* = B$. Let us consider a city of a million people and a pathogen with an $R_0 (= \beta)$ of five:

```
paras = c(B = 800, beta = 5, alpha = 0.97, N = 1e+06)
eq = with(as.list(paras), c(S = B^(1 - alpha) * N/beta,
    I = B))
```

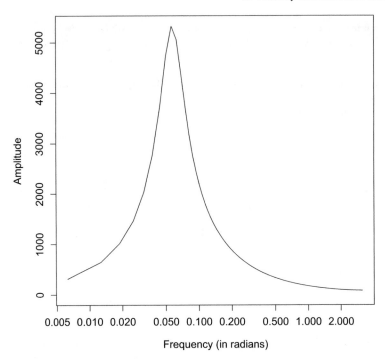

Fig. 10.5: The full power spectrum of the SIR model with stochasticity in β as predicted from the transfer functions of the linearized system

Evaluating the relevant matrices (assuming randomness in β):

```
#states
states=c("S", "I")
#equations
elist = c(Seq = quote(S-beta * S * I^alpha/N+B),
    Ieq = quote(beta * S * I^alpha/N))
#matrices
JJ = jacobian(states = states, elist = elist,
    parameters = paras, pts = eq)

a1 = D(elist$Seq, "beta")
a2 = D(elist$Ieq, "beta")
A = with(as.list(c(paras, eq)),
    matrix(c(eval(a1), eval(a2)), ncol = 1))
Id = diag(2)
```

Recalling that for discrete-time models with dominant eigenvalues being a conjugate pair of $a \pm b\iota$, the resonant period is $2\pi/\arctan(b/a)$:

```
evs = eigen(JJ)$values
2 * pi/atan2(Im(evs[1]), Re(evs[1]))
```

```
## [1] 112.9908
```

The parameterized model using the deterministic resonant period predicts an inter-epidemic period of 113 disease generations. For the full stochastic spectrum, the transfer function is

```
wseq = seq(0, pi, length = 500)
Fr = vector("list", 500)   #Set up empty list of matrices

# Loop to fill those matrices with Fourier
# transforms
for (i in 1:500) {
    # Solve gives matrix inverse
    Fr[[i]] = matrix(solve(Id - exp((0+1i) * wseq[i]) *
        JJ) %*% A, ncol = 1)
}
# Power spectrum
PS = matrix(NA, ncol = 2, nrow = 500, dimnames = list(1:500,
    c("S", "I")))
# Power spectra from real and imaginary parts
for (i in 1:500) {
    PS[i, ] = sqrt(Re(Fr[[i]])^2 + Im(Fr[[i]])^2)
}
# Peak in spectrum
2 * pi/wseq[which.max(PS[, 2])]
```

```
## [1] 110.8889
```

The peak in the power spectrum from the transfer function is around 111 genera-tions, so the resonant period is in good agreement with the broader stochastic anal-ysis.

To compare the predicted power spectrum from the transfer functions against a simulation, we can use the `tsirSim` function introduced in Chap. 8. Assuming a standard deviation in β of one and simulating for 100 years (assuming the generation time is a week), the first 20 years of the simulation is shown in Fig. 10.6. The figure suggests a transient period of a couple of years before the dynamics settles down to stochastically excited recurrent epidemics.

```
out = tsirSim(B = 800, beta = 5, sdbeta = 1, N = 1e+06,
    IT = 100 * 52, I0 = 10, S0 = 0.3)
plot(out$I[1:1040], xlab = "Biweek", ylab = "Incidence",
    type = "l")
```

The spectrum estimated from the simulation using the periodogram (discarding the first two years of data) is

```
sfit = spectrum(out$I[-c(1:104)])
```

As discussed in Sect. 7.4, the classic Schuster periodogram estimates the spec-tral density of a time series at the canonical frequencies, but with the drawback that it is not a "consistent" method. In statistics, a consistent method is one where the

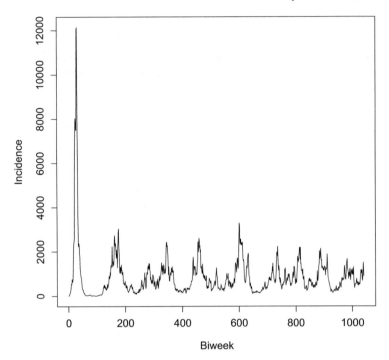

Fig. 10.6: Twenty years of simulated incidence from the TSIR model with stochasticity in transmission

estimate converges on the truth as the sample size increases. For the Schuster periodogram, the spectral density is estimated at T/2 frequencies, and thus doubling the length of the time series doubles the number of parameters, which defies consistency. Various window-smoothing approaches have been proposed to ameliorate this (see for example Priestley, 1981). An alternative to smoothing is to estimate the spectral density using Kooperberg et al.'s (1995) log-spline method with the lspec function of the polspline package. Figure 10.7 shows the empirical estimates and the transfer function predicted spectra for the TSIR model. Theory based on the linearized system provides an excellent approximation to the empirical estimates for the stochastically excited but asymptotically stable system (Fig. 10.7).[8]

```
require(polspline)
sfit2 = lspec(out$I[-c(1:104)])
plot(wseq, PS[,2], type = "l", ylab = "Amplitude",
     xlab = "Frequency (in radians)", xlim = c(0, 0.6))
lines(pi * sfit$freq/0.5,
      5000 * sfit$spec/max(sfit$spec), col = 2)
par(new = TRUE)
```

---

[8] In addition to the discussions in Chap. 6, Chap. 11 will elaborate on the many ways linearized predictions break down when strong nonlinearities govern epidemic clockworks.

```
plot(sfit2, col = 3, xlim = c(0, 0.6), axes = FALSE)
legend("topright", c("Transfer fn", "Periodogram",
    "Log-spline"), lty = c(1, 1, 1), col = c(1, 2, 3))
```

10.9 (Even More) Advanced: Transfer Functions and Delay Coordinates

While a bit esoteric with respect to the current text, the Hamilton–Caley theorem shows that any stochastic, autonomous (i.e., unforced), linear, discrete-time multi-state d-dimensional system can be rewritten as an ARMA (Sect. 7.3) delay-coordinate system. The significance of this jargon is that any linear(ized) vector system of the form

$$\mathbf{X}_t = \mathbf{J}\mathbf{X}_{t-1} + \mathbf{A}\varepsilon_t, \tag{10.12}$$

where ε_t is a stochastic term and other notations, as above, can be rewritten in an equivalent delay form:

$$x_t = c + \underbrace{b_1 x_{t-1} + b_2 x_{t-2} + \ldots + b_d x_{t-d}}_{\text{autoregressive}} + \varepsilon_t + \underbrace{a_1 \varepsilon_{t-1} + \ldots + \alpha_q \varepsilon_{t-q}}_{\text{moving average}}. \tag{10.13}$$

This is useful for understanding how dynamics can induce delayed feedbacks and how the echo of stochastic perturbations propagates through time. It also provides an alternative route for analyzing systems for which only a subset of variables (e.g., one) has been measured. The theorem says it can always be done, but in practice it can be tedious because of the equivalence between finite AR processes and infinite MA processes and vice versa. It turns out that transfer functions (Sect. 10.8) are very helpful for such calculations (Priestley, 1981; Bjørnstad et al., 2004). In its general analytic form, the discrete-time transfer function takes the rational form:

$$T(\varpi) \propto \frac{1 + a_1 e^{-\iota\varpi} + \ldots + a_q e^{-q\iota\varpi}}{1 - b_1 e^{-\iota\varpi} - \ldots b_p e^{-p\iota\varpi}}, \tag{10.14}$$

where the a's and b's correspond exactly to the coefficients of the ARMA(p, q) delay-coordinate representation of the system. R does unfortunately not (yet?) have enough symbolic power to solve the transfer function analytically. However, a program such as Mathematica will show that the transfer functions for the I compartment of the linearized stochastic TSIR are

$$T_I(\varpi) = \frac{B}{1+\beta} \frac{1 + (B^\alpha(\beta-1)-1)e^{-\iota\varpi}}{1 - (1+\alpha-\beta B^\alpha\beta)e^{-\iota\varpi} + \alpha e^{-2\iota\varpi}}, \tag{10.15}$$

where B, α, and β are as defined for the TSIR model (Eqs. (8.1) and (8.2)). Theoretically, therefore, the model predicts an ARMA(2,1) delay-coordinate structure to the time series of incidence according to

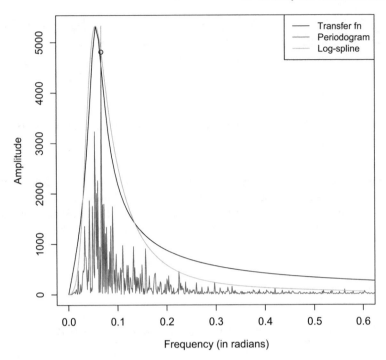

Fig. 10.7: The spectrum of the TSIR model with stochasticity in β as predicted from the transfer functions of the linearized system with the periodogram and log-spline density estimate from a simulation (Fig. 10.6) superimposed

$$I_{t+1} = \text{const} + (1 + \alpha - \beta B^\alpha \beta)I_t - \alpha I_{t-1} + \varepsilon_t + (B^\alpha(\beta - 1) - 1)\varepsilon_{t-1}, \quad (10.16)$$

thus lending some mechanistic underpinning to the analysis in Sect. 7.3.

Bjørnstad et al. (2001) used this so-called state-space/delay-coordinate equivalence to study how viruses and parasitoids structurally alter the pattern of delayed density-dependent feedbacks in the population dynamics of their insect host. Bjørnstad et al. (2004) provide some additional worked examples of using transfer functions to study population dynamics.

10.10 SEIRS and TSIR shinyApps

The `seirs.app` calculates the resonant periodicity for the SEIRS model, which is a slight elaboration of the model in Sect. 10.5. The `tsir.app` from Chap. 8 also calculates the power spectrum predicted from the transfer function for the TSIR model to ground-truth it with simulated data. To run:

```
require(epimdr2)
runApp(seirs.app)
runApp(tsir.app)
```

Bjørnstad et al. (2020b) provide an additional shinyApp to investigate the SEIRS
model that can be directly accessed from https://shiny.bcgsc.ca/posepi2/.

Chapter 11
Exotica

11.1 Too Nonlinear

Chapter 10 discussed how a linear approximation to the perennially nonlinear dynamics of infectious disease can provide important insights on invasion, stability, and resonant periodicity. As remarked by Nisbet and Gurney (1982) more generally, linear approximation can often provide remarkably useful insights for nonlinear ecological systems as long as they are not too nonlinear.

From a dynamical system's point of view, dynamics are considered (approximately) linear if the system does not "miss-behave" as it approaches (diverges) from its stable (unstable) fix-points. Thus, while the simple SIR model is mathematically speaking nonlinear (because of the $\beta SI/N$ term), its dynamics can be thought of as being "linear" because of its smooth inward spiraling toward the endemic equilibrium (the stable focus) and logistic divergence from the disease free equilibrium (the unstable node) when $R_0 > 1$. However, highly infectious immunizing diseases have the potential for exhibiting dynamics so nonlinear that crazy things can happen, things that require a different set of tools. The multiannual and chaotic fluctuations seen in the seasonally forced SEIR model and measles in the prevaccination USA (Sect. 6.4) are some such highly nonlinear phenomena. There are however other dynamic exotica that can arise when stochasticity and nonlinearity interacts, or when there are great perturbations (such as introduction of mass vaccination) to the nonlinear epidemic clockworks. The following sections explore this and discuss some useful tools.

This chapter uses the following R packages: deSolve, pomp and nlts.

O. N. Bjørnstad, *Epidemics*, Use R!, https://doi.org/10.1007/978-3-031-12056-5_11

11.2 Chaos

In nonlinear systems, a perturbation will either dissipate or expand as it interacts with the dynamic clockwork. The hallmark of a chaotic attractor is "sensitive dependence on initial conditions":[1] Two very nearby trajectories will diverge exponentially over time. The standard way to quantify this is through the dominant Lyapunov exponent

$$L_E = \lim_{T \to \infty} \frac{1}{T} \log(\prod_t^T \mathbf{J}_t \mathbf{U}_0), \qquad (11.1)$$

where $\mathbf{J}_t$ is the Jacobian matrix evaluated on the point of the attractor at time t, and for a 2D system (like the TSIR), $\mathbf{U}_0$ is the length two unit vector $\{1,0\}$. A chaotic attractor has $L_E > 0$. As an example, the Jacobian of the TSIR model is

$$\mathbf{J}_t = \begin{bmatrix} 1 - \beta_s I_t^\alpha/N & -\beta_s S_t(I_t^{\alpha-1}\alpha)/N \\ \beta_s I_t^\alpha/N & \beta_s S_t(I_t^{\alpha-1}\alpha)/N \end{bmatrix}. \qquad (11.2)$$

We can estimate the Lyapunov exponent numerically by simulating the TSIR a long time (Grenfell et al., 2002). As an example, consider the measles dynamics as estimated from the New York time series between 1920 and 1941 (Fig. 11.1) (Dalziel et al., 2016). We first fit the parameters using the protocol discussed in Chap. 8; the profile likelihood on $\overline{S}$ suggests a mean fraction of susceptibles of 0.051. We follow the estimation protocol of Chap. 8.

The first step is the susceptible reconstruction and correcting for underreporting:

```
data(dalziel)
NY = na.omit(dalziel[dalziel$loc == "NEW YORK", ])
NY = NY[NY$year %in% c(1920:1940), ]
plot(NY$decimalYear, sqrt(NY$cases), type = "b", xlab = "Year",
     ylab = "Sqrt(cases)")
# Susceptible reconstruction and correcting for
# underreporting
cum.reg = smooth.spline(cumsum(NY$rec), cumsum(NY$cases),
     df = 5)
D = -resid(cum.reg)   #The residuals
rr = predict(cum.reg, deriv = 1)$y
Ic = NY$cases/rr
Dc = D/rr
```

The second step is estimating the key parameters:

```
# Align lagged variables
seas = rep(1:26, 21)[1:545]
lInew = log(Ic[2:546])
lIold = log(Ic[1:545])
```

---

[1] Interestingly, Ruelle (1993) paraphrases Henri Poincaré as defining *chance* as sensitive dependence on *unknown* initial conditions as far back as 1908.

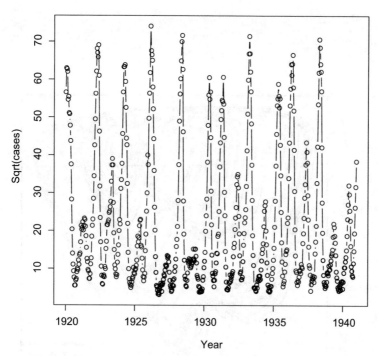

Fig. 11.1: Measles in New York city

```
Dold = Dc[1:545]
# TSIR fit
N = NY$pop
offsetN = -log(N[1:545])
lSold = log(0.051 * N[1:545] + Dold)
glmfit = glm(lInew ~ -1 + as.factor(seas) + lIold +offset(lSold +
    offsetN))
```

The tsirSim2 function from Chap. 8 allows simulation of a deterministic trajectory from the fitted model. The result is a highly erratic trajectory in the phase plane (Fig. 11.2).

```
sim2 = tsirSim2(beta = exp(glmfit$coef[1:26]), alpha = 0.98,
    B = rep(median(NY$rec), 5200), N = median(N),
    inits = list(Snull = exp(lSold[1]), Inull = Ic[1]),
    type = "det")
Sattr = sim2$S[2601:5200]
Iattr = sim2$I[2601:5200]
plot(Sattr, Iattr, log = "y", type = "l",
    xlab = "S", ylab = "I")
points(sim2$S[seq(2601, 5200, by = 26)],
```

```
sim2$I[seq(2601, 5200, by = 26)],pch = 19, col = "red")
legend("bottomright", c("Trajectory", "Strobe"),
pch = c(NA, 19), lty = c(1, NA) , col = c("black", "red"))
```

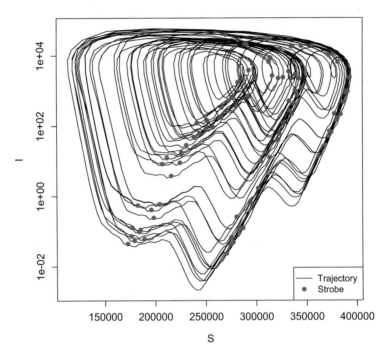

Fig. 11.2: The deterministic trajectory of the New York measles TSIR model. The black line represents the full trajectory. The red dots are the annual stroboscopic section

Calculating the Lyapunov exponent is a bit involved, so the best is to write a function to do it. Because we will be wanting to study the attractor in greater detail, we make the function both calculate the Lyapunov exponent and store all the Jacobian elements evaluated along the attractor.

```
tsirLyap = function(I, S, alpha, bt, N) {
    IT = length(I)
    s = length(bt)
    j11 = rep(NA, IT)
    j12 = rep(NA, IT)
    j21 = rep(NA, IT)
    j22 = rep(NA, IT)
    # initial unit vector
    J = matrix(c(1, 0), ncol = 1)
    # loop over the attractor
    for (i in 1:IT) {
```

```
        j11[i] = 1 - bt[((i - 1)%%s) + 1] * I[i]^alpha/N
        j12[i] = -(bt[((i - 1)%%s) + 1] * S[i] * (I[i]^(alpha -
            1) * alpha)/N)
        j21[i] = bt[((i - 1)%%s) + 1] * I[i]^alpha/N
        j22[i] = bt[((i - 1)%%s) + 1] * S[i] * (I[i]^(alpha -
            1) * alpha)/N

        J = matrix(c(j11[i], j12[i], j21[i], j22[i]),
            ncol = 2, byrow = TRUE) %*% J
    }
    res = list(lyap = log(norm(J))/IT, j11 = j11, j12 = j12,
        j21 = j21, j22 = j22, I = I, S = S, alpha = alpha,
        bt = bt, N = N)
    class(res) = "lyap"
    return(res)
}
```

The function applied to the last 100 years of the simulated dynamics is

```
nylyap = tsirLyap(I = Iattr, S = Sattr, alpha = 0.98,
    bt = exp(glmfit$coef[1:26]), N = median(N))
nylyap$lyap
```

```
  ## [1] 0.0134336
```

The exponent is positive indicating that the deterministic skeleton of the TSIR model for measles in New York is a chaotic attractor as concluded by Dalziel et al. (2016). This contrasts with the negative Lyapunov exponent of measles in London testifying to the stability of its biennial limit cycle (see below).

11.3 Local Lyapunov Exponents

Bailey et al. (1997) suggested that it is useful to study the *local* Lyapunov exponents to understand short-term predictability, and also how noise and nonlinearity will interact in epidemic systems. The idea is that regardless of whether dynamics is asymptotically stable, cyclic or chaotic, there is likely to be regions in the phase plane of expansion in which stochastic divergence will be amplified and regions of contraction where perturbations will be dampened. Grenfell et al. (2002) used local Lyapunov exponents to understand the remarkable predictability of prevaccination measles in London. Local Lyapunov exponents are similar in nature to the global exponent, except that rather than evaluating a product of Jacobians across the attractor, the Jacobians are evaluated locally. Armed with an object produced with the tsirLyap function, it is easy to write a second function to calculate local exponents across m-steps along the attractor (or anywhere else in the phase plane, such as along a "repellor"; see Sect. 11.5). Since the TSIR is a discrete-time model, contraction occurs if the largest eigenvalue of the Jacobian matrix is inside the unit circle—thus $\log(|\lambda|) < 0$ is the cut-off between contraction and expansion. The `tsirLlyap` function calculates the local Lyapunov exponents for outputs from the `tsirLyap` function. The parameter m controls the number of iterations along the attractor on which to calculate the product (Bailey et al., 1997).

```
tsirLlyap = function(x, m = 1) {
    llyap = rep(NA, length(x$I))
    for (i in 1:(length(x$I) - m)) {
        J = matrix(c(1, 0, 0, 1), ncol = 2)
        for (k in 0:(m - 1)) {
            J = matrix(c(x$j11[(i + k)], x$j12[(i + k)],
                x$j21[(i + k)], x$j22[(i + k)]), ncol = 2,
                byrow = TRUE) %*% J
        }
        llyap[i] = log(max(abs(eigen(J)$values)))/m
    }
    res = list(llyap = llyap, I = x$I, S = x$S)
    class(res) = "llyap"
    return(res)
}
```

For ease of use, we can also write a function to visualize the local exponents:[2]

```
plot.llyap = function(x, inches = .5){
    pm = x$llyap > 0
    plot(NA, xlim = range(x$S), ylim = range(x$I), xlab = "S",
        ylab = "I", log = "y")
    symbols(x$S[pm], x$I[pm], circles = x$llyap[pm],
        inches = inches, add = TRUE)
    symbols(x$S[!pm], x$I[!pm], squares = -x$llyap[!pm],
        inches = inches, add = TRUE, bg = 2)
}
```

We can study the measles NY attractor using the local Lyapunov exponents. Despite the overall attractor being chaotic, there are distinct areas of contraction associated with the collapse of epidemics and post-epidemic troughs in the phase plane (Fig. 11.3).

```
nyllyap = tsirLlyap(nyllyap, m = 5)
plot(nyllyap, inches = 0.15)
```

Section 8.3 provided TSIR transmission estimates for prevaccination measles in London and highlighted the limit-cycle nature of the dynamics. Biweekly transmission estimates were

```
beta = c(27.71, 43.14, 37.81, 33.69, 31.64, 32.1, 30.16,
    24.68, 30.19, 31.53, 30.31, 26.02, 26.57, 25.68, 23.21,
    19.21, 17.5, 20.5, 29.92, 35.85, 32.65, 28.34, 31.11,
    29.89, 26.89, 39.38)
```

---

[2] The formalism of S3 class programming will be discussed in a bit more detail in Sect. 14.2.

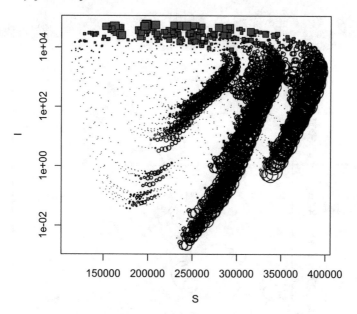

Fig. 11.3: Local Lyapunov exponents across the New York city measles attractor. Positive exponents are shown as open circles, and negative exponents as red squares

The median biweekly birth rate for London was 2083 during this time period, so the tsirSim2 function can trace out the attractor and calculate associated global and local Lyapunov exponents.

```
sim = tsirSim2(beta = beta, alpha = 0.98, B = rep(2083,
    5200), N = 3300000, inits = list(Snull = 133894, Inull = 474))
Sattr = sim$S[5149:5200]
Iattr = sim$I[5149:5200]
lonlyap = tsirLyap(I = Iattr, S = Sattr, alpha = 0.98,
    bt = beta, N = 3300000)
lonlyap$lyap

  ## [1] -0.004289374

lonllyap = tsirLlyap(lonlyap, m = 1)
```

The dominant Lyapunov exponent is negative testifying to the stability of the limit cycles. We can look in greater detail across the biennial attractor (Fig. 11.4). Interestingly, there is potential for significant divergence during the growth phase of the minor and major epidemics; however, the post-epidemic convergence is apparently strong enough to overcome this to result in a strongly dissipative cyclic attractor (Grenfell et al., 2002; Dalziel et al., 2016).

```
pm = (lonllyap$llyap > 0)
plot(NA, xlim = c(1, 52), ylim = range(Iattr), xlab = "Biweek",
    ylab = "I", log = "y")
symbols((1:52)[pm], Iattr[pm], circles = lonllyap$llyap[pm],
    inches = 0.3, add = TRUE)
```

```
symbols((1:52)[!pm], Iattr[!pm], squares = -lonllyap$llyap[!pm],
    inches = 0.3, add = TRUE, bg = 2)
```

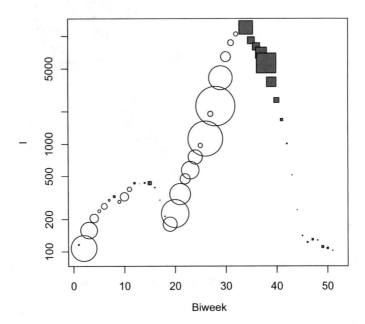

Fig. 11.4: Local Lyapunov exponents across the biennial London measles attractor. Positive exponents are shown as open circles, and negative exponents as red squares

To visualize the notion of dissipation more clearly, we can plot the long-term deterministic attractor with 20 stochastic simulation (assuming demographic stochasticity only) (Fig. 11.5). The simulations show that despite abundant variability—particularly during the minor epidemics—the trajectories exhibit long-term predictability, except for the rare stochastic trajectory that escapes onto the opposite-year coexisting attractor toward the end of the simulations. As an exemplar, Grenfell et al. (2001) show how the area around Norwich locked on to the opposite-year coexisting attractor compared to the rest of England and Wales for about 15 years following World War II before locking into step.

```
sim = tsirSim2(beta = beta, alpha = 0.98, B = rep(2083,
    520), N = 3300000, inits = list(Snull = 133894, Inull = 474),
    type = "det")
plot(sqrt(sim$I), ylab = "Sqrt(Cases)", xlab = "Biweek")
for (i in 1:20) {
    sim = tsirSim2(beta = beta, alpha = 0.98, B = rep(2083,
        520), N = 3300000, inits = list(Snull = 133894,
        Inull = 474), type = "stoc")
    lines(sqrt(sim$I))
}
sim = tsirSim2(beta = beta, alpha = 0.98, B = rep(2083,
    520), N = 3300000, inits = list(Snull = 133894, Inull = 474),
```

```
    type = "det")
points(sqrt(sim$I), col = 2)
```

During the first biweek of 1940, 23 cases of measles were reported in New York city. Given our estimate of the reporting rate of 22.54% in that biweek, a best guess of the incidence is 102; correspondingly, the best guess of the number of suscepti-bles is 402,153. To visualize the "sensitive dependence on initial conditions" of the chaotic New York measles attractor, we can forward simulate 10 years of dynamics, assuming there were either 5 more or fewer infecteds (and conversely susceptibles) during that biweek. The rapid deterministic divergence (Fig. 11.6) is a stark contrast to the long-term predictability of the London attractor (Fig. 11.5).

```
sim2 = tsirSim2(beta = exp(glmfit$coef[1:26]), alpha = 0.98,
    B = rep(median(NY$rec), 260), N = median(N),
    inits = list(Snull = 402153, Inull = 102))
sim3 = tsirSim2(beta = exp(glmfit$coef[1:26]), alpha = 0.98,
    B = rep(median(NY$rec), 260), N = median(N),
    inits = list(Snull = 402153-5, Inull = 102+5))
sim4 = tsirSim2(beta = exp(glmfit$coef[1:26]), alpha = 0.98,
    B = rep(median(NY$rec), 260), N = median(N),
    inits = list(Snull = 402153+5, Inull = 102-5))
plot(sim2$I[1:260], type = "l", ylab = "I",
    xlab = "Biweek (from 1940)")
lines(sim3$I[1:260], col = 2)
lines(sim4$I[1:260], col = 3)
```

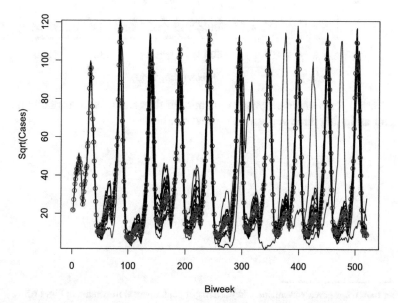

Fig. 11.5: Twenty years of deterministic dynamics (red circles) with 20 stochastic simulations of the biennial London measles attractor

11.4 Coexisting Attractors

Another nonlinear complication is how seasonally forced epidemic systems can exhibit coexisting attractors[3] as, for example, seen in the seasonally forced SEIR model (Sect. 6.6). Stochastic perturbation can push dynamics between different basins of attraction leading to erratic dynamics not predicted by basic theory.

One of the many puzzles about whooping cough dynamics is the apparent contradiction between historical herd immunity and historical multiannual epidemics versus current circulation in adults.[4] To reconcile these seemingly mutually exclusive facets of whooping cough epidemiology, Lavine et al. (2011) proposed an anamnestic hypothesis that immunity to whooping cough may wane over time, but re-exposure can boost immune memory. This premise leads to the following SIRWS

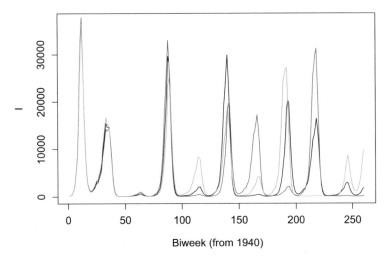

Fig. 11.6: 10 years of deterministic dynamics of the chaotic New York city measles attractor assuming three very similar initial conditions

---

[3] Other than the relatively mundane odd/even major peak reversal illustrated in Fig. 11.5.

[4] Modeling chickenpox, a herpes virus that can reactivate in older individuals in the form of zoster, Ferguson et al. (1996) showed that the SEIR model cannot sustain multiannual (or chaotic) childhood dynamics in the presence of "immigration" of the virus from an adult carrier group.

compartmental model in which W is a waning class that is under the influence of two competing processes: return to the S class at a rate of 2ω or boost back to the R class at a rate proportional to the force of infection ($\beta I/N$):

$$\frac{dS}{dt} = \underbrace{\mu(1-p)N}_{\text{recruitment}} - \underbrace{\beta IS/N}_{\text{infection}} - \underbrace{\mu S}_{\text{death}} + \underbrace{2\omega W}_{\text{wane in}} \tag{11.3}$$

$$\frac{dI}{dt} = \underbrace{\beta IS/N}_{\text{infection}} - \underbrace{\gamma I}_{\text{recovery}} - \underbrace{\mu I}_{\text{death}} \tag{11.4}$$

$$\frac{dR}{dt} = \underbrace{\gamma I}_{\text{recovery}} - \underbrace{2\omega R}_{\text{waning}} + \underbrace{\kappa\beta SW/N}_{\text{boosting}} + \underbrace{\mu pN}_{\text{vaccination}} - \underbrace{\mu R}_{\text{death}} \tag{11.5}$$

$$\frac{dW}{dt} = \underbrace{2\omega R}_{\text{waning}} - \underbrace{\kappa\beta SW/N}_{\text{boosting}} - \underbrace{2\omega W}_{\text{waning}} \tag{11.6}$$

In the absence of boosting, immunity will last for an average of $1/\omega$ year (and distributed according to a Gamma distribution with a shape parameter of two because it takes two transitions to move from R back to S; see Sect. 2.9). The parameter κ scales how sensitive boosting is relative to infection, and p is the fraction of children vaccinated at birth thus moving straight to R and thus discounting susceptible recruitment from births. A surprising finding is that, even in the absence of seasonality, parts of the parameter space harbor a limit cycle coexisting with a fix-point attractor. We can use the forward and backward bifurcation algorithm introduced in Sect. 6.6 to look at this. We first define the gradients (using the log-trick):

```
sirwmod = function(t, logy, parameters) {
    y = exp(logy)
    S = y[1]
    I = y[2]
    R = y[3]
    W = y[4]
    with(as.list(parameters), {
        dS = mu * (1 - p) * N - mu * S - beta * S * I/N +
            2 * omega * W
        dI = beta * S * I/N - (mu + gamma) * I
        dR = gamma * I - mu * R - 2 * omega * R + kappa *
            beta * W * I/N + mu * p * N
        dW = 2 * omega * R - kappa * beta * W * I/N -
            (2 * omega + mu) * W
        res = c(dS/S, dI/I, dR/R, dW/W)
        list(res)
    })
}
```

Assuming susceptible recruitment is reduced by vaccination, we can bifurcate on the p parameter (Fig. 11.7). The forward/backward bifurcation analysis reveals the coexistence of the fix-point and cyclic attractors when vaccination is in the 20–40% range.

```
require(deSolve)
start = log(c(S = 0.06, I = 0.01, R = 0.92, W = 0.01))
res = matrix(NA, ncol = 100, nrow = 5000)
p = seq(0.01, 1, length = 100)
# Forwards
for (i in 1:100) {
    times = seq(0, 200, by = 0.01)
    paras = c(mu = 1/70, p = p[i], N = 1, beta = 200,
        omega = 1/10, gamma = 17, kappa = 30)
    out = as.data.frame(ode(start, times, sirwmod, paras))
    start = c(S = out[20001, 2], I = out[20001, 3], R = out[20001,
        4], W = out[20001, 5])
    res[, i] = out$I[15002:20001]
    cat(i, "\r")
}
# Backwards
res2 = matrix(NA, ncol = 100, nrow = 5000)
start = c(S = -1.8, I = -5.8, R = 1.9, W = -1.9)
for (i in 100:1) {
    paras = c(mu = 1/70, p = p[i], N = 1, beta = 200,
        omega = 1/10, gamma = 17, kappa = 30)
    out = as.data.frame(ode(start, times, sirwmod, paras))
    start = c(S = out[20001, 2], I = out[20001, 3], R = out[20001,
        4], W = out[20001, 5])
    res2[, i] = out$I[15002:20001]
    cat(i, "\r")
}
plot(NA, xlim = range(p), ylim = range(res), ylab = "Log(I)",
    xlab = "p")
for (i in 1:100) points(rep(p[i], 2), range(res[, i]))
for (i in 1:100) points(rep(p[i], 2), range(res2[, i]),
    col = 2)
```

Figure 11.8 shows trajectories toward the two attractors assuming 20% vaccination but with different initial conditions. For the given parameters, the limit cycle is stable and has a period of 1.8 years, and the fix-point attractor is a stable focus with a damping period of 1.2 years. Using a seasonally forced version of the SIRWS model, Lavine et al. (2013) explored the hypothesis that the regime shifts in prevaccination whooping cough dynamics in Copenhagen (Fig. 11.12) were due to stochastic switching between a low-amplitude noisy annual attractor and a high-amplitude multiannual attractor. In the end, the best evidence suggests that the major recurrent outbreaks between 1915 and 1925 were instead a fly-by of an unstable multiannual "almost attractor" (Lavine et al., 2013, see Sects. 11.5 and 11.7).

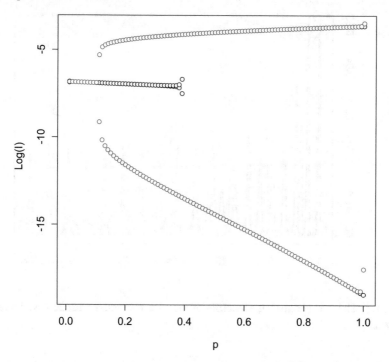

Fig. 11.7: The forward (black) and backward (red) bifurcation diagrams of the SIRWS model across the range of vaccination rates

```
paras = c(mu = 1/70, p = 0.2, N = 1, beta = 200, omega = 1/10,
    gamma = 17, kappa = 30)
start = c(S = -1, I = -5, R = 3.3, W = 0)
times = seq(0, 30, by = 1/52)
out = as.data.frame(ode(start, times, sirwmod, paras))
plot(out$time, exp(out$I), xlab = "Year", ylab = "I",
    type = "l", ylim = c(0, 0.05))
start = c(S = -1.8, I = -5.8, R = 1.9, W = -1.9)
times = seq(0, 30, by = 1/52)
out = as.data.frame(ode(start, times, sirwmod, paras))
lines(out$time, exp(out$I), col = 2)
```

11.5 Repellors/Almost Attractors

Rand and Wilson (1991) studied a seasonally forced SEIR model (Sect. 6.3) of chickenpox (assuming that shedding from zoster can be ignored). They assumed a latent period and infectious period of around 10 days and sinusoidally forced trans-

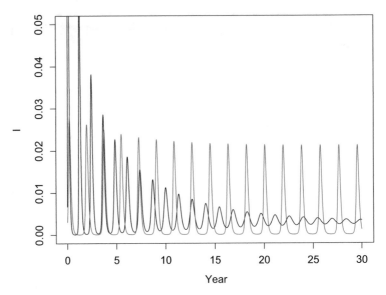

Fig. 11.8: The two coexisting attractors of the SIRWS model with 20% vaccination at birth

mission with a β_0 of 537/year, a β_1 of 0.3, and a birth rate of 0.02. In the absence of seasonality , we can use the Jacobian calculator from Sect. 6.8 to calculate the resonant period:

STEP 1 define state variables:

```
states = c("S", "E", "I", "R")
```

STEP 2 list of equations:

```
elist2 = c(dS = expression(mu * (N - S) - beta0 * S *
    I/N), dE = expression(beta0 * S * I/N - (mu + sigma) *
    E), dI = expression(sigma * E - (mu + gamma) * I),
    dR = quote(gamma * I - mu * R))
```

STEP 3 define parameter values:

```
cparas = c(mu = 0.02, N = 1, beta0 = 537, beta1 = 0.3,
    sigma = 36, gamma = 34.3)
```

STEP 4 evaluate endemic equilibrium:

```
R0 = with(as.list(cparas), sigma/(sigma + mu) * 1/(gamma +
    mu) * beta0)
Sstar = 1/R0
Istar = with(as.list(cparas), mu * (1 - 1/R0) * R0/beta0)
Estar = with(as.list(cparas), (mu + gamma) * Istar/sigma)
Rstar = cparas["N"] - (Sstar + Estar + Istar)
eq = list(S = Sstar, E = Estar, I = Istar, R = Rstar)
```

STEP 5 invoke calculator:

```
JJ = jacobian(states = states, elist = elist2,
    parameters = cparas, pts = eq)
round(eigen(JJ)$value, 2)

  ## [1] -70.41+0.00i   -0.12+2.26i   -0.12-2.26i   -0.02+0.00i

2 * pi/Im(eigen(JJ)$value[2])

  ## [1] 2.775299
```

So the damping period is 2.8 years. The seasonally forced differential equations, in contrast, predict robust annual epidemics (Fig. 11.9).

```
times = seq(0, 100, by = 1/120)
start = c(S = 0.06, E = 0, I = 0.001, R = 0.939)
cparas = c(mu = 0.02, N = 1, beta0 = 537, beta1 = 0.3,
    sigma = 36, gamma = 34.3)
out = as.data.frame(ode(start, times, seirmod2, cparas))
plot(out$time, out$I, type = "l", xlab = "Year", ylab =
    "Prevalence", xlim = c(91, 100), ylim = c(0, 0.0015))
```

The conundrum highlighted by Rand and Wilson (1991) is that stochastic simulations of the model (see Sect. 11.9 for coding details) exhibit dynamics with conspicuous regime shifts; periods with the expected somewhat variable annual outbreaks are interspersed with periods of violent multiannual cycles with a period of around 4 years (Fig. 11.10) that is seemingly completely unrelated to the above calculated resonant period of the SEIR model. This thus appears to be a dynamical phenomenon different to what we have studied previously.

For the stochastic simulations, we build a pomp object using Csnippet (King et al., 2015b). The Csnippet coding is a bit involved but is detailed in the chapter appendix (Sect. 11.9), but the final code for the stochastic simulation is

```
seirp = simulate(
    t0 = 0, times = seq(0, 500, by = 1/52),
    rprocess = euler(Csnippet(rproc), delta.t = 1/52/20),
    skeleton = vectorfield(Csnippet(skel)),
    rmeasure = Csnippet(robs),
    dmeasure = Csnippet(dobs),
    rinit = Csnippet(rinit),
    params = c(
```

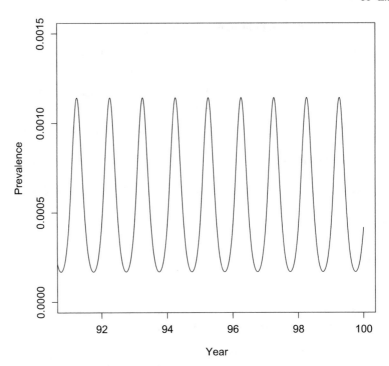

Fig. 11.9: Ten years of simulation of the forced SEIR model parameterized according to Rand and Wilson's (1991) chickenpox model predicts robust annual epidemics

```
        iota = 0, beta0 = 537, beta1 = 0.3, sigma = 36,
        gamma = 34.3, alpha = 0.015, rho = 0.6, theta = 1,
        b = 0.02, mu = 0.02, pop0 = 5e8,
        S0 = 0.06, E0 = 0, I0 = 0.001, R0 = 0.939
    ),
    paramnames = c("iota", "beta0", "beta1", "gamma",
        "sigma", "alpha", "rho", "theta", "b", "mu", "pop0",
        "S0", "E0", "I0", "R0"),
    statenames = c("S", "E", "I", "R", "inc", "pop"),
    obsnames = "reports",
    accumvars = "inc"
)
```

Simulated deterministic and stochastic trajectories are shown in Figs. 11.9 and 11.10.

```
detsim = trajectory(seirp, format = "data.frame")
plot(detsim$time, detsim$I/5e+08, type = "l", xlim = c(101,
    110), xlab = "year", ylab = "prevalence")
```

The annual stroboscopic section of the deterministic and stochastic simulation is shown in Fig. 11.10b.

```
par(mfrow = c(1, 2))
stocsim = as.data.frame(simulate(seirp, seed = 3495135,
    nsim = 1))
plot(stocsim$time, stocsim$I/5e+08, type = "l", xlim = c(150,
    250), xlab = "Year", ylab = "Prevalence")
sel = seq(105, length(stocsim$I), by = 52)
plot(stocsim$S[sel]/5e+08, stocsim$I[sel]/5e+08, log = "xy",
    xlab = "S", ylab = "I")
sel2 = sel[401:500]
points(detsim$S[sel2]/5e+08, detsim$I[sel2]/5e+08, col = 2,
    pch = 21, bg = 2)
```

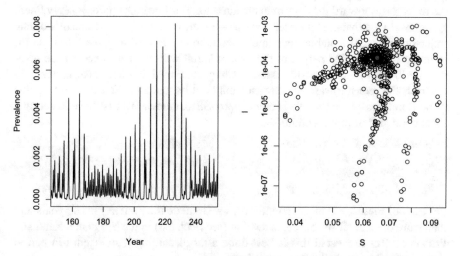

Fig. 11.10: (**a**) Hundred years of stochastic simulation of the forced SEIR model parameterized according to Rand and Wilson's (1991) chickenpox parameters assuming stochasticity in transmission. (**b**) Annual stroboscopic section of the stochastic simulation in the S–I phase plane

Rand and Wilson (1991) studied the apparent similarity of the stochastic trajectory in the S–I phase plane (Fig. 11.10) to the quasi-periodic chaotic attractor of the parametrically nearby model of Sect. 6.4 and Fig. 6.5. They stipulated that the stochastic dynamics of the deterministically annual system is intermittently governed by the weakly unstable ghost of the nearby 4-year quasi-periodic chaotic attractor which they termed a repellor, and Eckmann and Ruelle (1985) had previously dubbed an "almost attractor." To study this further, we turn to the notion of invasion orbits.

11.6 Invasion Orbits

Studying highly nonlinear, stochastic dynamical systems is complicated by the in-
termingling of two different sources of dynamic variability: the variability due to
deterministic instability and the variability due to stochastic forcing (Bjørnstad &
Grenfell, 2001). In order to elucidate this complexity, we may think of the stochastic forcing as a perturbation to the nonlinear system whose laws subsequently will
attempt to return the system to the deterministic attractor. In Sect. 6.3, we discussed
how to study the long-term asymptotic behavior of the seasonally forced SEIR system through numeric integration from arbitrary initial conditions and discarding
the initial transient dynamics to provide a bifurcation analysis. Invasion orbits are
the flip-side of this (Rand & Wilson, 1991); systematically distribute initial conditions across the phase plane and numerically integrate the transients to describe
the trajectories toward the deterministic attractor. For linear or approximately linear
systems—in the dynamical systems sense—the invasion orbits will trace monotonic
trajectories toward a stable node and smooth spirals toward a stable focus (as for
example Fig. 2.5). The period of the inward spiral will be determined by the resonant period of the focus as discussed in Chap. 10. For highly nonlinear systems, in
contrast, the return toward the attractor may not be smooth. We can illustrate this
using Rand and Wilson's (1991) chickenpox SEIR model. We first have to set up a
systematic grid of initial conditions:

```
starts = expand.grid(S = seq(0.02, 0.1, length = 10),
    E = seq(1e-08, 0.0125, length = 10), I = seq(1e-08,
        0.005, length = 10))
starts$R = 1 - apply(starts, 1, sum)
```

For each of these 1000 initial conditions, we simulate the system for 100 years and
then store the annual stroboscopic section (see Sect. 6.5) in the S–I plane. Rand and
Wilson (1991) suggested this is best done after discarding a short burn-in period
(here 5 years) to study the invasion orbits.

```
#times for integration
itimes  = seq(0, 100, by = 1/52)
#points for stroboscopic section
isel = seq(1, length(itimes), by = 52)
#list to fill with results
cporbs = list(S = matrix(NA, ncol = dim(starts)[1],
    nrow = length(isel)), I = matrix(NA,
    ncol = dim(starts)[1], nrow = length(isel)))
```

Next integrate to obtain the 1000 invasion orbits:

```
for (i in 1:dim(starts)[1]) {
    out2b = as.data.frame(ode(as.numeric(starts[i, ]),
        itimes, seirmod2, cparas))
    cporbs$S[, i] = out2b[, 2][isel]
    cporbs$I[, i] = out2b[, 4][isel]
}
```

Finally, the plot of the stroboscopic section of the invasion orbits in the S–I phase
plane with the deterministic attractor superimposed (Fig. 11.11) reveals that the

stochastic simulation is largely governed by the unstable highly nonlinear structure in the phase plane dubbed variously a "repellor," a "chaotic saddle," or an "unstable manifold." Eckmann and Ruelle (1985) first referred to this as an "almost attractor."

```r
# Invasion orbits
plot(as.vector(cporbs$S[-c(1:5), ]), as.vector(cporbs$I[-c(1:5),
    ]), pch = 20, cex = 0.25, log = "xy", ylab = "I",
    xlab = "S")
# Stochastic simulation
sel = seq(105, length(stocsim$I), by = 52)
points(stocsim$S[sel]/5e+08, stocsim$I[sel]/5e+08, col = 2)
# Deterministic attractor
times = seq(0, 1000, by = 1/120)
start = c(S = 0.06, E = 0, I = 0.001, R = 0.939)
out = as.data.frame(ode(start, times, seirmod2, cparas))
sel = seq(120 * 100, length(times), by = 120)
points(out$S[sel], out$I[sel], pch = 21, col = "white",
    bg = "white")
```

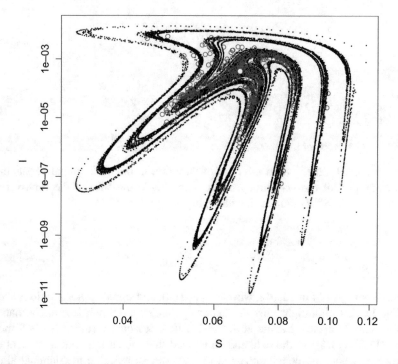

Fig. 11.11: The stroboscopic section of the invasion orbits of the forced SEIR model traces out the ghost of a chaotic attractor that has lost stability in the region of parameter space that (Rand & Wilson, 1991) used for their chickenpox model. The white central circle is the annual deterministic attractor, and the red open circles are annual strobes from a stochastic simulation

Rohani et al. (2002) discussed how the multiannual cycles in whooping cough following vaccination may be explained as the dynamics chasing a periodic almost attractor akin to Lavine et al.'s (2013) conclusion regarding pertussis regime shifts in prevaccination Copenhagen.

11.7 Stochastic Resonance

Whooping cough in prevaccination Copenhagen generally exhibited low-amplitude fuzzy annual epidemics, with the exception of a 10-year period of violent triannual epidemics starting around 1915 (Fig. 11.12). We can use a wavelet analysis with the crazy climber ridge finding algorithm (Sect. 7.5) to characterize the transitions in dynamics (Lavine et al., 2013).

```
data(pertcop)
require(Rwave)
# Wavelet decompostion
no = 8
nv = 16
a = 2^seq(1, no + 1 - 1/nv, by = 1/nv)
wfit = cwt(sqrt(pertcop$cases), no, nv, plot = FALSE)
wspec = Mod(wfit)
# Crazy climber
crcinc <- crc(wspec, nbclimb = 10, bstep = 100)
fcrcinc <- cfamily(crcinc, ptile = 0.5, nbchain = 1000,
    bstep = 10)

  ## There are 1 chains.
```

Lavine et al. (2013) used the ratio of variation in the multiannual versus high-frequency part of the wavelet spectrum as a simple measure of the time-varying signal-to-noise (SNR) ratio in the whooping cough dynamics.

```
sigind = which((a/52) > 3 & (a/52) < 4)
noiseind = which((a/52) < 0.5)
snr = apply(wspec[, sigind], 1, sum)/apply(wspec[, noiseind],
    1, sum)
```

A composite plot of incidence, wavelet spectrum, and signal-to-noise ratio is shown in Fig. 11.12 to highlight how the major epidemics are much less noisy than the low-amplitude cycles. Lavine et al. (2013) fit a seasonally forced SIRWS model (Eqs. (11.3)–(11.6)) to the data and concluded that the curious run of violent epidemics of whooping cough appeared to trace out an unstable multiannual almost attractor.

```
par(mfrow = c(3, 1), mar = c(0, 4, 2, 1))
layout(matrix(c(1, 1, 2, 2, 2, 3), ncol = 1))
#Top panel
plot(as.Date(pertcop$date), pertcop$cases, xlab = "",
```

```
    ylab = "Sqrt(cases)", type = "l", bty = "l",
    xlim = c(as.Date("1901-01-01"),
    as.Date("1938-01-01")), xaxt="n", yaxt="n")
axis(2, at = seq(0, 200, by = 100), labels = FALSE)
axis(2, at = seq(50, 250, by = 100), labels = TRUE)
#Mid panel
par(mar = c(0, 4, 0.25, 1))
image(x = as.Date(pertcop$date, origin = "1900-01-07"),
    wspec, col = gray((30:10)/32), y = a/52, ylim = c(0,5),
    ylab = "Period (year)", main = "", xaxt = "n", yaxt = "n")
contour(x = as.Date(pertcop$date, origin = "1900-01-07"),
    wspec, y = a/52, ylim = c(0,5),
    zlim = c(quantile(wspec)[4], max(wspec)), add = TRUE)
axis(2, at = 0:4)
ridges = fcrcinc[[1]]
ridges[which(ridges < 1.5 * 10^-5)] = NA
image(x = as.Date(pertcop$date, origin = "1900-01-07"),
    y = a/52, z = ridges, add = TRUE, col = "black")
#Bottom panel
par(mar = c(3, 4, 0.25, 1), tcl = -0.4)
plot(x = as.Date(pertcop$date, origin = "1900-01-07"), snr,
    type = "l", bty = "l",xaxt = "n", yaxt = "n", ylab = "SNR")
axis.Date(1, at = seq(as.Date("1900-01-01"),
    as.Date("1938-01-01"), "years"))
```

In addition to highlighting the potential influence of unstable manifolds in disease dynamics, prevaccination Copenhagen whooping cough hints at another *exotic* feature of certain nonlinear dynamical systems: increased stochasticity can sometimes *increase* predictability through a process dubbed stochastic resonance in the dynamic systems literature (e.g., Wiesenfeld & Moss, 1995; Gammaitoni et al., 1998). We can illustrate this phenomenon with the stochastically excited seasonally forced SEIR model introduced in Sect. 11.5. The somewhat involved Csnippets for pomp are detailed in Sect. 11.9. We simulate 500 years of weekly data across a range of 126 transmission variances between 0 and 0.025 (given by the alpha vector). The dynamics is prone to stochastic extinction so, for each parameter set, we change the pseudorandom seed until a 500-year persistent time series is produced (using the while loop).

```
dat = data.frame(time = seq(0, 500, by = 1/52), reports = NA)
sds = rep(NA, 126)
alpha = seq(0,0.025, by = 0.0002)
Smat = Imat = matrix(NA, nrow = 26001, ncol = 126)
for(i in 1:126){
    seirp = simulate(t0 = 0, times = seq(0,500,by=1/52),
        rprocess = euler(Csnippet(rproc),delta.t = 1/52/20),
        skeleton = vectorfield(Csnippet(skel)),
        rmeasure = Csnippet(robs), dmeasure = Csnippet(dobs),
        rinit = Csnippet(rinit),
        params = c(iota = 0, beta0 = 537, beta1 = 0.3,
            sigma = 36, gamma = 34.3, alpha = alpha[i],
            rho = 0.6, theta = 1, b = 0.02, mu = 0.02, pop0 = 5e8,
```

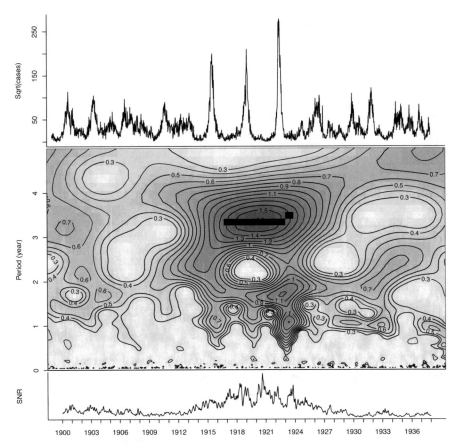

Fig. 11.12: (**a**) Incidence of whooping cough in Copenhagen. (**b**) The wavelet spectrum reveals a 10-year run of significant 3-year cycles starting around 1915. (**c**) The three-year cycles are associated with increased signal-to-noise (SNR) ratio in the wavelet spectrum

```
            S0 = 0.06, E0 = 0, I0 = 0.001, R0 = 0.939),
   paramnames = c("iota", "beta0", "beta1", "gamma",
       "sigma", "alpha", "rho", "theta", "b", "mu", "pop0",
       "S0", "E0" ,"I0", "R0"),
   statenames = c("S", "E", "I", "R", "inc", "pop"),
   obsnames="reports", accumvars = "inc")

stocsim <- list()
stocsim$I[26001] = 0
j = -1
while(stocsim$I[26001]==0){
    j = j + 1
    stocsim = as.data.frame(simulate(seirp,
```

```
        seed = 3495131 + j, nsim = 1))
    sds[i] = 3495131 + j
    }
    Imat[, i] = stocsim$I
    Smat[, i] = stocsim$S
}
```

To study stochastic resonance, we simulate the model across a range of stochastic variabilities in the transmission rate. Following Lavine et al. (2013), we use wavelet analysis to quantify "predictability" as a function of stochasticity (Fig. 11.13).[5]

```
predn = rep(NA, 126)
#Set the number of "octaves" and "voices"
no = 8; nv = 10
#then calculate the corresponding periods
a = 2^seq(1, no + 1 - 1 / nv, by = 1 / nv)
sel2 = a < 39 & a < 260 #Multiannual signal
sel = a < 39 #High frequency noise
for(i in 1:126){
    wfit = cwt(sqrt(Imat[, i]), no, nv)
    wspec = Mod(wfit)
    predn[i] = sum(wspec[, sel2])/sum(wspec[sel])
}
plot(alpha, predn, xlab = "Noise variance",
     ylab = "'Predictability'")
```

The wavelet signal-to-noise ratio indicates the curious phenomenon that "predictability" increases with noise up to a point and then decays (Fig. 11.13). The effect comes about because with low noise variance, the system rarely interacts with the high-amplitude quasi-periodic almost attractor and at high noise variance the stochasticity breaks the epidemiological clockwork, but at intermediate perturbation levels the repellor governs the dynamics.

Stochasticity can also push a dynamical system toward an almost stable multiannual cycle, as Lavine et al. (2013) argued was the case of prevaccination whooping cough in Copenhagen, or toward an almost stable fix-point. The latter for which perhaps the clearest biological illustration is provided by laboratory colonies of cyclic populations of the flour beetle *Tribolium castaneum* (Cushing et al., 1998; Bjørnstad & Grenfell, 2001). The notion that stochasticity can push a system toward an almost stable chaotic manifold (as is the case of the seasonally forced chickenpox model of Rand and Wilson (1991)) led to an interesting discussion of the meaning of "noise-induced chaos" between Yao and Tong (1994), Dennis et al. (2003), and Ellner and Turchin (2005).

---

[5] "Predictability" is deliberately written in quotes here because the mid-pass amplitude is not a true measure of predictability. Section 11.8 will elaborate on this.

11.8 Predictability: Empirical Dynamic Modeling

The "predictability" measure used in the previous section is not truly a measure of the level of determinism of the dynamics. Various researchers have proposed to use some form of nonparametric autoregression—sometimes called nonlinear forecasting (Tong, 1995; Fan et al., 1996) and recently empirical dynamic modeling (Ye et al., 2015)—in combination with leave-one-out cross-validation to quantify predictability in empirical time series. These approaches have used nearest-neighbor methods (Sugihara et al., 1990), kernel regression (Yao & Tong, 1998), and local polynomials (Fan et al., 1996). The ntls package has implementations of the local polynomial approaches proposed by Tong and co-workers (Cheng & Tong, 1992; Fan et al., 1996; Yao & Tong, 1998) building on the locfit package of Loader (2006). The function ll.order calculates the cross-validation error across a range of kernel bandwidths and autoregressive lags.[6]

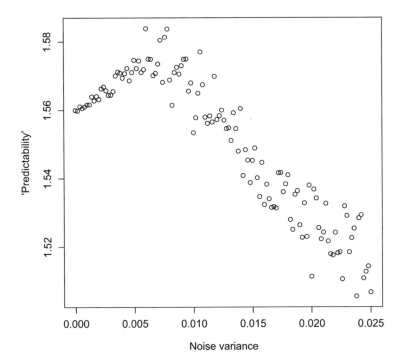

Fig. 11.13: "Predictability" measured as the ratio of the wavelet spectrum that falls in the multiannual region versus the high-frequency region as a function of the stochastic variance in the transmission rate for the seasonally forced SEIR model

---

[6] The method was originally proposed as a nonparametric method to estimate what time series statisticians call the "order" and dynamical systems theorists call the "embedding dimension" (Cheng & Tong, 1992; McCaffrey et al., 1992; Tong, 1995).

Consider the chickenpox SEIR model across a range of stochasticities in transmission and use `ll.order` to calculate the cross-validation predictability in annually strobed versions of the weekly simulations (discarding the first 10 years).

```
require(nlts)
llcv = rep(NA, 126)
for (i in 1:126) {
    llfit = ll.order(sqrt(Imat[seq(521, 26001, by = 52),
        i]), step = 1, order = 1:5, bandwidt = seq(0.5,
        1.5, by = 0.5), cv = FALSE)
    llcv[i] = min(llfit$grid$GCV)
}
plot(llcv ~ alpha, ylab = "GCV", xlab = "Noise variance")
```

The action of stochastic resonance due to the almost attractor is readily visible, as the generalized cross-validation error is lowest for intermediate noise variances (Fig. 11.14).

In an early application to epidemiology, Sugihara et al. (1990) proposed to use nonparametric forecasting error as a function of prediction lag to distinguish deterministic chaos from noisy limit cycles in measles epidemics. Nonparametric autoregression is a completely mechanism-free time series model for the disease dynamics (as in contrast to for example the chain binomial or TSIR). We can use the `ll.edm` function to check that the method produces dynamics that are in rough correspondence to the empirical patterns. Consider for example a 10-year segment of the weekly simulation using the 10th parameter set. We use order (embedding dimension) 3 because this is indicated as best fit based on the order-consistent estimator (`ll.order`). The resultant empirical dynamic model has roughly appropriate dynamics, though the period is slightly too short (Fig. 11.15).

```
x = sqrt(Imat[seq(521, 1040, by = 1), 10])
sim = ll.edm(x = x, order = 3, bandwidth = 0.8)
plot(x, type = "b", ylab = "Prevalence", xlab = "Week")
lines(sim, col = 2)
legend("topright", legend = c("Simulation", "EDM"), lty = c(1,
    1), pch = c(1, NA), col = c("black", "red"))
```

11.9 Appendix: Making a Pomp Simulator

Doing the computations involved in Sects. 11.5 and 11.7 is computationally expensive. The pomp package includes a Csnippet function that will compile C code on the fly to speed up calculations (King et al., 2015b). The following provides the C code used in the simulations of the stochastic SEIR model.

```
require(pomp)
```

The Csnippet for the deterministic skeleton is

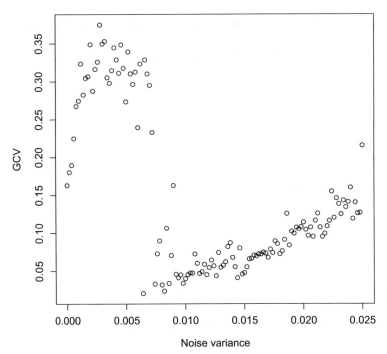

Fig. 11.14: Predictability measured as the generalized cross-validation error of the optimized nonparametric autoregression as a function of the stochastic variance in the transmission rate for the seasonally forced chickenpox SEIR model

```
"
double rate[8]; // transition rates
double trans[8]; // transition numbers

double beta = beta0*(1+beta1*cos(2*M_PI*t)); //transmission
double lambda = (iota+I*beta)/pop; // force of infection

// transition rates
rate[0] = b*pop; // birth of S
rate[1] = lambda; // infection of S
rate[2] = mu;  // death of S
rate[3] = sigma; // latent period  of E
 rate[4] = mu; // death of E
 rate[5] = gamma; // recovery of I
 rate[6] = mu; // death of I
 rate[7] = mu; // death of R

// compute the transition numbers
trans[0] = rate[0];
trans[1] = rate[1]*S;
trans[2] = rate[2]*S;
```

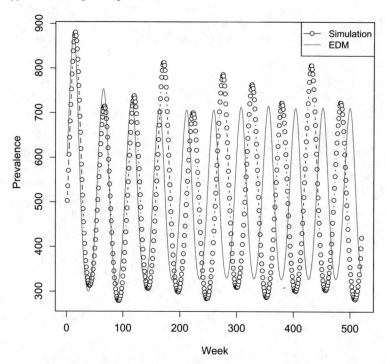

Fig. 11.15: Model simulation and dynamics predicted by the nonparametric autore-gressive (empirical dynamic) model

```
trans[3] = rate[3]*E;
trans[4] = rate[4]*E;
trans[5] = rate[5]*I;
trans[6] = rate[6]*I;
trans[7] = rate[7]*R;

// balance the equations
DS = trans[0] - trans[1] - trans[2];
DE = trans[1] - trans[3] - trans[4];
DI = trans[3] - trans[5] - trans[6];
DR = trans[5] - trans[7];
Dinc = trans[5]; // incidence from cumulative recovery
Dpop = trans[0] - trans[2] - trans[4] - trans[6] - trans[7]
" -> skel
```

The Csnippet for the stochastic simulator is

```
"
double rate[8]; // transition rates
double trans[8]; // transition numbers

double beta = beta0*(1+beta1*cos(2*M_PI*t)); // transmission
```

```
double dW = rgammawn(alpha,dt);   // white noise
double lambda = (iota+I*beta*dW/dt)/pop;

// transition rates
rate[0] = b*pop; // birth of S
rate[1] = lambda; // infection of S
rate[2] = mu; // death of S
rate[3] = sigma; // end of latency
rate[4] = mu; // death of E
rate[5] = gamma; // recovery of I
rate[6] = mu; // death of I
rate[7] = mu; // death of R

// compute the transition numbers
trans[0] = rpois(rate[0]*dt); // births are Poisson
reulermultinom(2, S, &rate[1], dt, &trans[1]);
reulermultinom(2, E, &rate[3], dt, &trans[3]);
reulermultinom(2, I, &rate[5], dt, &trans[5]);
reulermultinom(1, R, &rate[7], dt, &trans[7]);

// balance the equations
S += trans[0] - trans[1] - trans[2];
E += trans[1] - trans[3] - trans[4];
I += trans[3] - trans[5] - trans[6];
R += trans[5] - trans[7];
inc += trans[5];   // incidence from cumulative recovery
   pop = S + E + I + R;
" -> rproc
```

pomp wants Csnippets for the observational process also (even if we only use the object for simulation).

```
## Observation model simulator (negative binomial)
"
double mean = rho*inc;
double size = 1/theta;
reports = rnbmodinom_mu(size,mean);
" -> robs

## Observation model likelihood  (negative binomial)
"
double mean = rho*inc;
double size = 1/theta;
 reports = rnbinom_mu(size,mean);
" -> dobs
```

We need initial conditions:

```
"
S = nearbyint(pop0*S0);
E = nearbyint(pop0*E0);
I = nearbyint(pop0*I0);
R = nearbyint(pop0*R0);
```

```
pop = S+E+I+R;
 inc = 0;
" -> rinit
```

Finally, the built pomp object is

```
seirp = simulate(
   t0 = 0, times = seq(0,500,by=1/52),
   rprocess = euler(Csnippet(rproc),delta.t = 1/52/20),
   skeleton = vectorfield(Csnippet(skel)),
   rmeasure = Csnippet(robs),
   dmeasure = Csnippet(dobs),
   rinit = Csnippet(rinit),
   params = c(
    iota = 0,beta0 = 537,beta1 = 0.3,sigma = 36,
    gamma = 34.3,alpha = 0.015,rho = 0.6,theta = 1,
    b = 0.02,mu = 0.02,pop0 = 5e8,
    S0 = 0.06,E0 = 0,I0 = 0.001,R0 = 0.939),
    paramnames = c("iota", "beta0", "beta1", "gamma",
         "sigma", "alpha", "rho", "theta", "b", "mu",
         "pop0", "S0", "E0", "I0", "R0"),
   statenames = c("S", "E", "I", "R", "inc", "pop"),
  obsnames="reports",
  accumvars = "inc"
)
```

The pomp package has numerous functions to simulate deterministic and stochastic trajectories from pomp objects (King et al., 2015b).

Part II
Space

Chapter 12
Spatial Dynamics

12.1 Introduction

Space adds an additional axis to the richness of infectious disease dynamics. For example, Gog et al. (2014) detailed the diffusive nature of the spread of influenza A/H1N1pdv and Lau et al. (2017) characterized the geographic spread of the West African 2014–2015 Ebola outbreak. Walsh et al. (2005) calculated that Ebola was spreading through gorilla and chimpanzee populations at 50 km/year. Moreover, Grenfell and Harwood (1997) and Keeling et al. (2004) outlined how spatial spread may permit long-term persistence through metapopulation dynamics. This part of the monograph explores the spatial and spatiotemporal dimensions to infectious disease dynamics. The current chapter introduces the basics of modeling spatial disease dynamics. Chapter 13 introduces a range of geostatistical methods that are useful for quantifying spatial and space-time patterns from surveillance data. Chapter 14 discusses how in addition to geographic space, social space (as eluded to in Sect. 3.8) can be analyzed and modeled using network methods. Finally Chap. 15 will attempt to bring a synthesis of Part I and Part II of this monograph through consideration of invasion, persistence, and eradication of infectious diseases.

12.2 Dispersal Kernels

Pathogens move in space because of movement of transmission stages and infected/susceptible hosts. Spatial patterns arise from landscape heterogeneities, dispersal and reaction-diffusion dynamics among spatially dispersed susceptible and infected individuals. The probability distribution that governs dispersal distances is often referred to as the dispersal kernel. A variety of functional forms have been pro-

---

This chapter uses the following R packages: ncf, animation and plotly.
A five minute epidemics MOOC on spatial spread is: https://www.youtube.com/watch?v=WPjsAdyD1Gg

O. N. Bjørnstad, *Epidemics*, Use R!, https://doi.org/10.1007/978-3-031-12056-5_12

posed in the ecological and epidemiological literature (e.g., Mollison, 1991; Clark, 1998; Bjørnstad & Bolker, 2000; Smith et al., 2002a). From the point of view of basic theory, it is often assumed that dispersal takes an exponential (the probability of dispersing a distance $d \propto \exp(-d/u)$, where u is the range) or Gaussian ($\propto \exp(-(d/u)^2)$) shape. The exponential model arises, for example, if we assume dispersal happens in a constant direction with a constant stopping rate. The Gaussian model arises if the stopping rate is constant but movement direction changes randomly like a Brownian motion. However, other kernels are relevant; Broadbent and Kendall (1953) calculated the movement probabilities of infectious larvae of a gut nematode of sheep, *Trichostrongylus retortaeformis*, that performs a random walk until it encounters a leaf of grass. Assuming the location of the leaves are according to a spatially random point process, they showed that the random walk leads to a dispersal distance distributions that follows a Bessel K_0 function. Ferrari et al. (2006b) used this kernel in a model of pollinator-vectored plant pathogens. Empirical dispersal distributions of free-living organisms typically have an overrepresentation of rare long-range jumps that are improbable according to these kernels; they are the so-called fat-tailed kernels (Clark, 1998), which have important consequences for the speed of spatial spread (Kot et al., 1996).

For human infections, spatially contiguous, diffusive kernels are often a poor fit to empirical patterns because spread often follows a characteristic hierarchical fashion (Grenfell et al., 2001, see Sect. 12.9). Infections usually appear in big cities early, thereafter the timing of epidemics on average happens in an order of descending size and increasing isolation. This chapter is focused on inferring the shape of the spread kernel from spatial patterns over time, and then investigate the dynamical consequences of such spread. We start with considering the simpler diffusive kernels and then consider the more complicated patterns arising from human mobility.

12.3 *Filipendula* Rust Data

Jeremy Burdon and Lars Ericson surveyed presence/absence of a fungal pathogen on a wild plant, *Filipendula ulmaria*, across islands in a Swedish archipelago (Smith et al., 2003). The filipendula data contains observations for 1994 ($y94) and 1995 ($y95), with spatial coordinates $X and $Y. There are additionally a large number of descriptive covariates for each site. Smith et al. (2003) used the data to estimate the most likely dispersal kernel of the rust. The host plant is an herbaceous perennial with pathogen spores overwintering on dead tissue. The infections in 1995 thus arose from the spores produced in 1994.

If spores disperse according to, say, an exponential function with range, u, then the spatial force of infection on any location, i, will be $\propto \sum_j z_j u^{-1} \exp(-d_{ij}/u)$, where z_j is the disease status (0/1) in the previous year and d_{ij} are the distances to other locations. The idea is that in each spring, every local group of hosts will be in the accumulated spore shadow of last year's infected individuals. This leads to a metapopulation incidence function model (Hanski, 1994) for the presence/absence

of rust among all locations from year to year. Figure 12.1 shows the spatial layout
and disease status of the host plants.

```
data(filipendula)
symbols(filipendula$X, filipendula$Y, circles = rep(1,
    162), inches = 0.1, bg = filipendula$y95 + 1, xlab = "X",
    ylab = "Y")
symbols(filipendula$X, filipendula$Y, circles = rep(1,
    162), inches = 0.05, bg = filipendula$y94 + 1, add = TRUE)
legend("topright", c("infected 94", "infected 95"), pch = c(21,
    21), pt.cex = c(1, 2), pt.bg = c(2, 2))
```

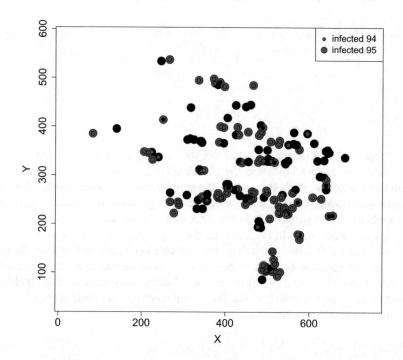

Fig. 12.1: Presence/absence of the rust on its *Filipendula ulmaria* host plant in 1994
(large symbols) and 1995 (small symbols). Red is infected. Black is uninfected

As for the basic catalytic (Chap. 4) and TSIR (Chap. 8) models, we can use the
`glm` framework to estimate the parameters. Since the response variable is binary,
we use logistic regression to calculate a profile likelihood for u. First calculate the
distance matrix among the 162 locations:

```
dst = as.matrix(dist(filipendula[, c("X", "Y")]))
```

Arbitrarily assuming a value of u of 10m, the 1995 FoI on each location will be
proportional to:

```
u = 10
foi = apply(exp(-dst/u) * filipendula$y94, 2, sum)
```

The glm function evaluates the likelihood. Recall the deviance of the glm object is 2 times the negative log-likelihood.

```
lfit = glm(y95 ~ foi, family = binomial(), data = filipendula)
lfit$deviance/2
```

```
   ## [1] 69.8527
```

Figure 12.2 shows the likelihood profile across candidate values for *u*.

```
u = seq(1, 20, length = 1001)
llik = rep(NA, length(u))
for (i in 1:length(u)) {
    foi = apply(exp(-dst/u[i]) * filipendula$y94, 2, sum)
    lfit = glm(y95 ~ foi, family = binomial(), data = filipendula)
    llik[i] = lfit$deviance/2
}
plot(u, llik, type = "l", ylab = "Neg. log-like")
abline(h = min(llik) + qchisq(0.95, 1)/2)
```

The comparison of the best kernel model with a non-spatial model assuming a homogenous risk among hosts use the likelihood ratio test introduced in Sect. 9.4; recall that for nested glm's (i.e., where the simpler model is nested within the more complicated model), the difference in deviances is $\chi^2(\Delta p)$-distributed, where Δp is the number of extra parameters in the more complex model. The anova function provides this calculation in R. Since the above calculations first profiled on *u* and then used the value $\hat{u}$ that minimized the negative log-likelihood—which the glm object has no memory of—the spmod object has to be corrected for the residual degrees of freedom ($df - 1$) of the spatial model to get the correct likelihood ratio test. The calculations show that the spatial model gives a significantly better fit than the non-spatial null model.

```
uhat = u[which.min(llik)]
foi = apply(exp(-dst/uhat) * filipendula$y94, 2, sum)
spmod = glm(y95 ~ foi, family = binomial(), data = filipendula)
nullmod = glm(y95 ~ 1, family = binomial(), data = filipendula)
# correct the df of the spmod
spmod$df.residual = spmod$df.residual - 1
anova(nullmod, spmod, test = "Chisq")
```

```
   ## Analysis of Deviance Table
   ##
   ## Model 1: y95 ~ 1
   ## Model 2: y95 ~ foi
   ##   Resid. Df Resid. Dev Df Deviance  Pr(>Chi)
   ## 1       161     222.10
   ## 2       159     109.48  2   112.63 < 2.2e-16 ***
   ## ---
   ## Signif: 0 '***' 0.001 '**' 0.01 '*' 0.05 '.' 0.1 ' ' 1
```

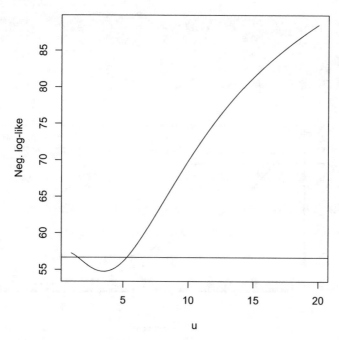

Fig. 12.2: The likelihood profile for the u parameter of the exponential dispersal kernel. The horizontal line represents the 95% cutoff for the $\chi^2(1)/2$ deviation from the minimum

The alternative Gaussian dispersal kernel takes the form proportional to $\exp(-(d_{ij}/u)^2)$:

```
llik2 = rep(NA, length(u))
for(i in 1:length(u)){
    foi2 = apply(exp(-(dst/u[i])^2) * filipendula$y94, 2, sum)
    lfit2 = glm(y95 ~ foi2, family = binomial(),
        data = filipendula)
    llik2[i] = lfit2$deviance/2
}
uhat2 = u[which.min(llik2)]
foi2 = apply(exp(-(dst/uhat2)^2) * filipendula$y94, 2, sum)
spmod2 = glm(y95 ~ foi2, family = binomial(),
    data = filipendula)
spmod2$df.residual = spmod2$df.residual - 1
```

Figure 12.3 depicts the shape of the competing probability kernels (using appropriate scaling for power exponential functions; the θ-power exponential scales according to $\Gamma(1/\theta)\exp(x)^\theta$).

```
curve((2 / (uhat2 * gamma(1/2))) * exp(-((x/uhat2)^2)), 0, 10,
    col = 2, lty = 2, ylab = "Probability", xlab="Meters")
curve((1/(uhat) * gamma(1)) * exp(-x/uhat), 0, 10, add = TRUE)
legend("topright", c("Exponential", "Gaussian"),
    lty = c(1, 2), col = c(1, 2))
```

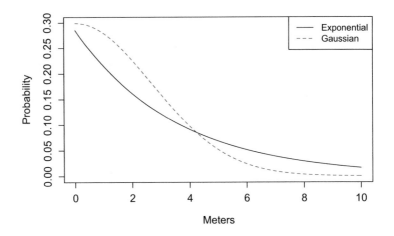

Fig. 12.3: The estimated exponential versus Gaussian kernels for the filipendula rust data

The two spatial models are not nested[1] but can be less formally ranked according to their AICs that supports the exponential model over the Gaussian:

```
spmod$aic
```

```
## [1] 113.4775
```

```
spmod2$aic
```

```
## [1] 116.6538
```

12.4 Simulation

In addition to being a statistical method, the binomial spatial model also represents a metapopulation model for presence/absence of the rust.[2] Given the assumed logistic

---

[1] As discussed in Sect. 9.4 these two models are not nested in the sense that one model is a simpler version of the other so formal likelihood ratio test does not apply.

[2] Just like the chain-binomial model in Sects. 3.4 and 3.5, the spatial logistic can be used both as a statistical method and as a stochastic simulator.

model (the default for the binomial-family), the regression provides estimates for $logit(p) = c_0 + c_1\phi$, where c_0 is the logistic intercept and c_1 is the slope on the spatial force of infection (ϕ). The inverse link is $p = \exp(c_0 + c_1\phi)/(1 + \exp(c_0 + c_1\phi))$ as previously discussed in Sect. 5.2.

A simulator that stochastically projects the epidemic metapopulation forwards in time (assuming a fixed host plant distribution) initiated with the state of the system in 1995 is:

```
zprev = filipendula$y95
x = filipendula$X
y = filipendula$Y
c0 = spmod$coef[1]
c1 = spmod$coef[2]
```

Infection probabilities for next year are:

```
foi = apply(exp(-dst/uhat) * zprev, 2, sum)
logitp = c0 + c1 * foi
p = exp(logitp)/(1 + exp(logitp))
```

And a stochastic realization is:

```
znew = rbinom(162, 1, p)
symbols(x, y, circles = rep(1, 162), bg = znew + 1, inches = 0.1,
    xlab = "X", ylab = "Y")
```

The following code animates a stochastic realization for another 100 years (if un-commented, the `Sys.sleep` argument makes the computer go to sleep for 0.1s to help on-screen visualization:

```
simdat = matrix(NA, ncol = 100, nrow = 162)
for(i in 1:100){
    zprev = znew
    foi = apply(exp(-dst/uhat) * zprev, 2, sum)
    logitp = c0 + c1 * foi
    p = exp(logitp)/(1 + exp(logitp))
    znew = rbinom(162, 1, p)
    simdat[, i] = znew
    #Code for in-line animation:
    #symbols(x, y, circles = rep(1,162), bg = znew + 1,
    #inches = 0.1, xlab = "X", ylab = "Y")
    #Sys.sleep(0.1)
}
```

Figure 12.4 shows the predicted relative spatial risk from the stochastic simulation. The `spatial.plot` function in the ncf package is a wrapper for `symbols` that plots values larger (smaller) than the mean as red circles (black squares). It shows that spatial configuration alone can result in heterogenous infection risk across the metapopulation.

```
require(ncf)
mprev = apply(simdat, 1, mean)
spatial.plot(x, y, mprev, ctr = TRUE)
```

A corollary to this simulation is how specialist plant pathogens may regulate the spatial distribution of host plant recruitment through locally frequency-dependent mortality and thus promote species diversity according to the Janzen-Connell hypothesis (e.g., Clark & Clark, 1984; Petermann et al., 2008). Janzen (1970) and Connell (1971) were both pondering the ecological conundrum of how very many species of trees can coexist in tropical forests given the tenet of Gause's competitive exclusion principle (see e.g., Hardin, 1960). This essentially can be paraphrased as saying that if two species have the same resource requirements one will outcompete the other.[3] Their hypothesis was that if a specialist natural enemy such as a plant pathogen cast a local spatial shadow-of-mortality on seedlings of a particular species, then exclusion may not happen because death rates will be positively frequency-dependent in the neighborhood defined by the spatial kernel.

12.5 Gypsy Moth

Various viruses and parasitoids cause population instabilities and cycles in their insect hosts (see Chap. 16 for additional examples). The 5–10 year cycles in the gypsy moth (*Lymantria dispar*) are caused by the ldNPV multicapsid nuclear polyhedrosis virus (Elkinton & Liebhold, 1990). Larvae get infected when ingesting viral occlusion bodies while feeding on leaves. The virus subsequently kills the larvae to release more of these infectious particles. There is a strong delayed density-dependent feedback loop in this system because when hosts are rare very few viral occlusion bodies are produced leading to negligible transmission; whereas when hosts are abundant the force of infection becomes very high. USDA Forest Service conducts surveys each year of defoliation by the gypsy moth across the Northeastern USA to reveal complex spatiotemporal patterns of locally synchronous but regionally asynchronous outbreaks (see Sect. 13.10). A web-optimized animated GIF of the annual defoliation across between 1975 and 2002 can be viewed from https://tinyurl.com/3kp8wm8t.

Spatiotemporal models can help to better understand such dynamics. There are specialized models for both the local and spatiotemporal dynamics of the gypsy moth (Dwyer et al., 2000, 2004; Abbott & Dwyer, 2008; Bjørnstad et al., 2010). Section 12.10 provides a spatially extended gypsy moth model, which, because of its biological detail, is quite specific to this system and therefore left as an appendix (Sect. 12.10). Here we instead consider a simpler spatially extended SIR model.

---

[3] This is closely related to Tilman's (1976) R^* theory of competitive dominance discussed in Sects. 3.1 and 3.12.

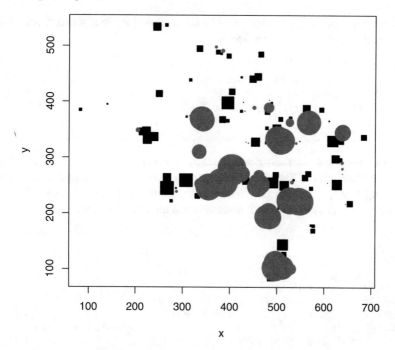

Fig. 12.4: Plot of predicted relative risk of rust infection from the metapopulation model. Risks larger (smaller) than the mean are shown as red circles (black squares). The size of the symbols reflects the deviation from the mean

12.6 A Coupled Map Lattice SI Model

Coupled map lattice models (CMLs) are constructed by assuming that spatiotemporal dynamics happens in two steps (Kaneko, 1993; Bascompte & Solé, 1995).[4] First, local growth according to some model, for example, the seasonally forced (discrete time) SI model. Followed, second, by spatial redistribution of a fraction, m, of all individuals to other neighboring patches.

Because R is a vectorized language one can simulate CMLs very compactly with a function for the local SI dynamics according to the expectation from the chain-binomial formulation (Sect. 3.4) followed by matrix-based redistribution. If we assume a birth/death rate of μ and sinusoidal forcing on the transmission rate according to $\beta_0 + \beta_1 \cos(2 * \pi * t/26)$ (so there are 26 time steps in a year) and infected individuals stays infected and infectious for one time step the function to

---

[4] The name refers to how the most stylized of these models assumes a lattice (checker board) of locations at which local numbers change from one generation to the next according to some "mapping" rule of onward local change such as the discrete logistic, the Nicholson-Baily model (see Chap. 16) or, in this case, a discrete-time seasonally forced SI model, followed by spatial redistribution via some spatial coupling rule.

simulate dynamics is the below `local.dyn`. Note, here that S and I are vectors representing numbers across the locations.

```
local.dyn = function(t, S, I, b0, b1, mu, N) {
    beta = b0 * (1 + b1 * cos(2 * pi * t/26))
    I = S * (1 - exp(-beta * I))
    S = (1 - mu) * S + mu * N - I
    list(S = S, I = I)
}
```

The next generates the redistribution matrix among the nx–by–ny locations (the below assumes a 30×30 lattice). Nearest neighbors will be < 2 spatial units apart. Assuming that the fraction that disperses to neighboring patches is $m = 0.25$ and that movement is independent of disease status the redistribution matrix is:

```
m = 0.25
ny = nx = 30
# generate coordinates
xy = expand.grid(x = 1:nx, y = 1:ny)
# make distance matrix
dst = as.matrix(dist(xy))
# make redistribution matrix with zeros
redist = matrix(0, nrow = ny * nx, ncol = ny * nx)
# populate the matrix so each of the 8 neighbors
# gets their share
redist[dst < 2] = m/8
# the remaining fraction stays put
diag(redist) = 1 - m
```

The S and I matrices will hold the results from the simulation. Twenty years of simulation represents `IT=520` iterations of the CML model. Assuming that all patches have `S0 = 100` susceptibles and that 1 infected is introduced in location $\{x = 10, y = 14\}$ (which is row 400 in the `xy` coordinate matrix) in the first year initial conditions are:

```
IT = 520
S = I = matrix(NA, nrow = ny * nx, ncol = IT)
S[, 1] = 100
I[, 1] = 0
I[400, 1] = 1
```

The remaining parameters necessary for the local dynamics are:

```
b0 = 0.04
b1 = 0.8
mu = 0.2/26
N = 100
```

To simulate the CML model, recalling from Sect. 4.4 that the `%*%` operator represents matrix multiplication, so the matrix multiplication of a vector of abundances with the redistribution matrix will move all individuals appropriately the code is:

```
for (t in 2:IT) {
    # local growth:
    tmp = local.dyn(t, S = S[, t - 1], I = I[, t - 1],
        b0 = b0, b1 = b1, mu = mu, N = N)

    # spatial movement
    S[, t] = redist %*% tmp$S
    I[, t] = redist %*% tmp$I
    # progress monitor
    cat(t, " of ", IT, "\r")
}
```

The simulation can be visualized as an in-line animation. The predicted incidence from the spatial SI model varies so widely it is useful to transform incidence (using a fourth-root transform) so that low values shows up better.

```
x = xy[, 1]
y = xy[, 2]
scIcubed = I^(1/4)/(max(I[, 10:IT]^(1/4)))
```

```
for (k in 1:IT) {
    symbols(x, y, fg = 2, circles = scIcubed[, k], inches = FALSE,
        bg = 2, xlab = "", ylab = "")
    Sys.sleep(0.05)
}
```

Analyses of a variety of host-parasit(oid) CML models (Hassell et al., 1991; Bjørnstad et al., 1999b; Earn et al., 2000a) have revealed a variety of emergent spatiotemporal patterns including complete synchrony, waves, spatial chaos , and frozen Turing patterns named after Alan Turing's seminal work on "The mathematics of biological pattern formations" published in 1953 and reprinted in the Bulletin of Mathematical Biology in 1990 (Turing, 1990). The latter is the term used when spatially heterogenous but static patterns arise despite identical temporal laws of diffusion across each location. The emergent spatiotemporal pattern in any given system depends on the local dynamics and mobility. Chapter 16 will visit on these other CML models further.

12.7 Making Movies

Permanent animations can be made by writing the plots to a sequence of images and then use an open-source utility like ImageMagick to convert the sequence to a movie.[5]

---

[5] The system() function in R passes the convert and rm calls to the command line. A web-optimized version of the animated GIF can be viewed on https://git.io/JMnHk. While not using base R syntax the plotly package is very effective for generating browser-rendered animations. An example can be found in the nbspat.app shinyApp in Chap. 16.

```
for(k in 100:IT){
png(filename = paste("m", 1000 + k,".png", sep = ""))
    symbols(x, y, fg = 2, circles = scIcubed[, k],
    inches = FALSE, bg = 2, xlab = "",ylab = "")
    dev.off()
}
system("convert m*.png -delay 1x8 -coalesce -layers
    OptimizeTransparency simovie.gif")
system("rm m*.png")
#For mp4-animation:
#system("convert -delay 5 m*.jpg simovie.mp4")
```

Alternatively R's animation package will bypass writing the intermediate image files, but with the downside that the resultant file may be less optimized and therefore larger and render less well.

```
require("animation")
ani = function(xy, data) {
    x = xy[, 1]
    y = xy[, 2]
    for (i in 1:dim(data)[2]) {
        dev.hold()
        symbols(x, y, fg = 2, circles = scIcubed[, i],
            inches = FALSE, bg = 2, xlab = "", ylab = "")
        ani.pause()
    }
}

ani(xy = xy, data = scIcubed)

saveGIF(ani(xy = xy, data = scIcubed))
```

12.8 Covariance Functions for Spatiotemporal Data

Keeling et al. (2002) discuss how we may understand the emergent complicated spatiotemporal dynamics of natural enemies in terms of the spatial variance (or associated autocorrelation) and covariance of the interacting species.[6] Bjørnstad and Bascompte (2001) proposed to calculate auto- and cross-correlation functions from simulated or real data. We can use the Sncf function in the ncf package to calculate the multivariate spatial correlation function (Bjørnstad et al., 1999b) among time series (see Chap. 13 for further details on this and other geostatistical methods). We can further look at the spatial cross-correlation function between susceptibles and infected (Fig. 12.5). The background synchrony for both compartments (of around 0.3) is due to the common seasonal forcing. The locally higher autocorrelation at shorter distances is due to emergence of dispersal-induced aggregations

---

[6] Seabloom et al. (2005) provide similar calculations for spatial plant competition models.

of infected individuals. The negative local cross-correlation is due to the local S-I cycles.

```
fitI = Sncf(x = xy[, 1], y = xy[, 2], z = sqrt(I[, 261:520]),
    resamp = 500)
fitS = Sncf(x = xy[, 1], y = xy[, 2], z = sqrt(S[, 261:520]),
    resamp = 500)
fitSI = Sncf(x = xy[, 1], y = xy[, 2], z = sqrt(S[, 261:520]),
    w = sqrt(I[, 261:520]), resamp = 500)
par(mfrow = c(1, 3))
plot(fitI, ylim = c(-0.1, 1))
plot(fitS, ylim = c(-0.1, 1))
plot(fitSI, ylim = c(-0.2, 0.2))
```

One interesting additional application is the time-lagged spatial correlation function (Bjørnstad et al., 2002a). This method may help quantifying wave-like spread. For example, if considering the spatiotemporal relationship among infected at five time step lag (Fig. 12.6). The peak in correlation is offset from the origin by somewhere between five and 10 units. This makes sense, since we assume nearest-neighbor dispersal so the leading edge should move 5 units vertically/horizontally and $5 * \sqrt{2} = 7.1$ units diagonally during 5 time steps.

```
fitIlag = Sncf(x = xy[, 1], y = xy[, 2], z = I[, 261:515],
    w = I[, 266:520], resamp = 100)
plot(fitIlag, ylim = c(-0.2, 0.2))
```

Bjørnstad et al. (2002b) used time-lagged spatial correlation functions to show that parasitoid-host interactions (see Chap.16) lead to diffusive waves of larch tree defoliation that travels at 210 km per year in a north-easterly direction across the European Alps. Traveling waves have also been documented in the dynamics of dengue (Cummings et al., 2004) and the 2009 influenza A/H1N1pdm pandemic (Gog et al., 2014).

12.9 Gravity Models

Regional spread of human pathogens rarely forms a simple diffusive pattern because human mobility patterns are more complex; movement may be distant dependent, but overall flow between any two communities also typically depends on the size (and desirability) of both donor and recipient locations (Fotheringham, 1984; Erlander & Stewart, 1990). Grenfell et al. (2001), for example, showed that the spatiotemporal dynamics of measles across all cities and villages in prevaccination England and Wales exhibited hierarchical waves, in which the timing of epidemics relative to the big urban conurbations (the donors) depended negatively on distance but positively on the size of the recipient. Viboud et al. (2006) demonstrated similar hierarchical spread of seasonal influenza across the states of continental USA. Xia et al. (2004) and Viboud et al. (2006) showed that metapopulation models where

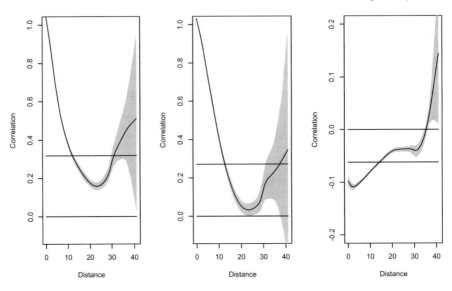

Fig. 12.5: Spatial correlation of (**a**) Infected, (**b**) Susceptibles, and (**c**) S-I cross-correlation as a function of distance. Grey shaded polygons represent the 95% confidence envelopes

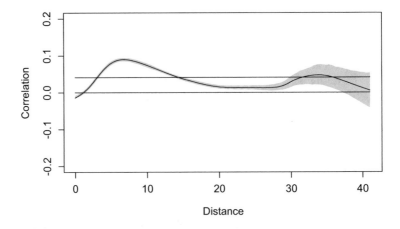

Fig. 12.6: A five-step time-lagged spatial cross-correlation function of predicted prevalence of the SIR coupled map lattice model

movement among communities follows a generalized gravity formulation approximate the spatial dynamics of measles and seasonal influenza. The gravity model is a model of mobility from transportation science that posits that transportation volume between two communities depends inversely on distance, d, but bilinearly on the size, N, of the communities (Fotheringham, 1984; Erlander & Stewart, 1990). Gravity-like models have since been applied to study the spatial dynamics of a variety of human infection settings (e.g., Mari et al., 2012; Truscott & Ferguson, 2012; Gog et al., 2014). The generalized gravity model quantifying the spatial interaction between locations i and j takes the form $\theta N_i^{\tau_1} N_j^{\tau_2} d_{ij}^{-\rho}$, where θ, τ_1, τ_2, and ρ are non-negative parameters shaping the topology of the spatial interaction network. The gravity model has at least two important special cases: $\rho = 0, \tau_1 = \tau_2 = 1$ representing a mean field model and $\tau_1 = \tau_2 = 0$ representing simple spatial diffusion. Viboud et al. (2006) proposed a stochastic multipatch SIR model for the spread of seasonal influenza among the states of continental USA. Here consider a simpler SIR version of the model (ignoring susceptible recruitment):[7]

$$\frac{dS_i}{dt} = -(\underbrace{\beta I_i}_{\text{local foi}} + \underbrace{\sum_{j \neq i} \iota_{j,i} I_j}_{\text{spatial foi}}) S_i / N_i \qquad (12.1)$$

$$\frac{dI_i}{dt} = \underbrace{(\beta I_i + \sum_{j \neq i} \iota_{j,i} I_j) S_i / N_i}_{\text{transmission in } i} - \underbrace{\gamma I_i}_{\text{recovery}} \qquad (12.2)$$

$$\frac{dR_i}{dt} = \underbrace{\gamma I_i}_{\text{recovery}}, \qquad (12.3)$$

where $\iota_{j,i} I_j$ is the gravity-weighted force of infection exerted by state j on state i. The corresponding code (subsuming the N_i denominator into a state-specific β parameter for computational convenience) is:

```
sirSpatmod = function(t, y, parameters) {
    L = length(y)/3
    i = c(1:L)
    S = y[i]
    I = y[L + i]
    R = y[2 * L + i]
    with(parameters, {
        beta = beta[i]
        dS = -(beta * I + m * G %*% I) * S
        dI = (beta * I + m * G %*% I) * S - gamma * I
        dR = gamma * I
        list(c(dS, dI, dR))
    })
}
```

Here G is the spatial interaction matrix, m is an overall scaling factor, and y is a vector of length 3L with initial values for all the location. The first 1–L represents

---

[7] Note that this formulation assumes that spatial transmission does not dilute local transmission. Keeling and Rohani (2002) provide a discussion of this issue. Section 15.7 also considers a model for which spatial transmission dilutes local transmission.

initial S's, $(L+1)-2L$ are initial I's, and the last $(2L+1)-3L$ are initial R's. Combining state-level influenza-like ILI data with county-level commuter census data, Viboud et al. (2006) estimated the gravity parameters to be $\tau_1 = 0.3$, $\tau_2 = 0.6$, and $\rho = 3$.[8] The usflu data contains coordinates and populations for each of the contiguous lower 48 states plus the District of Columbia. The gcdist function of the ncf package generates spatial distance matrices from the latitude/longitude data.

```
require(ncf)
data(usflu)
usdist = gcdist(usflu$Longitude, usflu$Latitude)
```

Define a function to generate the spatial interaction matrix given parameters and distances:

```
gravity = function(tau1, tau2, rho, pop, distance) {
    gravity = outer(pop^tau1, pop^tau2)/distance^rho
    diag(gravity) = 0
    gravity
}
G = gravity(0.3, 0.6, 3, usflu$Pop, usdist)
```

Finally define initial conditions and parameters scaling β by the N_i denominator such that R_0 is the same in all states (cf. Sect. 4.1). Viboud et al. (2006) were interested in exploring spread in a pandemic setting. Accordingly we assume that everybody is susceptible except for 1 initial index case arriving in New York.

```
gamma = 1/3.5
R0 = 1.8
beta = R0 * gamma/usflu$Pop
m = 1/1000/sum(usflu$Pop)
parms = list(beta = beta, m = m, gamma = gamma, G = G)

S = usflu$Pop
R = I = rep(0, length(usflu$Pop))
I[31] = 1
inits = c(S = S, I = I, R = R)
```

With this the sirSpatmod function can simulate a spatial SIR pandemic across the USA:

```
require(deSolve)
times = 0:200
out = ode(inits, times, sirSpatmod, parms)
L = length(usflu$Pop)
matplot(out[, 50 + (1:L)], type = "l", ylab = "Prevalence",
    xlab = "Day")
```

The outbreak peaks are predicted to be staggered because of the hierarchical diffusion of infection across the continent (Fig. 12.7).

---

[8] Viboud et al. (2006) showed that the commuter flows has a fatter tailed kernel (Sect. 12.2) than predicted by this gravity model which we, for expedience, ignore.

12.10 Appendix: A Spatial Gypsy Moth Model

Spatiotemporal outbreaks of the gypsy moth are an interesting case study of pathogen-host spatiotemporal dynamics because of the richness of data (Sects. 12.5 and 13.10), fascinatingly complex dynamics (Dwyer et al., 2004; Bjørnstad et al., 2010), and detailed mathematical models. Dwyer et al. (2000) combined field and laboratory measurements to propose a model that captures how the host (N) has one generation each year with eggs hatching in April–June, while the virus (Z), which kills infected larvae to produce viruses encased in environmentally long-lived protein crystals, has a fast transmission cycle during the larval season. Following the sort of mathematics underlying the final epidemic size equation in Sect. 2.4, Dwyer et al. (2000) derived an implicit equation for the within season death toll, f, for this host/pathogen system:

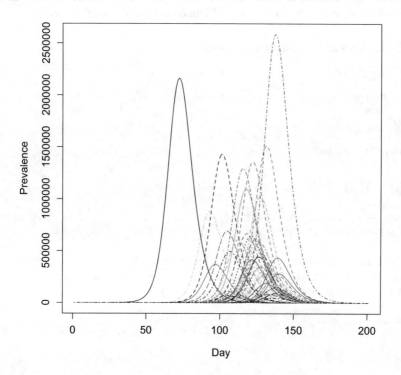

Fig. 12.7: Simulated influenza dynamics across the continental USA using a multipatch SIR model with gravity coupling parameterized according to Viboud et al. (2006)

$$f = 1 - \left(1 + \frac{\hat{v}}{\mu k}(Nf + \rho Z)\right)^{-k},$$

(12.4)

where μ is loss of infectiousness of dead larvae, $\hat{v}$ is mean infectiousness, related to total viral particles in a cadaver, $1/k$ is the coefficient of variation in infectiousness, and ρ is relative susceptibility of small versus large larvae. Local inter-annual virus–host dynamics is accordingly:

$$N_{t+1} = \lambda N_t(1-f) \tag{12.5}$$

$$Z_{t+1} = gN_t f, \tag{12.6}$$

where g is the compound variable of total number of occlusion bodies per cadaver discounted by their overwinter survival probability.

Because of the need to solve the implicit equation (Eq. (12.4)), the coding of the gypsy moth spatiotemporal model is a bit more involved than in Sect. 12.6. However, it still follows the same basic recipe: (i) generate the redistribution matrix, (ii) define the function for local dynamics and provide parameter values, and (iii) forward iterate cyclically between local transmission and spatial spread . . .

STEP 1: Generate the redistribution matrix.

```
ny = nx = 50
# generate coordinates
xy = expand.grid(x = 1:nx, y = 1:ny)
# make distance matrix
dst = as.matrix(dist(xy))
# make redistribution matrix with zeros
redist = matrix(0, nrow = ny * nx, ncol = ny * nx)
# populate the matrix so each of the 8 neighbors
# gets their share
m = 0.05
redist[dst < 2] = m/8
# the remaining fraction stays put
diag(redist) = 1 - m
```

STEP 2: Local dynamics. The code is a bit laborious because the implicit final epidemic equation coded in the `fn` and `ffn` functions need to be vectorized (thus the `split(...)` and `unlist(lapply(...))`).

```
local.dyn = function(NZ) {
    # fn implicit function
    fn = function(x, paras) {
        nu = 0.9
        mu = 0.32
        k = 1.06
        rho = 0.8
        with(as.list(paras), (1 - (1 + nu * (N * x + rho *
            Z)/(mu * k))^(-k) - x))
    }
    # ffn function to numerically solve for in-year
    # epidemic size at each location:
    ffn = function(params) {
        uniroot(fn, lower = 0, upper = 1, tol = 1e-09,
```

```
                        paras = params)$root
        }
        # code for forward iteration of host and virus
        sp = split(NZ, 1:dim(NZ)[1])
        ff = unlist(lapply(sp, ffn))
        lambda = 74.6
        g = 2000
        Nnew = lambda * NZ$N * (1 - ff)
        Znew = g * NZ$N * ff
        return(list(N = Nnew, Z = Znew))
}
```

STEP 3: Finally simulate the spatiotemporal host-virus dynamics:

```
IT = 500
N = Z = matrix(NA, nrow = ny * nx, ncol = IT)
N[, 1] = runif(ny * nx)
Z[, 1] = runif(ny * nx)

for (t in 2:IT) {
    # local growth:
    tmp = local.dyn(data.frame(N = N[, t - 1], Z = Z[,
        t - 1]))
    # spatial movement
    N[, t] = redist %*% tmp$N
    # Assuming negligible viral dispersal but virus
    # initially present (otherwise redist%*%tmp$Z):
    Z[, t] = tmp$Z
    # progress monitor cat(t,' of ', IT, '\r')
}

par(mfrow = c(1, 2))
symbols(xy[, 1], xy[, 2], fg = 2, circles = sqrt(N[, 150]),
    inches = 0.1, bg = 2, xlab = "", ylab = "")
symbols(xy[, 1], xy[, 2], fg = 2, circles = sqrt(N[, 350]),
    inches = 0.1, bg = 2, xlab = "", ylab = "")
```

Depending on parameter values, the initial spatially random map is predicted to give way to outbreaks that produces waves across the landscape (Fig. 12.8a) that over time erodes into highly clustered but spatially erratic outbreaks (Fig. 12.8b). The following code provides a `plotly` animation of the model.

```
N2 = as.data.frame(N)
N2$x = xy[, 1]
N2$y = xy[, 2]
longN = reshape(N2, direction = "long", varying = 1:IT,
    v.names = "N")

require(plotly)
anim = ggplot(longN, aes(x = x, y = y, frame = longN$time)) +
    geom_point(size = 4 * longN$N/max(longN$N))
ggplotly(anim)
```

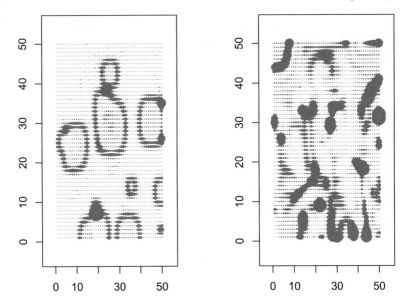

Fig. 12.8: Snapshots from the gypsy moth coupled map lattice model from (**a**) early and (**b**) late in the simulation

Chapter 13
Spatial and Spatiotemporal Patterns

13.1 Spatiotemporal Patterns

Spatial and spatiotemporal data analysis is of great importance in disease dynamics for a number of reasons such as looking for space-time clustering, hotspot detection, characterizing invasion waves, and quantifying spatial synchrony. Spatial synchrony—the level of correlation in outbreak dynamics at different locations—is of particular significance to acute immunizing infections, because asynchrony may permit regional persistence of infections despite local chains-of-transmission breaking during post-epidemic troughs (Keeling et al., 2004, see Sect. 15.7). Conversely, spatial synchrony can exacerbate the economic and public health burden because the resulting regionalized outbreaks can overwhelm logistical capabilities as was evident in the early part of the 2013–2014 West African Ebola outbreak and the 2020–2021 SARS-CoV-2 pandemic. Spatial statistics is also important in order to correct for the problem of spurious associations between incidence and environmental data because spatial autocorrelation violates the assumption of independence. This is further discussed in Sect. 18.2.

13.2 A Plant-Pathogen Case Study

Pathogenic fungi are generally not very important pathogens of mammals, though a virulent species of *Pseudogymnoascus* emerged in North America in 2007 to cause white-nose syndrome and exert major mortality events of bats (Blehert et al., 2009; Hoyt et al., 2021). In humans they cause ringworm and several opportunistic infections such as aspergillosis and candidiasis that are of minor importance except for in immunocompromised people. In various non-vertebrate animal case studies fungal pathogens have been shown to cause major epizoonoses. For example, *Aspergillus sydowii* has recently decimated Caribbean sea fan corals (Bruno et al.,

This chapter uses the following R package: ncf.

© The Author(s), under exclusive license to Springer Nature Switzerland AG 2023
O. N. Bjørnstad, *Epidemics*, Use R!, https://doi.org/10.1007/978-3-031-12056-5_13

2011) and fungal infections frequently slaughter their way through insect popula-tions (Hajek & St. Leger, 1994). Fungi are very common pathogens of plants on which non-systemic pathogens are often called rust. Systemic infections cause dev-astating disease like Dutch elm disease and chestnut blight. The latter completely altered the nature of North American hardwood forests when emerging during the first decade of the twentieth century (Anagnostakis, 1987).

While a bit idiosyncratic, the spatial dataset from Jennifer Koslow's experiment on a foliar, non-systemic rust fungus (*Coleosporium asterum*) that infects the flat-top goldenrod (*Euthamia graminifolia*) provides useful illustrations of various geo-statistical methods. The euthamia data present the severity of rust disease expres-sion ($score, from 0 to 10) on host-plants planted within mesocosms ($plot) in an old field near Ithaca in New York State. The mesocosms were in a checkerboard grid with locations specified by coordinates $xloc and $yloc. Each mesocosm contained 3 focal *E. graminifolia* plants. The field also contained naturally occur-ring *E. graminifolia*, as well as several other hosts of the rust, most notably the Canada goldenrod (*Solidago canadensis*). Two different treatments, species com-position ($comp, with three levels) and watering treatment ($water, with two levels), were applied to the mesocosms in a fully factorial design. Finally, to ac-count for spatial variation the field were divided into four blocks with treatment combinations randomly assigned within each block.

For some of the analyses we need jittered coordinates because the three plants within each plot were not given separate coordinates. Figure 13.1 shows the spatial layout of the study. The vertical lines mark the predefined blocks.

```
data(euthamia)
euthamia$jx = jitter(euthamia$xloc)
euthamia$jy = jitter(euthamia$yloc)
symbols(y = euthamia$xloc, x = euthamia$yloc,
    circles = euthamia$score, inches = 0.1,
    xlab = "y", ylab = "x")
abline(v = 47.5, col = 2)
abline(v = 97.5, col = 2)
abline(v = 147.5, col = 2)
```

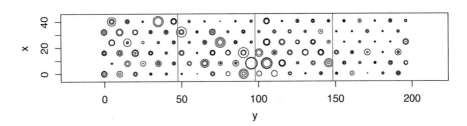

Fig. 13.1: Rust scores from Keslow's experiment

13.3 Spatial Autocorrelation

Spatial statistics is a very rich field. This chapter focuses on a subset of methods that are commonly used in epidemiology involving the notion of spatial autocorrelation. Legendre (1993) is a great introduction to the use of spatial autocorrelation statistics in ecological studies in general. While all the methods discussed—such as Mantel tests, parametric and nonparametric correlation functions, local indicators of spatial association, etc.—come in canned packages (this chapter uses the `ncf` package), it is useful to spend a bit of time on the underlying ideas.

Many geostatistical methods to describe spatial pattern are focused on either spatial variance (Gary's C) or spatial correlation (Moran's I). This chapter largely focuses on the family of correlational methods. The regular (Pearson's) product-moment correlation (ρ) between two random variables, Z_1 and Z_2, is defined as:

$$\rho_{12} = \frac{(Z_1 - \mu_1)}{\sigma_1} \frac{(Z_2 - \mu_2)}{\sigma_2},$$

where μ's are expectations and σ's are standard deviations.[1] The *auto*correlation has exactly the same definition and is used when the Z's are measurements of the same quantity (e.g., prevalence, incidence, presence/absence, etc.) at different spatial locations (or different times; Sect. 7.2).

The calculation needs to know (or have an estimate of) the values of the μ's and σ's. In the case of single snapshot spatial data the marginal mean and marginal standard deviation is normally used.[2] For the `euthamia` rust data (Fig. 13.1) these quantities are:

```
n = length(euthamia$score)
# marginal mean:
mu = mean(euthamia$score)
# marginal MLE  sd:
sig = sd(euthamia$score) * (n - 1)/n
```

Using the `outer` function that provides all pairwise products of two vectors, the estimated autocorrelation matrix (`rho`) among all 360 plants is then:

```
# rescale Zs
zscale = (euthamia$score - mu)/sig
# autocorrelation  matrix
rho = outer(zscale, zscale)
```

Note that while the individual pairwise values are not constrained to be between -1 and 1, as correlations need to be, the various geostatistical methods discussed in the following involves manipulations of this matrix to normalize values. Most

---

[1] It is, again, unfortunate that these Greek symbols as used in statistics take a different meaning than their previous usage in epidemiology, but it cannot be helped since the study of epidemics leans on so many different fields of science.

[2] Note that the geostatistical methods usually use the maximum likelihood estimator of σ rather than the best linear unbiased (BLUE) estimator; the denominator is n rather than $n - 1$.

of the methods also require some sort of associated spatial distance matrix. Most commonly used are the Euclidian distance for UTM coordinates or the <u>great-circle distance</u> for latitude/longitude coordinates. The Euclidean distance matrix among all 360 plants in the euthamia dataset is:

```
dst = as.matrix(dist(euthamia[, c("xloc", "yloc")]))
```

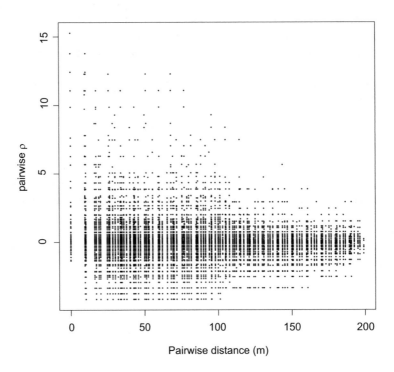

Fig. 13.2: Scatterplot of pairwise ρ against pairwise distance

To understand the different geostatistical methods, consider the plot of the paired autocorrelations as a function of their spatial distance (Fig. 13.2).

```
plot(dst, rho, cex = 0.1, ylab = expression("pairwise " *
    rho), xlab = "Pairwise distance (m)")
```

With this it is easy to erect a conceptual understanding of many different geostatistical methods.

- **Mantel test:** An overall test for whether there is any significant relationship between the elements in the two matrices. This is essentially a test for significant correlation between ρ and distance.
- **Correlogram:** The most classic tool of testing how autocorrelation depends on distance without assuming any particular function. Hack the distance x-axis into

segments (given by specifying some distance increment) and calculate the average ρ within each distance class.[3]

- **Parametric correlation functions:** Assume the relationship follows some parametric relationship—such as Exponential, Gaussian, or Spherical functions—and do the appropriate nonlinear regression of ρ on distance. Section 18.2 provides an example of such fitting via the lme function of the nlme library.
- **Nonparametric correlation function:** Fit a nonparametric regression (usually a smoothing spline or a kernel smoother) to the relationship (Hall & Patil, 1994). This also goes by the name of the spline correlogram (Bjørnstad & Falck, 2001).
- **Local indicators of spatial association (LISA):** A test for hotspots (Anselin, 1995) specifying a neighborhood size and for each location calculates the average ρ with all the other locations that belongs to its neighborhood to find areas of significant above average values.

There are a bunch of other named methods that are variations of these. Several of which are extensions to when there is multiple observations at each location (such as a spatial panel of time series), in which case it is natural to estimate the autocorrelation matrix using the regular correlation matrix. The modified correlogram of Koenig (1999) is the multivariate extension of the correlogram (see also Bjørnstad et al., 1999b). The time-lagged spatial cross-correlation function has been used to study waves of spread (see below and Sect. 12.8). Various other versions allow the spatial correlation function to vary by cardinal direction (so-called anisotropic correlograms) to investigate directional patterns (Bjørnstad et al., 2002b).

13.4 Testing and Confidence Intervals

An important reason why specialized methods are needed for these analyses, despite most being conceptually simple, is because while the n original data points may (or may not) be statistically independent the n^2 numbers in the autocorrelation matrix is obviously very statistically non-independent and the interdependence is very intricate (as nicely discussed and visualized by Rousseeuw and Molenberghs, 1994). None of the usual ways of testing for significance or generating confidence intervals is therefore applicable. Testing is usually done using permutation tests under the null hypothesis of no spatial patterns. The correlogram (or Mantel test, or ...) of the real data should look no different than that of a random re-allocation of observations to spatial coordinates if the null hypothesis is true. Statistical significance is calculated by comparing the observed estimate to the distribution of estimates for, say, 999 different randomized datasets.[4] If the observed is more extreme than 950 (990) of the randomized data we conclude that there is significant deviation from

---

[3] The variogram is similar to the correlogram but instead of using the autocorrelation similarity measure it uses the semivariance dissimilarity measure: $(Z_i - Z_j)^2/2$.

[4] This produces a total of 1000 known possible outcomes; the 999 we randomly generated plus the one nature provided.

spatial randomness at a nominal 5%-level (1%-level). For some of the methods it is possible to generate confidence envelopes using bootstrapping (resampling with replacement; Bjørnstad and Falck, 2001). All the above methods are available in the `ncf` package.

```
require(ncf)
```

13.5 Mantel test

We continue using the `euthamia` data as a case study:

```
test1 = mantel.test(M1 = rho, M2 = dst, quiet = TRUE)
test1

  ## $correlation
  ## [1] -0.04603662
  ##
  ## $p
  ## [1] 0.000999001
  ##
  ## $call
  ## [1] "mantel.test(M1 = rho, M2 = dst, quiet = TRUE)"
  ##
  ## attr(,"class")
  ## [1] "Mantel"
```

There is a significant negative association between similarity and distance showing that the rust data are not spatially random. The Mantel test is a crude tool but it does reveal that locations near each other tend to be more similar in disease status than those separated by a greater distance. If instead of having two matrixes have spatial coordinates and observations the syntax is:

```
mantel.test(x, y, z, latlon = FALSE)
```

In this case coordinates can either be Euclidian or latitude/longitude if `latlon` = TRUE.

13.6 Correlograms

The correlogram shows how the autocorrelation is a function of distance (Fig. 13.3). The shape of the correlogram can indicate random, diffusive, or clinal patterns. Random patterns show up as a flat non-significant correlogram, diffusive patterns will have significantly positive values at short distances that tapers off to zero, and gradient patterns will have significantly positive values at short distances and significantly negative values at long distances.[5] Legendre and Fortin (1989) provide visual probes for patterns using various characteristics of the correlogram. The illustration using the `euthamia` data is:

```
test2 = correlog(x = euthamia$xloc, y = euthamia$yloc,
    z = euthamia$score, increment = 10)
plot(test2)
```

The first distance class is significantly positive and the estimated distance to which the local positive value decays to zero (the x-intercept) is 44 meters indicative of significant local similarity. There is further evidence of significantly negative auto-correlation at long distances suggestive of a gradient across the field (Fig. 13.3).

13.7 Nonparametric Spatial Correlation Functions

Finer resolution and confidence intervals can be found using the nonparametric spatial covariance function (Hall & Patil, 1994; Bjørnstad & Falck, 2001):

```
test3 = spline.correlog(x = euthamia$xloc, y = euthamia$yloc,
    z = euthamia$score, quiet = TRUE)

summary(test3)$estimate

    ##                   x          e          y
    ## estimate 36.53666 5.981457 0.5824953

summary(test3)$quantiles

    ##               x           e                y
    ## 0       17.82638  0.005531342 -0.003692403
    ## 0.025   27.34768  0.409260018  0.126207964
    ## 0.25    32.96260  3.119520264  0.295493112
    ## 0.5     36.03922  5.992822095  0.391821835
    ## 0.75    39.95760  8.451637015  0.517451204
    ## 0.975   44.19246 12.655055265  0.778859891
    ## 1       59.30986 15.005569404  1.200445017
```

The `spline.correlogram` returns a bunch of stuff; in fact all the summary statistics I thought might be of relevance in some previous spatial analyses (Bjørnstad & Falck, 2001). These are:

- `estimates`: A vector of benchmark statistics.

---

[5] Inhibitory processes such as the Janzen-Connell effect discussed in Sect. 12.4 will produce significantly negative values at short distances that tapers off.

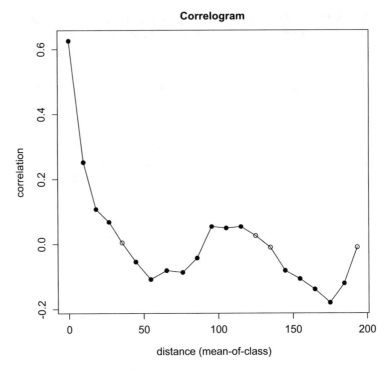

Fig. 13.3: The spatial correlogram for the `euthamia` rust data. Values that significantly deviates from that expected under the null hypothesis of complete spatial randomness are represented by filled black circles

- x: The lowest value at which the function is $= 0$.[6]
- e: The lowest value at which the function is $= 1/e$ (i.e., the spatial scale parameter in the presence of exponential or Gaussian spatial correlation; recall Sect. 12.2).
- y: The extrapolated value at $x = 0$.
- `quantiles`: A matrix summarizing the quantiles in the bootstrap distributions of the benchmark statistics. The 2.5- and 97.5-percentiles represent the 95% confidence interval.

```
plot(test3)
```

---

[6] If correlation is initially negative, the distance calculated appears as a negative measure. This may seem a little strange, but some locally inhibitory processes predict significant negative local auto- or cross-correlation (e.g., Seabloom et al., 2005).

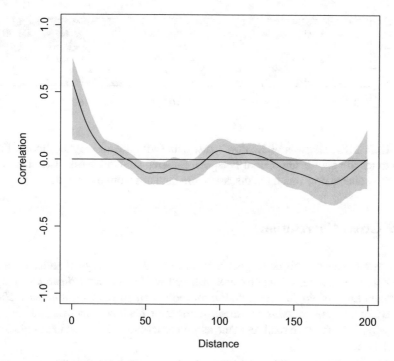

Fig. 13.4: The spline correlogram of the `euthamia` rust data. The grey polygon represents the 95% bootstrap confidence envelope

Figure 13.4 shows the estimated correlation function with its bootstrap 95% confidence envelope. The confidence envelope allows comparisons of correlation functions for different datasets to look for significant differences (Bjørnstad et al., 1999a).

13.8 LISA

The previous methods average across all locations to study how similarity depends on distance. Local indicators of spatial association (Anselin, 1995) quantify how similar observations are within neighborhoods of each observation. This can be used to test for significant spatial hot/cold-spots of disease (Fig. 13.5). For this we have to define the radius of the neighborhood. Spatial dependence in the `euthamia` data decay to zero at around 40m (Fig. 13.4), so we use 20 meters.

```
test4 = lisa(x = euthamia$yloc, y = euthamia$xloc,
      z = euthamia$score, neigh = 20)

plot(test4)
```

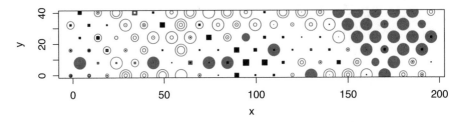

Fig. 13.5: LISA analysis of Koslow's rust data (with a 20m neighborhood). Filled red circles are significant spatial hotspots. Squares are cold-spots. The size of the symbols reflects how much the disease-score deviates from the mean

13.9 Cross-Correlations

Janis Antonovics and his colleagues have done roadside surveys of antler smut disease counting number of healthy and diseased wild campions (*Silene alba*) at the Mountain Lake Biological field station for more than 20 years (Antonovics, 2004). The `silene` data contains the mean number of healthy `$hmean` and diseased `$dmean` plants for each road segment, as well as latitude `$lat` and longitude `$lon` (Fig. 13.6).

```
data(silene)
symbols(silene$lon, silene$lat, circles = sqrt(silene$dmean),
    inches = 0.2, xlab = "Longitude", ylab = "Latitude")
```

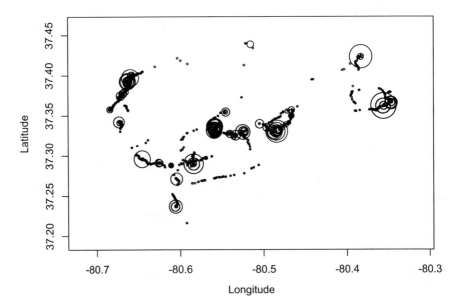

Fig. 13.6: Burden of antler smut on wild campion at the Mountain Lake field station (Antonovics, 2004)

Most geostatistical methods can be extended to consider spatial *cross*-correlation between different variables. As an example we can use the `silene` dataset to investigate if prevalence is spatially cross-correlated with abundance using the spline cross-correlogram (Fig. 13.7).

```
silene$ab = silene$dmean + silene$hmean
silene$prev = silene$dmean/(silene$dmean + silene$hmean)
```

The square-root transform of the abundance measure helps normalize the variance of the count data. There is significant positive cross-correlation within a 1 km range (95% CI: {0.6, 2.9} km) meaning that where the host tends to be abundant, the pathogen tends to be prevalent.

```
testcc = spline.correlog(x = silene$lon, y = silene$lat,
    z = silene$prev, w = sqrt(silene$ab), latlon = TRUE,
    na.rm = TRUE)
plot(testcc)
```

We can use a spatial cross-correlogram (using 25m distance increments) to study if presence/absence of rust is spatiotemporally cross-correlated between 1994 and 1995 in the filipendula dataset discussed in Sect. 12.3.

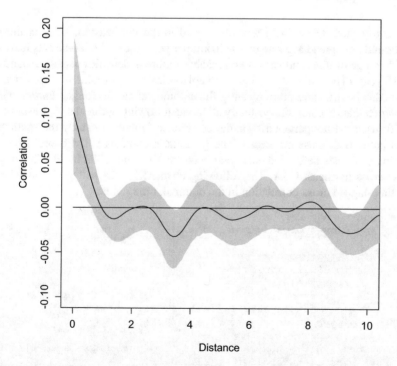

Fig. 13.7: Spatial cross-correlation of prevalence and abundance in the `silene` dataset

```
data(filip)
testcc2 = correlog(x = filip$X, y = filip$Y, z = filip$y94,
    w = filip$y95, increment = 25)
```

The local inter-year correlation (corr0) is 0.75 and the first cross-correlation is significantly positive with a cross-correlogram x-intercept of 148m:[7]

```
testcc2$corr0

  ## [1] 0.7651124

testcc2$x.intercept

  ## (Intercept)
  ##    148.939
```

Locations heavily affected in 1994 were thus also heavily affected in 1995 testifying to the importance of local contagion and/or habitat heterogeneity in infection risk. This is an example of a time-lagged cross-correlogram (Bjørnstad et al., 2002b).

13.10 Gypsy Moth

The gypsy moth (Sect. 12.5) was introduced to the northeastern USA in the late 1860s and has spread at a rate of 10–20 km per year since. The larvae eats leaves of a wide range of trees and shrubs and reaches outbreak densities usually around every 10 years. The outbreaks end through epizootics of the *Lymantria dispar* nuclear polyhedrosis virus and more recently the entomopathogenic fungus *Entomophaga maimaiga* that together kills virtually all larvae following outbreaks. Bjørnstad et al. (2010) used the nonparametric spatial covariance function to study the spatiotemporal patterns in these outbreaks. The gm dataset contains UTM coordinates and fraction of forests defoliated each year between 1975 and 2002 in 20×20 km grid cells across northeast USA. The following characterize the patterns of synchrony and time-lagged cross-correlation in the outbreak time series:

```
data(gypsymoth)
sel = apply(gypsymoth$defoliation[,2:28], 1, sum)!=0
#Synchrony:
fit1 = Sncf(gypsymoth$xy[sel, 1]/1000, gypsymoth$xy[sel, 2]/1000,
    gypsymoth$defoliation[sel, ], resamp = 500)
#Lag 1 cross-correlation
fit2 = Sncf(gypsymoth$xy[sel, 1]/1000, gypsymoth$xy[sel, 2]/1000,
    z = gypsymoth$defoliation[sel, 1:27],
    w = gypsymoth$defoliation[sel, 2:28], resamp = 500)
#Lag 2 cross-correlation
fit3 = Sncf(gypsymoth$xy[sel, 1]/1000, gypsymoth$xy[sel, 2]/1000,
    z = gypsymoth$defoliation[sel, 1:26],
    w = gypsymoth$defoliation[sel, 3:28], resamp = 500)
```

---

[7] The spline cross-correlogram would give bootstrap confidence intervals on these quantities.

The outbreaks are highly synchronized out to 200 km, with a regional average outbreak correlation of around 0.2. The time-lagged cross-correlogram show significant local cross-correlation at the 1-year lag but not 2-year lag, indicating that outbreaks tend to persist spatially for 2 years before collapsing (Fig. 13.8):

```
par(mfrow = c(1, 3))
plot(fit1, ylim = c(-0.1, 1))
title("Lag 0")
plot(fit2, ylim = c(-0.1, 1))
title("Lag 1")
plot(fit3, ylim = c(-0.1, 1))
title("Lag 2")
```

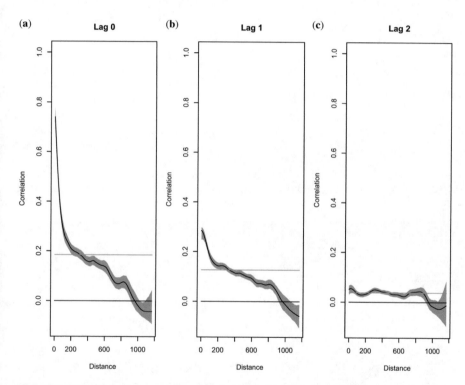

Fig. 13.8: The (a) nonparametric spatial covariance function, (b) lag one and (c) lag two cross-correlation function of gypsy moth outbreak data from northeastern USA between 1975 and 2002

Chapter 14
Transmission on Networks

14.1 Social Heterogeneities

Following the initial exploration of the simplest SIR model in Chap. 2, various chapters have explored a number of elaborations that are important in order to understand many aspects of infectious disease dynamics such as age-structure, seasonality, and more complex compartmental flows among individuals within a community. In addition to such heterogeneities which can be categorized according to covariates/cofactors (age, month, hospital versus community, etc.), there is often substantial variation that defies such classification. Lloyd-Smith et al. (2005), for example, identified significant heterogeneities from superspreading events during the 2003 SARS outbreak. Woolhouse et al. (1997) suggested a 80/20 rule-of-thumb: for many infections a core of 20% of infected accounts for 80% of onwards transmission. In various previous analyses (such as Chaps. 8 and 9) we obtained good fits to data using models that ignores such heterogeneities. This begs the question of what situations allow omission of such variabilities and what situations necessitate their inclusion. Highly transmissible acute directly transmitted pathogens may punch through most heterogeneities to conform more closely to homogenous epidemic models (Grenfell et al., 2006; Bansal et al., 2007). This chapter considers how one may use network models to think more carefully about social heterogeneities.

As an initial motivator we may consider the subset of the network of 749 sex-workers/clients from the survey from the so-called P90 project that mapped sexual contacts among 5,493 individuals in Colorado springs between 1988 and 1990. The study was motivated by the need to assess spread of STDs from risky sexual activities in the face of the then rising HIV pandemic (Klovdahl et al., 1994; Woodhouse et al., 1994). The cspring data on participation role in the network (cspring$role: 1=client, 2=worker, 3=both) and the 749-by-749

This chapter uses the following R packages: statnet and vioplot.
Five minute epidemics MOOC introductions to social networks are:
Structure of networks https://www.youtube.com/watch?v=hLwasjKxFoc
Networks and control https://www.youtube.com/watch?v=GBQqhtGAzGc

binary matrix (`cspring$cm`) mapping of contacts among the subset are included in the data list. The `statnet` package has comprehensive tools for network analysis and visualization for network data.

```
require(statnet)
data(cspring)
# convert contact matrix to network object
csnwrk = network(cspring$cm, matrix.type = "adjacency",
    directed = FALSE)
# set individual attributes to network
set.vertex.attribute(csnwrk, "role", cspring$nodes$type)
network.vertex.names(csnwrk) = c("client", "worker", "both")
plot(csnwrk, vertex.col = cspring$nodes$type)
legend("bottomleft", c("client", "worker", "both"), col = 1:3,
    pch = 21, pt.bg = 1:3)
```

Figure 14.1 uses the network plotting function in the `statnet` package to show contacts among the 749 individuals.

A key feature of a social network is the individual level heterogeneity in number of contacts, because it determines the "individual level reproduction number" (Lloyd-Smith et al., 2005) that socially underlies the emergence of 80/20-like phenomena.[1] The violin plot is a very useful visualization of distributional heterogeneities. Figure 14.2a shows the number of links of clients and workers. The workers have on average nearly 10 clients and clients just over two sex partners. Conspicuously, the distribution is heavily skewed. A small number of people has a disproportionate number of contacts (Fig. 14.2b).

```
require(vioplot)
par(mfrow = c(1, 2))
# violin plot
vioplot(apply(cspring$cm, 2, sum) ~ cspring$nodes$type,
    ylab = "partners", xlab = "(a)", h = 3)
legend("topleft", c("1: client", "2: worker", "3: both"),
    box.lty = 0)
# log-log plot
dd = table(apply(cspring$cm, 2, sum))
plot(as.numeric(names(dd)), dd, log = "xy", ylab = "frequency",
    xlab = "(b)")
```

14.2 S Preamble: Objects, Classes, and Functions

There is much coding throughout this monograph on infectious disease dynamics so it is useful to take a pause to visit a bit more formally on the programming. The S language which is the foundation of R was constructed using an object-based logic where each object is assigned a `class`. The class, in turn, controls printing,

---

[1] Though other heterogeneities like variability in infectiousness (e.g., Leynaert et al., 1998) and duration of the infectious period and long-term carriage (e.g., Brooks, 1996) are obviously very important additional contributing factors.

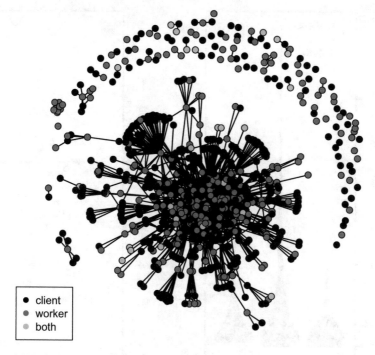

Fig. 14.1: A depiction of the Colorado springs sex worker and client network

plotting, and summarizing each object. There are many excellent introductions to
S programming (e.g., Venables & Ripley, 2013). This chapter uses basic S3 class
programming to streamline analysis of epidemics on networks. The basic idea is
this: if the result of some calculation is labeled as class foo, then R will look for
functions print.foo, summary.foo, and plot.foo functions in the search
path when further interacting with the result of the calculation. To illustrate with a
silly example:

```
foo = function(x) {
    res = x
    class(res) = "foo"
    return(res)
}

print.foo = function(x) {
    cat("foo is:\n", x)
}

summary.foo = function(x) {
    cat("In summary, foo is:\n", x)
}

plot.foo = function(x) {
```

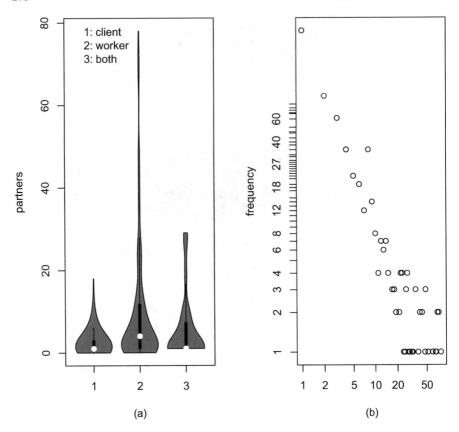

Fig. 14.2: Contact distribution in the Colorado springs sex worker and client network. (**a**) Violin plot of number of sexual partners for each category. (**b**) Log-log
plot of frequency of number of sexual partners across the network

```
plot(NA, type = "n", ylim = c(0, 1), xlim = c(0, 1),
    ylab = "")
text(x = seq(0.1, 0.9, by = 0.1), y = seq(0.1, 0.9,
    by = 0.1), as.character(x))
}
```

The result is a fully functional S3 class of R objects:[2]

<hr>

[2] Though, for a disseminated `plot` function there should be an opportunity for user customization
through a ... argument:

plot.foo=function(x, ...){
args.default=list(xlab = "x", ylab = "y", ylim = c(0,1),
xlim = c(0,1))
args.input=list(...)
args=c(args.default[!names(args.default) %in% names(args.input)], args.input)
do.call(plot, c(list(NA, type = "n"), args))

```
zz = foo("pibble")
```

which can print,

```
zz
```

```
## foo is:
##   pibble
```

summarize,

```
summary(zz)
```

```
## In summary, foo is:
##   pibble
```

and plot (Fig. 14.3):

```
plot(zz)
```

And that is the very basics of S3 class programming.

14.3 Networks

Transmission on social networks bears conceptual similarities to spatial transmission. The difference being that in spatial models transmission occurs among neighbors in space, and transmission on networks occurs among neighbors in social space. We can thus use the type of compact code used for CML models (Sect. 12.6) to simulate epidemics on networks. Two key determinants of invasibility and speed of spread are the average and the variance (*viz.* Fig. 14.2) in the number of contacts on a network (Newman, 2002; Keeling & Eames, 2005; Bansal et al., 2007). As we saw in the network of spread of gonorrhea (Sect. 3.8) and the Colorado springs network (Sect. 14.1) there is often substantial variation in the number of social contacts due to variation in individual behavior. Recall also Sect. 4.3 which highlighted strong age-specific variation in contact rates. Social networks tend to change over time because of seasonal behavioral changes (Eames et al., 2011); however, for this chapter it is easiest to consider the static network—networks for which contact patterns do not change during the duration of an epidemics—and for which the contact pattern is more easily characterized by the degree distribution (e.g., Fig. 14.2b) in which contacts are mapped as edges, and individuals are nodes.[3] The degree of an individual is its number of edges in the network.

```
text(x = seq(0.1, 0.9, by = 0.1), y = seq(0.1, 0.9, by = 0.1),
as.character(x))}
plot(zz, xlab="stupid plot", xlim=c(-0.1, 0.8)).
```

[3] The `statnet` family of packages (Handcock et al., 2008) have methods for considering dynamic networks.

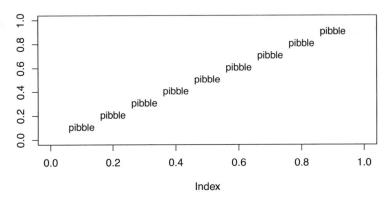

Fig. 14.3: A plot of objects of class foo

14.4 Models of Networks

In the previous spatial coupled map lattice models (Sect. 12.6), transmission was assumed restricted to the eight nearest neighbors on the lattice, so we can think of this as an example of a network with a fixed degree of 8. In network theory, an analogous fixed degree network is constructed as a ring lattice. The associated matrix that flags neighbors is a particular type of Toeplitz matrix. We can define a ringlattice function to generate such networks with N nodes and 2K degrees. Employing the S3 class logic label the result to be of class cm (short for contact matrix):

```
ringlattice = function(N, K) {
    # N is the number of nodes K is the number of
    # neighbors on each side to which each node is
    # connected so degree = 2K
    CM = toeplitz(c(0, rep(1, K), rep(0, N - 2 * K - 1),
        rep(1, K)))
    class(CM) = "cm"
    return(CM)
}
```

To further illustrate S3 class programming, the plot.cm function uses basic trigonometry to visualize a ring network or any other object that is defined as class cm. The following function lays nodes out in a circle and connect them by their mutual edges.

```
plot.cm = function(CM){
    N = dim(CM)[1]
    theta = seq(0, 2 * pi, length = N + 1)
    x = cos(theta[1:N])
    y = sin(theta[1:N])
    symbols(x, y, fg = 0, circles = rep(1, N),
```

```
        inches = 0.1, bg = 1, xlab = "", ylab = "", axes = FALSE)
    segx1 = as.vector(matrix(x, ncol = length(x),
        nrow = length(x), byrow = TRUE))
    segx2 = as.vector(matrix(x, ncol = length(x),
        nrow = length(x), byrow = FALSE))
    segy1 = as.vector(matrix(y, ncol = length(x),
        nrow = length(x), byrow = TRUE))
    segy2 = as.vector(matrix(y, ncol = length(x),
        nrow = length(x), byrow = FALSE))
    segments(segx1, segy1, segx2,
        segy2, lty = as.vector(CM))
}
```

Figure 14.4a depicts a ring lattice with 20 individuals and a fixed degree of four. In network science there are a number of important models of connectivity.

```
cm = ringlattice(N = 20, K = 2)
plot(cm)
```

Watts-Strogatz Networks: Real life social networks typically have heterogeneities in contact rates and usually exhibit much lower social separation than predicted by the ring lattice. In the study of small-world networks, Watts and Strogatz (1998) proposed an algorithm for generating more realistic networks by randomly rewiring a fraction Prw of the edges of a ring lattice.

```
wattsStrogatz = function(N, K, Prw) {
    # Build a Watts-Strogatz contact matrix from a
    # ring lattice, Prw is the rewiring probability
    CM = ringlattice(N = N, K = K)
    CMWS = CM
    tri = CM[upper.tri(CM)]
    Br = rbinom(length(tri), 1, Prw)  # Break edges
    a = 0
    for (i in 1:(N - 1)) {
        for (j in (i + 1):N) {
            a = a + 1
            if (Br[a] == 1 & CMWS[i, j] == 1) {
                # If 'Br == 1'
                CMWS[i, j] = CMWS[j, i] = 0  # break edge
                tmp = i
                tmp2 = c(i, which(CMWS[i, ] == 1))
                # new edge, if already present try
                # again
                while (any(tmp2 == tmp)) {
                    tmp = ceiling(N * runif(1))
                }
                CMWS[i, tmp] = CMWS[tmp, i] = 1  # make new edge
            }
        }
    }
}
```

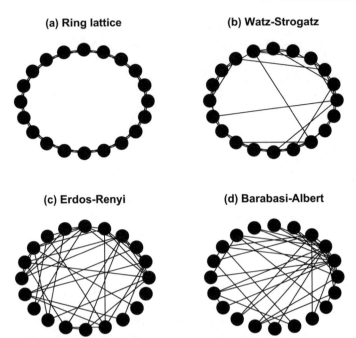

(a) Ring lattice   **(b) Watz-Strogatz**

(c) Erdos-Renyi   **(d) Barabasi-Albert**

Fig. 14.4: Contact matrix plots of 20 node networks of degree 4. (**a**) A ring lattice,
(**b**) a Watts-Strogatz small-world network, (**c**) an Erdős-Rényi random network, and
(**d**) a Barabási-Reka scale-free network

```
        class(CMWS) = "cm"
        return(CMWS)
}
```

Figure 14.4b depicts a Watts-Strogatz network with 20 individuals, a mean degree
of 4 and a rewiring probability of 0.3.

```
cm2 = wattsStrogatz(N = 20, K = 2, Prw = 0.3)
plot(cm2)
```

We can extend the notion of writing generic functions for class cm objects, to define a summary function that calculates and optionally plots (Fig. 14.5) the degree
distribution.

```
summary.cm = function(x, plot = FALSE) {
    x = table(apply(x, 2, sum))
    res = data.frame(n = x)
    names(res) = c("degree", "freq")
    if (plot)
        barplot(x, xlab = "degree")
    return(res)
}
```

```
cm2b = wattsStrogatz(N = 20,  K = 4,  Prw = 0.3)
summary(cm2b, plot = TRUE)

  ##   degree freq
  ## 1       6    1
  ## 2       7    5
  ## 3       8    8
  ## 4       9    5
  ## 5      10    1
```

The Watts-Strogatz model can scale the degree distribution of theoretical networks from the fixed (ring lattice) through small-world (low, but non-zero rewiring) through to the Erdős-Rényi random graph (Fig. 14.4c) when the rewiring probability is one (Erdős & Rényi, 1959). The random graph corresponds to a network with completely unstructured contact patterns and has a Poisson distributed degree distribution. The small-world networks (Fig. 14.4b) highlight how a few connections across a ring lattice will greatly reduce the overall social distancing among individuals.

Barabási-Albert Networks: The Watts-Strogatz model can at most have Poisson-like variance in degree distribution, so it cannot mimic heavy-tailed distributions seen in many empirical networks. Barabási and Albert (1999) proposed that such behavior arises from preferential attachment (rich-get-richer) dynamics. A function that generates a scale-free network with N nodes and mean degree $2K$ is:

```
barabasiAlbert = function(N, K) {
    CM = matrix(0, ncol = N, nrow = N)
    CM[1, 2] = 1
```

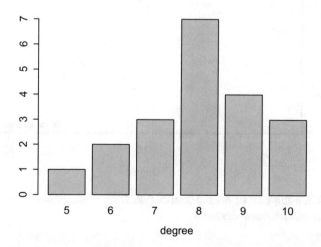

Fig. 14.5: The degree distribution of the Watts-Strogatz network with 20 individuals, a mean degree of 8 and a rewiring probability of 0.3 as generated by the summary(..., plot=TRUE) function

```
CM[2, 1] = 1
for (i in 3:N) {
    probs = apply(CM, 1, sum)
    link = unique(sample(c(1:N)[-i], size = min(c(K,
        i - 1)), prob = probs[-i]))
    CM[i, link] = CM[link, i] = 1
}
class(CM) = "cm"
return(CM)
}
```

Figure 14.4d shows a scale-free network among 20 individuals with mean degree 4. To better visualize the power law heterogeneity in contacts predicted by the Barabási-Albert model Fig. 14.6 shows a log-log plot for 200 individuals with a mean degree of 8.

```
cm3 = barabasiAlbert(200, 4)
ed = summary(cm3)
plot(as.numeric(ed$degree), ed$freq, log = "xy", xlab = "Degree",
    ylab = "Frequency")
```

For large networks the plotting functions in the statnet package introduced in Sect. 14.1 provides fancier visualization. The network function in the statnet

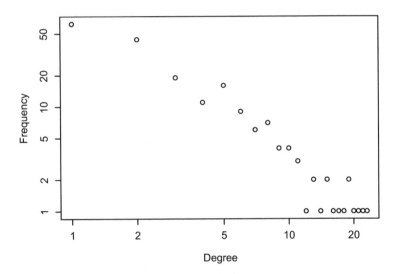

Fig. 14.6: A log-log plot of degree distribution from a Barabási-Albert network of 200 individuals with mean degree 8

package converts the contact matrix (of class cm) to a plottable network class object (Fig. 14.7).

```
require(statnet)
plot(network(cm3, directed = FALSE))
```

14.5 Epidemics on Networks

SIR-like epidemics can be simulated across networks by assuming that an infection is transmitted across an S–I edge with a probability, τ, per time step (Barbour & Mollison, 1990; Ferrari et al., 2006a). Following the Reed-Frost version of the chain-binomial model (Abbey, 1952), the probability of any given susceptible becoming infected in a given serial interval is $p = 1 - (1 - \tau)^y$ where y is the number of infected neighbors. If infected are removed with a constant probability, γ, the infectious period will be geometrically distributed. The `sirNetmod` function will simulate a closed SIR epidemic on arbitrary contact matrices and return an object of class `netSir`.

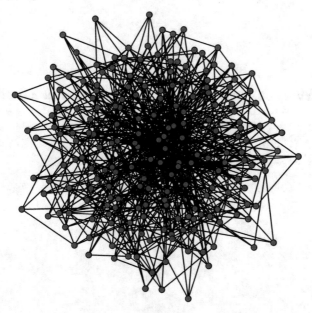

Fig. 14.7: Visualization of a Barabási-Albert network among 200 individuals with mean degree 8 using the `statnet` package

```
sirNetmod = function(CM, tau, gamma) {
    # generate SIR epidemic on a CM-network CM =
    # contact matrix tau = probability of infection
    # across an edge gamma = probability of removal
```

```
# per time step
N = dim(CM)[1]
I = matrix(rep(0, N), nrow = N, ncol = 1)    #First infecteds
S = matrix(rep(1, N), nrow = N, ncol = 1)    #First susceptibles
R = matrix(rep(0, N), nrow = N, ncol = 1)    #First removed
I1 = sample(1:N, size = 1)   #Pick first random infected
I[I1, 1] = 1
S[I1, 1] = 0
t = 1
while (sum(I[, t - 1]) > 0 | t == 1) {
    t = t + 1
    infneigh = CM %*% I[, t - 1]
    pinf = 1 - (1 - tau)^infneigh
    newI = rbinom(N, S[, t - 1], pinf)
    newR = rbinom(N, I[, t - 1], gamma)
    nextS = S[, t - 1] - newI
    nextI = I[, t - 1] + newI - newR
    nextR = R[, t - 1] + newR
    I = cbind(I, nextI)
    S = cbind(S, nextS)
    R = cbind(R, nextR)
}
res = list(I = I, S = S, R = R)
class(res) = "netSir"
return(res)
}
```

The summary.netSir and plot.netSir functions for the netSir class are:

```
summary.netSir = function(x){
    t = dim(x$S)[2]
    S = apply(x$S, 2, sum)
    I = apply(x$I, 2, sum)
    R = apply(x$R, 2, sum)
    res = data.frame(S = S, I = I, R = R)
    return(res)
}

plot.netSir = function(x){
    y = summary(x)
    plot(y$S, type = "b", xlab = "time", ylab = "", ylim = range(y))
    lines(y$I, type = "b", col = "red")
    lines(y$R, type = "b", col = "blue")
    legend("left", legend = c("S", "I", "R"),
        lty = c(1, 1, 1), pch = c(1, 1, 1),
        col = c("black", "red", "blue"))
}
```

Figure 14.8 shows stochastic epidemic spread on scale-free, Watts-Strogatz, random, and ring lattice networks.

```
cm1 = barabasiAlbert(N = 200, K = 2)
cm2 = wattsStrogatz(N = 200, K = 2, Prw = 0.1)
```

```
cm3 = wattsStrogatz(N = 200, K = 2, Prw = 1)
cm4 = ringlattice(N = 200, K = 2)
sim1 = sirNetmod(cm1, 0.3, 0.1)
sim2 = sirNetmod(cm2, 0.3, 0.1)
sim3 = sirNetmod(cm3, 0.3, 0.1)
sim4 = sirNetmod(cm4, 0.3, 0.1)
plot(apply(sim1$I, 2, sum), type = "l", xlab = "Time",
    ylab = "Infected")
lines(apply(sim2$I, 2, sum), type = "l", col = "red")
lines(apply(sim3$I, 2, sum), type = "l", col = "red",
    lty = 2)
lines(apply(sim4$I, 2, sum), type = "l", col = "blue")
legend("topright", legend = c("RL", "WS(0.1)", "ER", "BA"),
    lty = c(1, 2, 1, 1), col = c("blue", "red", "red",
        "black"))
```

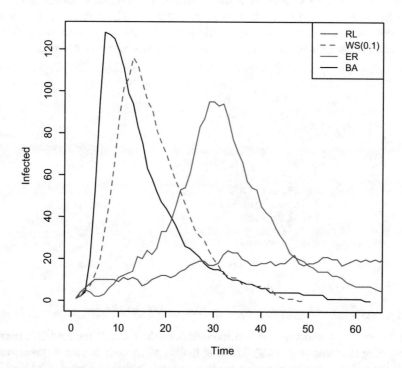

Fig. 14.8: Simulated stochastic epidemics on mean degree 4 ring lattice, Watts-Strogatz, Erdős-Rényi and Barabási-Reka networks

14.6 Epidemic Size Distribution

As analyzed in Sect. 2.4, the closed epidemic SIR model predicts the fraction of
individuals likely to be infected during the course of an outbreak in a randomly
mixed population. Given such mixing this fraction is substantial even for a moderate R_0 with the approximate expectation that only $\exp(-R_0)$ will escape infection.
However, as alluded to in Sect. 3.8 this final epidemic size prediction is strongly
dependent on the random mixing assumptions. Also as discussed in Sect. 9.2, even
randomly mixing supercritical ($R_0 > 1$) infections can stochastically burn out during the early phase of an emergence leading to a bimodal size distribution of either
a minor stutter or a major outbreak. From a probabilistic point of view this was
discussed already in Bailey's (1957) and Bartlett's (1960a) treatises on infectious
disease dynamics.

House et al. (2013) provide a useful overview of various mathematical approaches to understanding epidemic size distributions. The netSirmod function
provides a simple tool to look at stochastic epidemic size distributions in the face of
the various conceptualizations of social heterogeneities introduced above.

```
fs = matrix(NA, ncol = 4, nrow = 1000)
for (i in 1:1000) {
    cm4 = ringlattice(N = 200, K = 2)
    cm3 = wattsStrogatz(N = 200, K = 2, Prw = 0.1)
    cm2 = wattsStrogatz(N = 200, K = 2, Prw = 1)
    cm1 = barabasiAlbert(N = 200, K = 2)
    sim1 = sirNetmod(cm4, 0.15, 0.1)
    sim2 = sirNetmod(cm3, 0.15, 0.1)
    sim3 = sirNetmod(cm2, 0.15, 0.1)
    sim4 = sirNetmod(cm1, 0.15, 0.1)
    fs[i, 1] = tail(summary(sim1), 1)[1, 3]
    fs[i, 2] = tail(summary(sim2), 1)[1, 3]
    fs[i, 3] = tail(summary(sim3), 1)[1, 3]
    fs[i, 4] = tail(summary(sim4), 1)[1, 3]
}
fs = data.frame(fs)
names(fs) = c("RL", "WS", "ER", "BA")
require(vioplot)
vioplot(fs/200, h = 0.3, ylab = "Final size", main = "")
```

The difference in epidemic size distributions is marked despite the epidemic parameters being the same (Fig. 14.9). The ring lattice, which only has local connections,
tends to produce smaller outbreaks due to the probabilistic build-up of local herd immunity (Ferrari et al., 2006a). The small-world Watts-Strogatz network has distinct
bimodal behavior that reflects how epidemics will either die out early through local
herd immunity unless it transmits across small-world bridges to percolate further
across the network. Random networks and scale-free networks tend to experience
major outbreaks affecting most of the population with the exception of a few chains
that experience early stochastic breaks. Thus supercritical ($R_0 > 1$) stochastic epidemics will either stutter early or progress close to the final epidemic size predicted
by the deterministic model (Sect. 2.4).

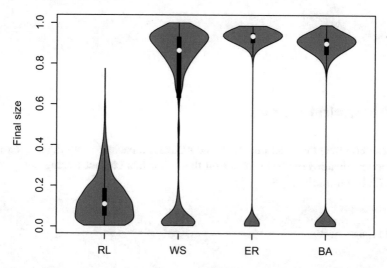

Fig. 14.9: Violin plots of the epidemic size distribution on 200 node networks of degree 4 with a transmission probability τ of 0.15 and a recovery probability γ of 0.1. Ring lattice (RL), Watts-Strogatz (WS) small-world network, Erdős-Rényi (ER) random network, and Barabási-Reka (BA) scale-free network

The difference in the mean size of the major epidemics of Fig. 14.9 as well as the difference in acuteness of spread depicted in Fig. 14.8 can be understood in terms of how network geometry molds R_0 even when all else (including transmission τ and recovery γ probabilities, and mean number of contacts) is constant. For network SIR models, like those introduced above, R_0 and thus spread of infections depends on both mean number of contacts $\overline{K}$ and heterogeneity in that number (quantified by $\overline{K^2}$) according to $R_0 = (\tau/(\tau+\gamma))(\overline{K^2} - \overline{K})/\overline{K})$ (Bansal et al., 2007). The term $(\overline{K^2} - \overline{K})/\overline{K}$ may be thought of as the inflation factor to the reproduction number due to the heterogeneities in social contacts. The `r0fun` function calculates R_0 for any given network. The greater the heterogeneity, the greater the cross-network reproduction number:

```
r0fun = function(CM, tau, gamma) {
    x = apply(CM, 2, sum)
    (tau/(tau + gamma)) * (mean(x^2) - (mean(x)))/mean(x)
}
r0fun(cm1, 0.3, 0.1) #BA

  ## [1] 5.138539

r0fun(cm2, 0.3, 0.1) #ER

  ## [1] 2.325

r0fun(cm3, 0.3, 0.1) #WS

  ## [1] 2.859375
```

```
r0fun(cm4, 0.3, 0.1) #RL
```

```
  ## [1] 2.25
```

14.7 Empirical Networks

One can combine the functionality of the `statnet` package with the above results
on network heterogeneity to revisit on the gonorrhea contact tracing study of De
et al. (2004) from Sect. 3.8.

```
data(gonnet)
nwt = network(gonnet, directed = TRUE)
x = degree(nwt)[2:89]
mean(x)
```

```
  ## [1] 1.920455
```

The mean degree is 1.92, but the inflation factor due to the network heterogeneity is
predicted to almost double the R_0 of a STD spreading across this network:

```
(mean(x^2) - (mean(x)))/mean(x)
```

```
  ## [1] 1.940828
```

To simulate an epidemic on the empirical contact tracing study from Sect. 3.8, we
first have to construct an undirected contact network among the 89 members and
next apply the `sirNetmod` model to plot a plausible stochastic time trajectory and
final infection status across the network:

```
# Undirected network
cmg = gonnet + t(gonnet)
# Simulate epidemic
cep = sirNetmod(cmg, tau = 0.3, gamma = 0.1)
sm = summary(cep)
par(mfrow = c(1, 2))
inf = ifelse(apply(cep$I, 1, sum) > 0, 2, 1)
nwt = network(cmg, directed = FALSE)
plot(nwt, vertex.col = inf)
matplot(sm, ylab = "Numbers")
legend("right", c("S", "I", "R"), pch = c("1", "2", "3"),
    col = c(1, 2, 3))
```

The simulated epidemic across the network (Fig. 14.10) reveals the feature that the
core group is likely to always be infected but peripheral individuals may escape infection by getting surrounded by removed individuals before getting exposed. Ferrari et al. (2006a) discuss how the geometry of a network shapes the likelihood of a
given individual escaping infection.

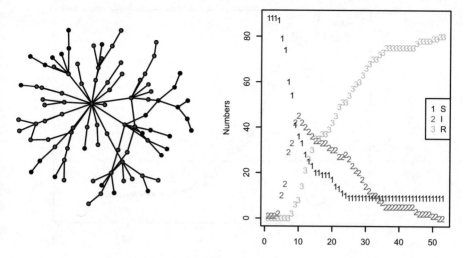

Fig. 14.10: A simulated closed epidemic on the gonorrhea contact tracing network (De et al., 2004). (**a**) Network infection history (red nodes = infected, black nodes = escapees). (**b**) Outbreak trajectory

To consider such effects more carefully, we can simulate an epidemic on the Colorado Springs network introduced in Sect. 14.1 and investigate the average degree (i.e., mean number of social links) of the infected individuals during the course of the simulation.

```
data(cspring)
csepi = sirNetmod(cspring$cm, 0.2, 0.1)
# which(csepi$I[,1] == 1): 415, degree=1 Number
# infected
inf = apply(csepi$I, 2, sum, na.rm = TRUE)
# Mean degree of infected
deg = apply(cspring$cm, 2, sum, na.rm = TRUE)
csepi$I[csepi$I == 0] = NA
mdeg = apply(csepi$I * deg, 2, mean, na.rm = TRUE)
symbols(x = 1:length(inf), y = inf, circles = mdeg, inches = 0.2,
    ylab = "I", xlab = "time")
legend("topleft", pch = 21, "mean\n degree")
```

If the first infected is at the periphery of the social network, the initial mean degree is low but it quickly explodes as the infection reaches an individual in the social core that results in accelerated dissemination among high-degree individuals (Fig. 14.11). The epidemic retreat is associated with transmission among less sociable individuals and, thus, a much reduced mean degree because the high-degree individuals were differentially depleted from the susceptible pool early on.

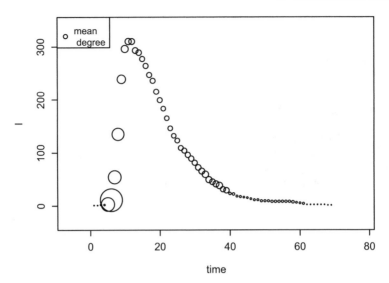

Fig. 14.11: A simulated trajectory of the average degree of infected individuals for a stochastically realized epidemic on the Colorado Springs network (Klovdahl et al., 1994; Woodhouse et al., 1994) with a per edge transmission probability $\tau = 0.2$ and per node recovery probability $\gamma = 0.1$ in a case where the random index case is in the periphery of the social network. Circle size is proportional to mean degree

14.8 Vaccinating Networks

Using social considerations for control of infectious diseases has a centuries long history, at least starting from the implementation of "quarantining"—the 40-day isolation of seamen on their ships before disembarkation—in the fifteenth century Italy in the wake of the black death. The complete lockdown of the city of Wuhan on 23 January 2020 in response to early spread of SARS-CoV-2 (Tian et al., 2020) is a recent example of attempted socio-spatial control of disease spread. Ring vaccination, a spatial network intervention, was used extensively to create immunological cordon sanitaire during the final years of smallpox eradication during which villages would be targeted as soon as a case was discovered (Henderson & Klepac, 2013). Cocooning—the idea of vaccinating all family members of at-risk children too young for immunization—is a social network intervention recommended to protect against whooping cough (e.g., Lavine et al., 2011).

In addition to these applications, there are multitudes of mathematical and computational studies on using social network consideration to think about vaccination strategies and vaccination deployment (Holme & Litvak, 2017). One amusing idea is "acquaintance vaccination" in the face of limited medical supply: pick random individuals in a network and ask them to identify a friend to be vaccinated. A friend of a random individual is likely to have a higher social connectivity and thus be more likely to contribute to onwards spread. A slightly less esoteric idea is to try to use social engineering of vaccine sentiments across a network. Fu et al. (2011) discussed this as "imitation dynamics", a form of social diffusion, where positive (or negative) opinions and adoption practices may spread to help toward herd immunity for voluntary vaccine programs. Sociologists have discussed how such dynamics depends on network homophily: The extent to which individuals with similar views assort preferentially. With strong assortment, diffusion of ideas and sentiments will be weak whereas with weak assortment influencers may sway general opinions. Homophily seems to have been an important factor during the SARS-CoV-2 spread in 2020–21 in the USA for which there was limited cross-talk among vaccine positive and vaccine skeptic segments of the population.

Models of networks and epidemics on networks are a vast literature, so the above should at best be considered a teaser. For example, it only considers static networks without births, deaths, or social reconfiguration. It does also not consider network modularity (Newman, 2006). Homophily is an obvious social process that leads to highly modular networks. The statnet project and associated `statnet` package have a rich set of resources for deeper explorations.

Chapter 15
Invasion and Eradication

15.1 Invasion

Pathogens invade new host niches all the time. The global invasion of the human niche by SARS-CoV-2 during the 2020–22 pandemic is the most recent example, but cross-species transmission is ubiquitous. In 2009 Influenza A/H1N1pdm09 emerged and spread globally most likely after a triple recombination of human, avian, and porcine viral segments (Smith et al., 2009a). The HIV-1 pandemic started in the mid-twentieth century probably from bushmeat spillover of chimpanzee simian immun-odeficiency virus, which itself is thought to have originated from spillovers from other primates, to go global in the 1970s (Hemelaar, 2012). Cross-species trans-mission is not just an issue of zoonotic spillover or anthropogenic spillback, it is equally important as spillover among animal species. Among the paramyxoviruses, Taber and Pease (1990) discuss how tissue tropism generally change more slowly than host specificity so that host switching is often more constrained by tissue sim-ilarity than host species identity. Phocine distemper virus, for example, is endemic to harp seals in the high arctic but have at least twice (in 1988 and 2002) invaded harbor seal populations of the North sea to cause catastrophic mortality (Hall et al., 2006).

Lloyd-Smith et al. (2009) provide a comprehensive classification of cross-species establishment of infectious diseases and thus invasion that recognizes three key stages:

- Stage II: Primary spillover wherein a pathogen cross the species border but with no onwards transmission in the secondary host. Human cases of old- and new-world hantaviruses, Bolivian hemorrhagic arenavirus fever, and Junin arenavirus are all exemplars of this.

This chapter uses the following R packages: scatterplot3d, raster, gdistance, maptools, rgdal, maps and ncf.
A five minute epidemics MOOC on spatial spread can be seen on YouTube: https://www.youtube.com/watch?v=WPjsAdyD1Gg

© The Author(s), under exclusive license to Springer Nature Switzerland AG 2023
O. N. Bjørnstad, *Epidemics*, Use R!, https://doi.org/10.1007/978-3-031-12056-5_15

- Stage III: Subcritical (i.e., $R_0 < 1$) establishment results in stuttering chains of transmission. Lassa fever virus for which Iacono et al. (2015) estimated that about 20% of cases are human-to-human and the rest are spillover from the multimammate mouse (*Mastomys natalensis*) is a good example. So also is another rodent-borne infection, monkey pox, for which Blumberg and Lloyd-Smith (2013b) estimated a human-to-human R_0 of 0.3 that has recently risen to 0.8. Other notorious examples are the Nipah virus and avian influenzas (Lloyd-Smith et al., 2009).
- Stage IV represents supercritical ($R_0 > 1$) establishment. To refine Lloyd-Smith et al.'s (2009) classification, it may be useful to distinguish type IVa which causes epidemics with failure of long-term establishment from type IVb which causes long-term endemism in the derived host. HIV, influenza A/H1N1pdm09, and SARS-CoV-2 are examples of the latter. In humans, Ebola and yellow fever are examples of the former. On the animal-to-animal side, phocine distemper virus (PDV) in harbor seals is an interesting example where outbreaks are so violent that the pathogen burns out of susceptibles to result in IVa dynamics.[1]

15.2 Stage III Branching Processes

The final epidemic size of Stage III subcritical spillover (sometimes called "cluster size") is usually modeled as a Galton-Watson branching process (Farrington et al., 2003). The model is quite general and can flexibly accommodate within-population heterogeneities (Blumberg & Lloyd-Smith, 2013b). For illustrative purposes we may consider the simplest case of subcritical spread in a homogenous host population. With homogeneity and assuming the population is sufficient large that susceptible depletion will not affect the stuttering chain, the offspring distribution (the number of onwards infected per infected) during a serial interval will follow a Poisson distribution with a mean of R_0 and the outbreak size distribution, O, will follow a Borel-Tanner distribution that depends on the initial number of infected, i_0 according to:

$$P(O = x | i_0) = \frac{i_0 x^{x-i_0-1} R_0^{x-i_0} e^{-xR_0}}{(x - i_0)!} \tag{15.1}$$

In addition to Stage III spillover, this model also applies to seeding of new chains from supercritical communities to communities that, through interventions, have achieved control. This was the case among areas of lockdown, partial lockdown, and no interventions during the early SARS-CoV-2 pandemic.[2] For illustration consider the predicted outbreak size distribution from an initial i_0 of five individuals in communities with subcritical R_0s of 0.5, 0.7 and 0.9:

---

[1] A kin to the failure of persistence of measles in human communities below the critical community size (Bartlett, 1960b; Grenfell & Harwood, 1997, Sect. 1.3).

[2] Engen et al. (2021) discuss an alternative diffusion approximation approach to study this issue.

```
R0 = 0.5
x = 1:50
i0 = 5
plot(i0 * x^(x - i0 - 1) * R0^(x - i0) *
    exp(-x * R0)/factorial(x - i0), xlab="Outbreak size",
    ylab="Probability", type="p")
R0 = 0.7
points(i0 * x^(x - i0 - 1) * R0^(x - i0) *
    exp(-x * R0)/factorial(x - i0), pch = 2)
R0 = 0.9
points(i0 * x^(x - i0 - 1) * R0^(x - i0) *
    exp(-x * R0)/factorial(x-i0), pch=3)
legend("topright", c("0.5", "0.7", "0.9"), pch = 1:3)
```

For these scenarios, some onwards transmissions are clearly happening with a cluster size mode of seven in the first scenario and 10 in the last scenario, but there is still a chance of seeing almost 20 cases in the former and 50 cases in the latter (Fig. 15.1).

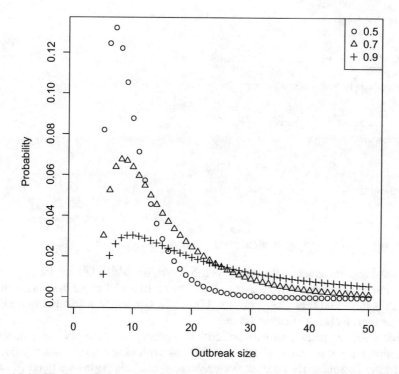

Fig. 15.1: Final epidemic size distributions predicted from the Galton-Watson branching process assuming a Poisson distributed offspring distribution and sub-critical spread with R_0s of 0.5, 0.7, and 0.9

Farrington and Grant (1999) used the branching process model to also study the distribution of lengths of stuttering chains. With the Poisson offspring distribution and a single introduction they derived that the probability that the chain will be shorter-or-equal to k generations (i.e., serial intervals) is:

$$f_k = P(G \leq k) \sim e^{-R_0} E_k(e^{R_0 e^{-R_0}}), \tag{15.2}$$

where $E_k(x)$ is the "iterated exponential function", $x^{x^{x \cdots}}$. So the interpretation of f_k is the cumulative probability of shortness. The distribution with i_0 introductions follows $f_k^{i_0}$. As a worked example the chain-length probability depends on i_0 for a pathogen with $R_0 = 0.9$ according to:

```
# Iterated exponential
Ek = function(k, x) {
    out = rep(NA, k + 1)
    out[1] = 1
    for (i in 2:(k + 1)) {
        out[i] = x^(out[i - 1])
    }
    return(out)
}


# cumulative from single introduction
R0 = 0.9
fk = exp(-R0) * (Ek(20, exp(R0 * exp(-R0))))[-1])
i0 = 1
# uncumulate
g = c(fk[1]^i0, diff(fk^i0))
plot(g, ylab = "Probability", xlab = "Length", log = "y",
    pch = 16)
# loop from 1 to 10 introductions
for (i0 in 1:10) {
    g = c(fk[1]^i0, diff(fk^i0))
    lines(g)
}
points(g, pch = 17)
legend("topright", c("1", "10"), pch = 16:17)
```

With a single introduction the modal length is one, but with a fair chance of getting secondary and maybe tertiary cases. With five or 10 initial cases the modal chain length is three and seven, respectively (Fig. 15.2). Obviously, a smaller R_0 leads to shorter typical chains of transmission.

For emerging pathogens with pericritical reproduction numbers above one, we sometimes see bimodal epidemic distributions with either minor clusters due to stochastic fadeout early on or major epidemics. Ebola is perhaps a good illustration with most of the several dozen reported outbreaks being small but two recent outbreaks in West Africa (2014–2015) and DRC (2016–2018) reaching into the thousands. Bailey (1957) and Bartlett (1960a) were among the first to study this bimodality from a theoretical point of view. This bimodality is also clearly seen in the predicted stochastic spread on social networks discussed in Sect. 14.6.

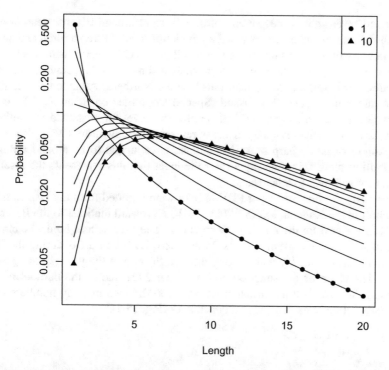

Fig. 15.2: Chain-length distributions predicted from the Galton-Watson branching process assuming a Poisson distributed offspring distribution and subcritical spread with $R_0 = 0.9$ and size of initial introduction varying from one to 10

15.3 Phocine Distemper Virus

There are two particularly well documented stage IVa animal-to-animal supercritical spillovers of PDV from arctic harp seals (*Pagophilus groenlandicus*) to North Sea harbor seals (*Phoca vitulina*) and grey seals (*Halichoerus grypus*) in 1998 and 2002. Using the type of next-generation formalism of structured transmission discussed in Sects. 3.9 and 10.7, Klepac et al. (2009) estimated the reproduction number in harbor seals during the invasion to be in the 2–2.5 range. Like other morbilliviruses, PDV causes mortality or lifelong immunity in its hosts. Thus, like for measles, susceptible recruitment through birth is critical for sustaining chains of transmission.[3] In prevaccination USA and UK the measles critical community size was around 300–500k (Fig. 1.2; see also Bartlett, 1960b; Grenfell & Harwood, 1997), which with a typical birth rate in these countries of around 20 births per thousand per year indicates that an annual recruitment of around 10k newborns is necessary to sustain local transmission. During 1920–40, New York city had a population size

---

[3] Though there are Cetacean morbilliviruses documented from rare species of toothed whales which mode of persistence is not understood (Van Bressem et al., 2014).

of around seven million people and birth cohorts of around 91k per year. London during the mid-twentieth century had a population size of three million and annual birth cohorts of 45k, so both cities were well above CCS recruitment levels. As a consequence both cities harbored violent sustained recurrent epidemics (Fig. 1.4).

Harbor seal communities ("haul-outs") in the Northeast Atlantic have numbers in the hundreds to several thousand (Special Commitee on Seals, 2002), so pup production is way under the critical recruitment level for sustained transmission particularly due to the seasonal pulsing of reproduction (Swinton, 1998). The annual birth cohort of arctic harp seals, in contrast, is estimated to be around a million (Hammill et al., 2021) thus supporting the tenet that this represents the reservoir species for spillover to other seals.

Curiously the first reports of PDV in both were reported from the Danish island of Anholt in the Kattegat sea ($55°20'N, 16°10'E$) toward the inlet to the Baltic sea that is far away from the Arctic PDV reservoir. The pdv dataset holds the number of dead seals washed ashore across 25 Northern European areas during the 2002 epidemic starting in May and running through the end of the year (Harding et al., 2002). The chain of transmission ended in late 2002 due to the burnout of susceptibles. To visualize the invasion we can map the date of early numbers using cumulative strandings of > 20 as a benchmark (Fig. 15.3).

```
require(rworldmap)
# Day to 20 deaths
inv = apply(pdv$ts[, -1] < 20, 2, sum)
newmap = getMap(resolution = "low")
plot(newmap, xlim = c(-7, 16), ylim = c(50, 61), asp = 1.5)
# Big circles are early invasion. The ^1.5 is to
# increase contrast of early vs late invasion
invsymsize = (-(inv - 275)/275)^1.5
symbols(pdv$coord$lon, pdv$coord$lat, circles = invsymsize,
    bg = gray(inv/275), inches = 0.15, add = TRUE)
```

Seals do not travel over land, so in terms of spatial spread of PDV some measure of seaway distance should be used. A quick search on rseek.org on converting a map into a "friction surface" can help identifying the paths of shortest seaway distance.[4] The recipe requires several geospatial R packages:

```
require(raster)
require(gdistance)
require(maptools)
require(rgdal)
require(maps)
# the wrld_simpl data set is from maptools package
data(wrld_simpl)
# make a default world projection
world_crs = crs(wrld_simpl)
world = wrld_simpl
```

---

[4] Manipulation of geospatial data is an enormous field and the R community has generated a lot of resources beyond the scope of this text. The code is adopted from stackoverflow.com/questions/69258889.

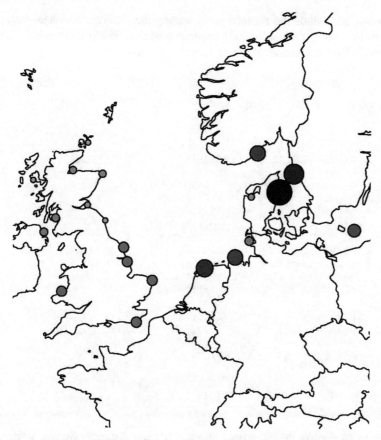

Fig. 15.3: A depiction of the day of > 20 cumulated strandings of harbor seals across 25 locales in Northeastern Europe from early May 2002 through the end of that year. Large dark circles represents earliest invasion. The largest circle is the Danish island of Anholt

```
worldshp = spTransform(world, world_crs)

# rasterize will set ocean to NA
ras = raster(nrow = 1000, ncol = 1000)
worldmask = rasterize(worldshp, ras)
worldras = is.na(worldmask)

# set land to very high friction
worldras[worldras == 0] <- 99
# create a friction object from the raster
tr = transition(worldras, function(x) 1/mean(x), 16)
tr = geoCorrection(tr, scl = FALSE)
```

The below code finds the shortest paths among the different seal haul-outs. This
calculation is computationally quite expensive so the friction surface distances are
included in the pdv dataset of the epimdr2 package.

```
dmat99sc = matrix(NA, ncol = 25, nrow = 25)
par(mfrow = c(1, 2))
plot(A, xlim = c(-10, 20), ylim = c(45, 65))
for(i in 1:25){
    # function accCost uses the transition object
    # and point of origin
    port_origin = structure(as.numeric(pdv$coord[i,3:2]),
        .Dim=1:2)
    port_origin = project(port_origin,
        crs(world_crs, asText = TRUE))
    A = accCost(tr, port_origin)
    for(k in i:25){
        port_destination= structure(as.numeric(pdv$coord[k,
            3:2]), .Dim=1:2)
        port_destination = project(port_destination,
            crs(world_crs, asText = TRUE))
        path = shortestPath(tr, port_origin, port_destination,
            output = "SpatialLines")
        t_path = shortestPath(tr, port_origin, port_destination)
        distance = costDistance(tr, port_origin, port_destination)
        lines(path, col = grey((i + 26)/56))
        dmat99sc[i, k] = dmat99sc[k, i] = distance[1, 1]
    }
}
plot(pdv$fs[1, ]/1000,as.vector(inv),
    xlab="Friction distance", ylab = "Day")
```

Figure 15.4a depicts the calculated shortest friction distances by sea between the
haul-outs and Fig. 15.4b shows days to > 20 dead seals against friction surface distance from Anholt. The strong positive relation to seaway distance testifies to the
spatially contagious nature of the spread of the virus. A similar pattern was seen
during the 1988 epizootic (Swinton et al., 1998).

15.4 Rabies

The eastern US invasion of rabies in raccoons first discussed in Sect. 10.1 is particularly well documented in Connecticut because the cases were geolocated to individual townships. The first reports were from the southwestern corner of the state in
March 1991. By January 1995 the virus had spread throughout the state. Smith et al.
(2002a) and Waller and Gotway (2004) provide a detailed statistical analysis of the

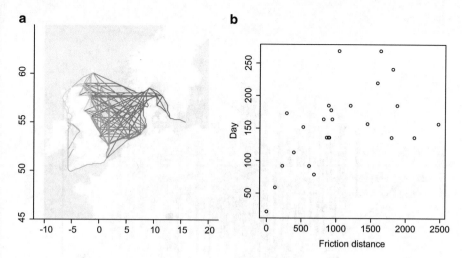

Fig. 15.4: (**a**) A depiction of the shortest sea distances between the 25 seal haul-outs that recorded significant die-offs during the 2002 PDV epizootic. (**b**) The day of report of > 20 dead seals against seaway friction surface distance from Anholt for each of the 25 well documented haul-outs

spatial spread. The data that represents the month of first appearance for each of the 168 townships are in the `waller` dataset.

```
data(waller)
head(waller)

##              x          y month
## 1 103.02200 68.71192       37
## 2  46.41953 28.43884       18
## 3 118.57160 88.25216       41
## 4  63.43697 76.50967       18
## 5  25.31975 91.60060       24
## 6  47.88734 35.93386       18
```

The x and y coordinates represent the geographic coordinates in kilometers from the southwestern corner. Following Waller and Gotway (2004) we can visualize the northeastward invasion of the virus (Fig. 15.5):

```
require(scatterplot3d)
s3d = scatterplot3d(waller$x, waller$y, waller$month,
    scale.y = 0.7, pch = 16, lwd = 2,
    color = gray(waller$month/max(waller$month)), type = "h",
    box = FALSE, xlab = "Easting", ylab = "Northing",
    zlab = "Month", angle = 120)
plane = lm(month ~ x + y, data = waller)
s3d$plane3d(plane)
```

Geolocated data on time-to-first-appearance (TFA) provides key information on rates and directions of spatial invasions of infectious diseases (Waller & Gotway,

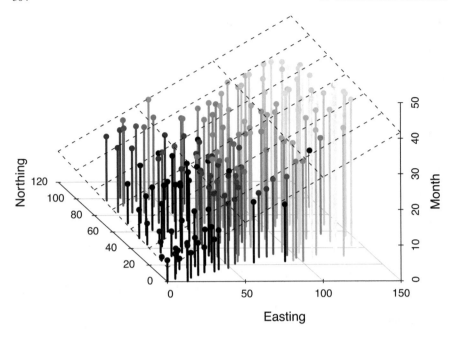

Fig. 15.5: Month of first report of raccoon rabies from March 1991 across 168 townships of Connecticut

2004) and other organisms of concern (Goldstein et al., 2019). A shallow smoothed surface of TFA across a landscape implies rapid range expansion, whereas slow spread results in a steep slope. If a spatial surface has a c_x slope in the x direction and a c_y slope in the y direction, then the steepest slope which reflect the spatial turnover is the geometric average of these and the invasion speed is the reciprocal. Thus, the speed of spread is $1/\sqrt{c_x^2 + c_y^2}$ and the dominant direction of spread (in radians) is $\arctan(c_y/c_x)$. For the raccoon rabies in Connecticut, the regression surface in Fig. 15.5 implies a speed of spread of about 4 km/month in a dominant 9° azimuth direction:

```
# speed
1/sqrt(plane$coef[2]^2 + plane$coef[3]^2)

   ##          x
   ## 3.927532

# direction
360 * atan2(plane$coef[3], plane$coef[2])/(2 * pi)

   ##          y
   ## 9.030879
```

In Eurasia the main host of rabies is the red fox. In Western and Central Europe a half century long enzootic of rabies started in the 1940s with a likely epicenter from Poland or Russia presumably as a spillover event from domestic dogs with subsequent spread throughout much of continental Europe. The virus was eventually eliminated[5] from Western Europe in 2008 through an EU-wide concerted effort of air-deployed oral vaccine baits (Freuling et al., 2013).[6] The European fox rabies enzootic have led to many important disease ecological insights such as the notion of a critical host density (Anderson et al., 1981) discussed in Sects. 3.1 and 10.7. Further important issues showcase how mathematical models can be used to understand and predict speed of spatial diffusion of infectious disease across a landscape once nuances in host biology are considered (Murray et al., 1986; van den Bosch et al., 1990; Mollison, 1991). From the initial epicenter, fox rabies spread at around 30–60km/year. Appropriate models for spatial spread of infection depend on the nature of the spatial transmission process such as "distributed contacts" versus "distributed infected" (Reluga et al., 2006). For spread of human infections parallel notions are often coined as commuter spread versus migration spread (Keeling & Rohani, 2002; Keeling et al., 2004).

The notion of spatial kernels introduced in Sect. 12.2 is central to predicting spatial diffusion rates. The study by van den Bosch et al. (1990) assumed that rabies transmitted among foxes with relatively stable home ranges (and thus a distributed contact scenario) and derived an approximate formula for the expected wave speed of $c = u\sqrt{2\log R_0}/V$, where u is the standard deviation of the spatial transmission kernel (in this case related to the size of each home range) and V is the serial interval. With a serial interval of about 33 days and a typical home range size, van den Bosch et al. (1990) predicted a wave speed of 45 km per year at low densities and 30 km/year at high densities, as long as the fox density is above the critical host density (Anderson et al., 1981, Sect. 10.7) of around 1 fox per km^2. Using a "distributed infecteds" scenario assuming foxes diffuse randomly across the landscape during the course of infection so u is related to the movement of foxes, Murray et al. (1986) predicted wave-like spread of rabies at a rate $c = u\sqrt{2(R_0 - 1/V)}$ (see also Mollison, 1991). With this calculation Murray et al. (1986) predicted a typical wave speed of around 50 km per year. In contrast to van den Bosch et al. (1990), the latter model predicts spread to increase with fox density. Mollison (1991) provides a discussion of different spread formulations, in general, and rabies and other case studies, in particular.

---

[5] Conventional usage is to use "eliminate" for regional control and "eradicate" for global control; smallpox and Rinderpest are the only two viruses that have been eradicated through vaccination.

[6] https://tinyurl.com/msszkdjw links to visualization of the invasion and elimination of fox rabies across Switzerland between 1967 and 1999.

15.5 Initial Control

The Spanish A/H1N1 influenza and SARS-Cov-2 pandemics are both exemplars of how overwhelmed hospital capacities lead to greatly exacerbated morbidity and mortality. For these, maxed out critical care units, respirators, and medical staff led to greatly increased individual severity from infection. Sudden outbreak calamities with associated breakdowns of health infrastructure also had important indirect consequences as, for example, seen in the cessation of routine vaccination against important childhood diseases during the 2013–14 West African Ebola epidemic (Takahashi et al., 2015). These examples clearly illustrate that containing the height of an initial epidemic peak is very important for individual health and overall public health burden. The mantra during the early part of the SARS-CoV-2 pandemic was to "flatten the curve." A vaccine is an obvious way to slow disease spread and other pharmaceutical interventions in the form of drugs may mitigate the stress on the health care system. In the absence of these, a number of non-pharmaceutical interventions (NPIs) were put in place in most countries.

As discussed throughout this text, the reproduction number is the transmission rate multiplied by the infectious period and for the closed epidemic (Sect. 3.1) the peak prevalence is $1 - (1 + \log R_0)/R_0$. Thus reducing the reproduction number will flatten the curve. It will also delay the timing of the peak (Bjørnstad et al., 2020a; Kröger et al., 2021) to allow for better preparedness. The various NPIs helped reduce the reproduction number in various ways; the transmission rate itself is the contact rate multiplied by the probability of infection given a contact, so social distancing reduce the rate and masking reduce the probability. Quarantining/self-isolation decrease both the contact rate and stunts the effective infectious period because infected individuals are not mixing with susceptibles. There are analytic approximations to the time to peak incidence but they are quite elaborate (Kröger et al., 2021), so a shortcut is to do numerical analyses using the sirmod function introduced earlier. Figure 15.6 shows how peak prevalence and the time of the peak is predicted to depend on the reproduction number.

```
ip = tp = rep(NA, 201)
R0 = seq(1.2, 2.5, length = 201)
for (i in 1:201) {
    times = seq(0, 365, by = 0.01)
    paras = c(mu = 0, N = 1, R0 = R0[i], gamma = 1/7)
    paras["beta"] = paras["R0"] * (paras["gamma"] + paras["mu"])
    start = c(S = 0.99999, I = 1e-05, R = 0) * paras["N"]
    out = ode(y = start, times = times, func = sirmod,
        parms = paras)
    out = as.data.frame(out)
    ip[i] = with(as.list(paras), 1 - (1 + log(R0))/R0)
    tp[i] = out$time[which.min(abs(out$I - ip[i]))]
}
par(mfrow = c(1, 2))
plot(R0, ip, type = "l", xlab = "Reproduction number",
    ylab = "Peak prevalence")
plot(R0, tp, type = "l", xlab = "Reproduction number",
```

```
ylab = "Peak day")
```

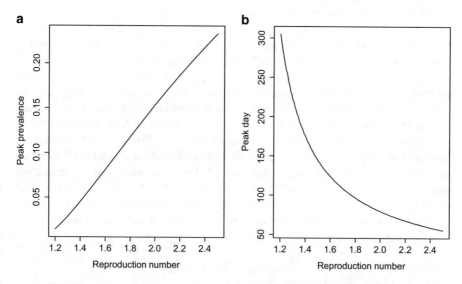

Fig. 15.6: The predicted (**a**) peak prevalence and (**b**) day of the peak as a function of the reproduction number assuming an infectious period of 7 days with a single initial infectious individual in a 100k population

Bjørnstad et al. (2020a) provide an interactive online shinyApp to do scenario analysis of NPI-reduced reproduction numbers, peak and time-of-peak prevalence.

15.6 Synchrony

Elimination—the local control of infectious disease—is generally a matter of locally deploying pharmaceutical and non-pharmaceutical interventions sufficient to push the reproduction number below one and thus break the chain of transmission. Eradication, in contrast, is a conceptually and practically tougher problem because it involves simultaneously breaking the chains everywhere. Section 1.3 visited on the notion that pathogens can persist regionally in host-pathogen metapopulations even if chains break during post-epidemic troughs (Grenfell & Harwood, 1997). As has been studied in great detail in general ecology, robust metapopulation persistence depends on spatial asynchrony among the coupled local populations (Hanski, 1998). With a high degree of synchrony, troughs will be aligned and there will be little opportunity for spatial rescue effects for a pathogen to evade eradication. Keeling et al. (2004) review how there is a tight interdependence between spatial coupling, synchrony, and regional persistence. It turns out all three may be strongly affected by vaccination. We can visit on this using the historical data from measles across England and Wales.

Grenfell and Harwood (1997) and Lau et al. (2020) outlined using measles as the exemplar the difference between source-sink metapopulations, locally coupled metapopulations, and globally coupled metapopulations. In the latter setting the coupling can either be spatially structured or spatially random. The CMLs discussed in Sects. 12.6 and 12.10 are examples of models of local coupling. The gravity model discussed in Sect. 12.9 is a spatially structured, globally coupled formulation. Prevaccination measles was a source-sink metapopulation in which for England and Wales some 5–10 large cities above the critical community size (Fig. 1.2) sustained chains of transmission through the troughs to fuel recurrent hierarchical waves of reintroduction to smaller communities (Grenfell et al., 2001). The m4494 dataset has the case counts and locations for each of 354 locations (cities and villages) that have been collated in a geographic fashion such that it represents spatially consistent time series for each week from 1944 through 1994 (Lau et al., 2020). We can use the nonparametric spatial covariance function discussed in Chap. 13 to study patterns of spatial synchrony in 1950–60 pre- and 1980–89, 1990–94 vaccination periods.

```
require(ncf)
data(m4494)
pre = m4494$year >= 50 & m4494$year < 60
post = m4494$year >= 80 & m4494$year < 90
late = m4494$year > 90
s5059 = Sncf(x = m4494$longlat[, 1], y = m4494$longlat[,
    2], z = m4494$measles[, pre], latlon = TRUE)
s8089 = Sncf(x = m4494$longlat[, 1], y = m4494$longlat[,
    2], z = m4494$measles[, post], latlon = TRUE)
s90 = Sncf(x = m4494$longlat[, 1], y = m4494$longlat[,
    2], z = m4494$measles[, late], latlon = TRUE)
plot(s5059, ylim = c(-0.1, 0.6))
plot(s8089, add = TRUE)
plot(s90, add = TRUE)
legend("topright", c("50-59", "80-89", "90+"), lty = 1,
    lwd = 3, col = c(gray(0.6), gray(0.8), gray(0.8)))
```

The covariance functions reveal local synchrony that decays with distance testifying to a dominance of local coupling particularly in the prevaccination period (Fig. 15.7). The local and hierarchical coupling is responsible for the gravity-like spread (Xia et al., 2004; Lau et al., 2020) discussed in Sect. 12.9 and recurrent spatial outbreak waves from large cities to surrounding conurbations (Grenfell et al., 2001). The relatively high region-wide average correlation of 0.25 (CI: {0.23, 0.27}) is partially due to the shared term-time forcing due to the yearly cycle of opening and closing of schools. The 1980–1989 period, which had an average vaccine cover of 73%, also exhibits evidence of distance decay and local coupling with a region-wide correlation of 0.14 (CI: {013, 0.15}]). In contrast, the epidemics during the 1990–94 period are completely decorrelated (correlation: 0.02) despite recording 56,765 cases during the period. In an elaborate statistical analysis, Lau et al. (2020)

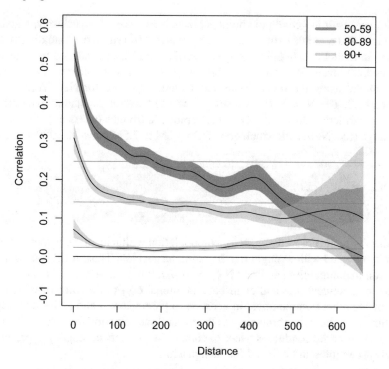

Fig. 15.7: The nonparametric spatial covariance functions of measles synchrony against separating distance for the 354 cities and villages in England and Wales in the 1950–59 prevaccine, 1980–89 early vaccine (mean cover: 71%) and the 90–94 late vaccine period (91% cover)

showed that the decorrelation is associated with a transition in the geometry of spatial coupling in the measles metapopulation. Whereas the probabilistic spread during the prevaccination era seems to adhere relatively well to predictions of the gravity model, this gave increasingly way to spatially random seeding of local epidemics as vaccine cover increased.

15.7 Coupling

Despite frequent local pathogen extinction, persistence may remain if there is spatial contagion among communities that exhibits asynchronous outbreaks. Thus, coupling and synchrony are key properties when it comes to the feasibility of eradication. The next section (Sect. 15.8) will attempt a more comprehensive synthesis pertaining to metapopulation persistence and eradication, but first consider these two factors. Intuition suggests that coupling is a two-edged sword: Too little spatial contagion will result in too infrequent recolonization and regional extinction, but too much may result in geographic homogenization and loss of asynchrony, alignment of troughs and regional extinction. Keeling et al. (2004) studied a spatially extended stochastic model of whooping cough to verify the idea of enhanced persistence at intermediate levels. We can revisit this analysis using a simple spatially extended TSIR model using the transmission parameters estimated for New York measles in Sect. 11.2. The New York case study is useful because its chaotic dynamics are prone to extinction during the deep post-epidemic troughs unless communities are very large (like New York which grew from 5.6M to 7.5M between 1920 and 1940).

```
# TSIR transmission coefficients
btny = c(32.552, 36.048, 43.163, 36.072, 37.459, 36.692,
     32.089, 35.116, 37.03, 29.915, 28.114, 20.413, 18.03,
     17.027, 15.855, 15.85, 18.87, 21.152, 26.08, 35.359,
     35.859, 34.128, 37.66, 34.19, 27.827, 38.87)
```

For simplicity the below assumes a metapopulation with p identical patches[7] that are globally coupled with strength c in a commuter fashion. Thus, if the local force of infection in community i at time t is $\phi_{i,t} = \beta_{i,t}I_{i,t}$, it will exert a pressure $(1-cp)\phi_{i,t}$ on the local susceptibles and contribute additional $c\phi_{i,t}$ to the force of infection in each of the other communities. In addition to parameters p and c, the tsirSpat function takes the same parameters as the tsirSim2 function from Sect. 8.6 except the list of initial conditions needs to contain two vectors of length p representing initial susceptibles and infected for each patch.

```
tsirSpat = function(beta, alpha, B, N, p, c, inits, type = "det"){
    type = charmatch(type, c("det", "stoc"), nomatch = NA)
    if(is.na(type))
        stop("method should be \"det\", \"stoc\"")
    IT = dim(B)[1]
    s = length(beta)
    lambda = matrix(NA, nrow = IT, ncol = p)
    I = matrix(NA, nrow = IT, ncol = p)
    S = matrix(NA, nrow = IT, ncol = p)

    I[1, ] = inits[[1]]
    lambda[1, ] = inits[[2]]
    S[1,] = inits$Snull
    cmat = matrix(c, ncol = p, nrow = p)
    diag(cmat) = 1 - c * p
    for(i in 2:IT) {
        lambda = beta[((i - 2) %% s) + 1]*cmat %*% (I[i -
            1,]^alpha)*S[i - 1,]/N
        if(type == 2) {
            I[i,] = rpois(p, lambda)
        }
        if(type == 1) {
            I[i, ] = lambda
        }
        S[i, ] = S[i - 1, ] + B[i, ] - I[i, ]
```

---

[7] The code is actually vectorized so can accommodate N as a vector of varying population sizes.

```
    }
    return(list(I = I, S = S))
}
```

As an illustration, assume five patches and draw initial conditions from the log-susceptible time series (lSold) and corrected infected time series (Ic) from Sect. 11.2.[8] The first run is assuming no spatial coupling and a simulation for 100 years:

```
p = 5
pinits = list(Snull = sample(exp(lSold), size = p),
    Inull = sample(Ic,size=p))
sim2 = tsirSpat(beta = btny, alpha = 0.98,
    B = matrix(median(NY$rec), ncol = p, nrow = 2600),
    N = median(N), p = p, c = 0, inits = pinits, type = "stoc")
mean(cor(sim2$I)[upper.tri(cor(sim2$I))])

    ## [1] NA

matplot(sim2$I, type="l", log="y", xlim=c(0,400),
    col = 1, xlab = "biweek", ylab = "I")
```

In the particular stochastic realization shown in Fig. 15.8 chains of transmission are all broken by about 10 years (260 biweeks). Armed with this general simulator one can study how spatial coupling affects local/global extinction rates and synchrony in the five patch system. The below looks at 100 stochastic realizations across a range of spatial contagion rates:

```
#coupling
coup = seq(0, 0.025, by = 0.0005)

sync = gext = lext = matrix(NA, ncol = length(coup), nrow = 100)
for(k in 1:length(coup)){
for(j in 1:100){
    sim2 = tsirSpat(beta = btny, alpha = 0.98,
        B = matrix(median(NY$rec), ncol = p, nrow = 2600),
        N = median(N), p = p, c = coup[k], inits = list(Snull =
            sample(exp(lSold), size = p),
        Inull = sample(Ic, size = p)), type = "stoc")
        #global extinction time
        gext[j, k] = 2600 - sum(apply(sim2$I, 1, sum) == 0)
        #fraction of local absence before extinction
        lext[j, k] = sum(sim2$I[1:gext[j,
            k], ] == 0) / (gext[j, k] * p)
        #synchrony
        sync[j, k] = mean(cor(sim2$I)[upper.tri(cor(sim2$I))])
    }
}
```

---

[8] So for this code to work the previous susceptible reconstruction must be available.

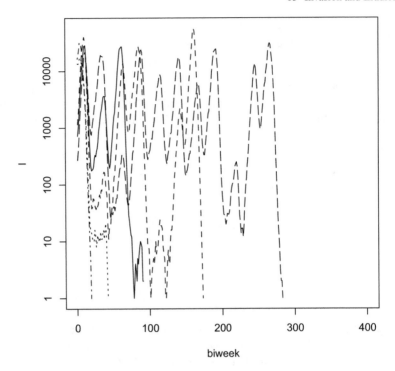

Fig. 15.8: A stochastic realization of the five patch spatial TSIR model assuming prevaccination New York transmission patterns and no spatial coupling. All chains of transmission broke within the first 5–10 years

The results (Fig. 15.9) verify the intuition. With low spatial contagion there is very little synchrony because of the underlying unstable dynamics and local extinction—here defined as the fraction of time of local absences among the communities while the pathogen is still circulating within the metapopulation—is frequent because spatial rescue is infrequent (Fig. 15.9a). As a consequence, the time to global extinction is short despite the substantial asynchrony (Fig. 15.9b). With strong coupling, time to global burnout is short and local extinction is relatively high because the spatial contagion leads to synchronization. There is a goldilocks zone for which most stochastic realizations predict regional persistence past the 100 year horizon (Fig. 15.9b).

```
boxplot(sync, outline = FALSE, xaxt = "n", xlab = "coupling",
    ylim = c(0, 1))
boxplot(lext, col = 0, outline = FALSE, , xaxt = "n",
    add = TRUE)
legend("right", c("Synchrony", "Local \n extinction"),
    pch = 22, pt.cex = 2, pt.bg = c("gray", 0), bty = "n")
boxplot(gext/26, xaxt = "n", xlab = "coupling")
legend("topright", c("Extinction\n time (yrs)"), pch = 22,
```

```
pt.cex = 2, pt.bg = c("gray"), bty = "n")
```

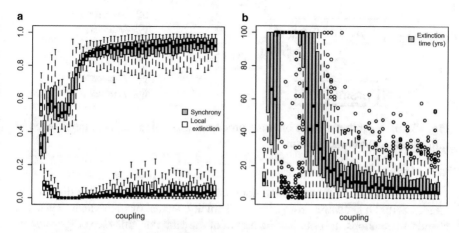

Fig. 15.9: (**a**) Boxplots of synchrony and local rates of extinction. Local rates of extinction is, here, defined as the fraction of time of local absences while the pathogen is still circulating within the metapopulation. (**b**) Time to global extinction as a function of coupling strength in the five patch metapopulation model. Open circles represent outlying outcomes among the simulations

15.8 A Synthesis

Eradication equates to regionalized metapopulation non-persistence. As alluded to in the previous sections forces influencing metapopulation persistence are multitude and are affected by both local and spatial processes. In the balance are local extinction, recolonization, coupling, and asynchrony. As a wrap-up of the main part of this monograph, the nuances and complexities are attempted summarized in Fig. 15.10.

Increased coupling ② will—all else being equal—enhance persistence because it leads to rescue from local breaks of chains of transmission (Metcalf et al., 2013). As highlighted above, this area has been explored in great depth in the general field of ecology (Hanski, 1998; Hanski & Gaggiotti, 2004). However, coupling in epidemic metapopulations also ① leads to loss of asynchrony and thus ④ reduce regional persistence as detailed in Sect. 15.7 and illustrated in Fig. 15.9 because of resultant diminished rescue effects.

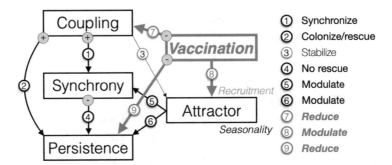

Fig. 15.10: A synthetic chart of some processes governing regional persistence as influenced by mass vaccination

Chapters 6 and 11 discussed the notion of attractors to characterize disease dynamics across a spectrum from stable endemicity, annual or multiannual cycles to chaotic fluctuations. It turns out the nature of the attractor influences regional persistence in two separate but important ways. When seasonality is strong enough to push dynamics into the erratic regime, ⑥ post-epidemic troughs tend to be very deep veering into the Atto-fox territory of (Mollison, 1991) leading to broken chains of transmission and reduced persistence (Ferrari et al., 2008). Though, as illustrated in Fig. 15.9 the associated asynchrony may prop up persistence. More curious ⑤ is the phenomenon of nonlinear phase-locking. The propensity for synchronization is sensitively dependent on the nature of the attractor (Bjørnstad et al., 1999b; Bjørnstad, 2000). Chaotic dynamics is usually hard to synchronize (Ruxton, 1994) and may therefore contribute to disease persistence. Stochastic, but asymptotically stable endemism, will generally inherit synchrony according to the strength of spatial coupling (Kendall et al., 2000). Local limit cycles, in contrast "yearn to synchronize" (Bjørnstad et al., 1999b; Bjørnstad, 2000) through the process of nonlinear phase-locking.[9] With low seasonality dynamics are asymptotically stable and synchrony is governed by coupling. With high seasonality the dynamics is erratic (Fig. 15.11b) but synchrony is comparable. In contrast, with intermediate seasonality which result in biennial cycles (Fig. 15.11b), spatial synchrony is almost perfect (Fig. 15.11a) due to the nonlinear phase-locking. Bjørnstad et al. (1999b) discuss this in general. Rohani et al. (1999) and Bjørnstad (2000) provides evidence that this is a true phenomenon in infectious disease dynamics. Rohani et al. (1999) showed that vaccination resulted in different changes in synchrony for whooping cough and measles. For whooping cough synchrony increased while for measles it decreased. For measles this was associated with vaccine-induced loss of cyclicity as per discussion in Sect. 6.6. For whooping cough Rohani et al. (2002) argued that the gain of cyclicity was due to the presence of the multiannual almost attractor discussed in Sect. 11.5.

---

[9] As described by watchmakers centuries ago who noted how clocks hanging on a common wall would lock-step.

We can use the spatial TSIR model to investigate the relation between attractor type and propensity for synchronization. As discussed in Chap. 6, increasing seasonality pushes dynamics from annual, to cyclic multiannual and to erratic epidemics. The following code simulates a 10-patch TSIR model assuming a coupling $c = 0.001$ and with varying degrees of seasonality for a 30 year time frame. The among-patch synchrony is assessed from the last 20 years of the simulation (Fig. 15.11a).

```
#Fig A
mbtny = mean(btny) #mean beta
p = 10 #number of patches
seasseq = seq(0, 0.3, by = 0.01) #seasonality
sync = gext = lext = matrix(NA, ncol = length(sdseq), nrow = 500)

for(k in 1:length(seasseq)) {#loop over seasonality
    for(j in 1:500) { #500 times
        bnty = exp(scale(log(btny)) * seasseq[k] + log(mbtny))
        sim2 = tsirSpat(beta = bnty, alpha = 0.98,
            B = matrix(median(NY$rec), ncol = p, nrow = 780),
            N = median(N), p = p, c = 0.001, inits =
            list(Snull = sample(exp(lSold), size = p), Inull =
            sample(Ic, size = p)), type = "stoc")
        gext[j, k] = 780 - sum(apply(sim2$I, 1, sum) == 0)
        lext[j,k]=sum(sim2$I[1:gext[j, k], ] ==
            0) / (gext[j, k] * p)
        #synchrony during year 10-30
        sync[j, k] = mean(cor(sim2$I[261:780, ])[upper.tri(
            cor(sim2$I[261:780, ]))])
    }
}
boxplot(sync, outline = FALSE, xaxt = "n", xlab = "Seasonality",
    ylab = "Synchrony")
```

In addition to charting the level of synchrony, it is instructive to plot annual stroboscopic sections as a bifurcation diagram (Fig. 15.11b). Because the TSIR is stochastic, the bifurcation lines are fuzzy; however, the transition from annual, biennial, and chaotic regimes are clear. The annual regime is associated with synchrony rising from 0.2. The chaotic regime is associated with synchrony of 0.4–0.5 because of increased shared seasonality. The biennial cycles are generally almost perfectly aligned despite the modest spatial coupling—The phenomenon of nonlinear phase-locking.

```
#Fig B
seasseq = seq(0, 0.3, by = 0.01) #seasonality
plot(NA, ylim = c(10, 1E4), xlim = range(seasseq),
    log="y", ylab="Infected", xlab="Seasonality")
    for(k in 1:length(seasseq)) {
        bnty = exp(scale(log(btny)) * seasseq[k] + log(mbtny))
        sim2 = tsirSpat(beta = bnty, alpha = 0.98,
            B = matrix(median(NY$rec), ncol = p,
            nrow = 52000 - 20), N = median(N), p = p, c=0.001,
```

```
    inits =  list(Snull = sample(exp(1Sold), size = p),
      Inull = sample(Ic, size = p)), type = "stoc")
    points(rep(seasseq[k], 2000 - 20), sim2$I[seq(from = 521,
      to = 52000, by = 26)], pch = 20, cex = 0.3)
}
```

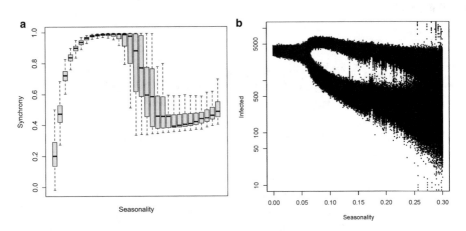

Fig. 15.11: (**a**) Synchrony versus seasonality. (**b**) Annual stroboscopic bifurcation diagram against seasonality

When it comes to introductions of mass-vaccination campaigns, there is an important notion of a honeymoon period during which diseases are seemingly fully controlled due to the background of substantial infection-induced immunity (Scherer & McLean, 2002; Klepac et al., 2013) after which substantial flare-ups may happen due to creeping buildup of susceptibility due to absence of circulation (Graham et al., 2019, Sect. 9.8). The metapopulation perspective adds to this by suggesting that in the aftermath of vaccine rollout there may be a period of infrequent spatial pathogen spread because of previous spatial epidemic synchrony. The subsequent change in spatial dynamics may over time give rise to more robust metapopulation persistence with increasing vaccine-induced asynchrony. Vaccination, thus, affects spatiotemporal dynamics in multiple ways. First, ⑦ it decreases spatial coupling because with lower numbers of susceptibles and infected there is less opportunity for spatial contagion. Second, ⑧ because it modulates dynamics toward greater or weaker cyclicity and so affects levels of synchrony and thus propensity for regional persistence. Finally, ⑨ vaccination generally reduces persistence because of the more frequent breaks in chains of transmission.

Part III
Miscellany

Chapter 16
Parasitoids

16.1 Introduction

This third part visits on a number of topics that are somewhat tangential to the main narrative of the monograph but that I have found useful for thinking on and analyzing data pertaining to infectious spread. The current chapter outlines how many of the ideas with regards to dynamics, persistence, and control carries over to other host/enemy systems of concern. Chapter 17 visits on multivariate methods to better characterize the in-host interactions among pathogens and the immune system that are ultimately responsible for shaping onwards transmission and epidemic flows. Chapter 18 is a brief sampler of how infectious disease processes in space and time generally lead to autocorrelated data that breach the classic statistical adage of "identically distributed, independent data" but for which a battery of modern methods can provide correct inference and additional insights.

16.2 Parasitoid-Host Dynamics

Many of the classic studies of the spatiotemporal dynamics of natural enemies and their hosts consider parasitoid-host interactions. Parasitoids represent a fascinating group of insect parasites. Adults are free-living and lay their eggs in larvae (or eggs) of host insects. Hosts die when the parasitoids complete their development and adults emerge from the infected hosts. From a dynamical system's point of view parasitoid-host interactions share many features with infectious disease dynamics. It is therefore instructive to cap the discussion of spatiotemporal dynamics with a discussion of this ecological interaction.

Burnett (1958) conducted a cage experiment involving greenhouse white flies (*Trialeurodes vaporariorum*) and its parasitoid *Encarsia formosa*. The population was followed for 21 generations (Fig. 16.1). The two populations oscillated in increasingly violent cycles until the parasitoid went extinct.

O. N. Bjørnstad, *Epidemics*, Use R!, https://doi.org/10.1007/978-3-031-12056-5_16

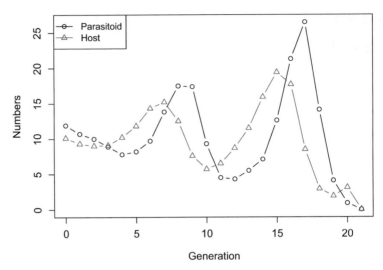

Fig. 16.1: Host-Parasitoid dynamics of *T. vaporariorum* parasitized by *E. formosa*

```
data(burnett)
plot(burnett$Generation,
    burnett$NumberofHostsParasitized,
    type = "b", ylab = "Numbers", xlab = "Generation")
lines(burnett$Generation,
    burnett$NumberofHostsUnparasitized,
    type = "b", col = 2, pch = 2)
legend("topleft", legend = c("Parasitoid", "Host"),
    lty = c(1, 1), pch = c(1, 2), col = c(1, 2))
```

Nicholson and Bailey (1935) developed the first mathematical model for this interaction. Assuming random search (with a searching efficiency a) by the parasitoids, the probability of escaping parasitation is $\exp(-aP_t)$ and the number of host, H, and parasitoids, P, in the next generation is:

$$H_{t+1} = RH_t \exp(-aP_t) \tag{16.1}$$

$$P_{t+1} = RH_t(1 - \exp(-aP_t)), \tag{16.2}$$

where R is the average number of offspring per hosts. A function for the host-parasitoid interaction is:

```
nbmod = function(R, a, T = 100, H0 = 10, P0 = 1) {
    # T is length of simulation (number of
    # time-steps) H0 and P0 are initial numbers
    H = rep(NA, T)   #Host series
    P = rep(NA, T)   #Parasitoid series
    H[1] = H0  #Initiating the host series
    P[1] = P0  #Initiating the parasitoid series
```

```
for (t in 2:T) {
    H[t] = R * H[t - 1] * exp(-a * P[t - 1])
    P[t] = R * H[t - 1] * (1 - exp(-a * P[t - 1]))
}

res = list(H = H, P = P)
return(res)
}
```

The Nicholson-Bailey model predicts that with density-independent growth of the host (in the absence of parasitism) and random search by the parasitoid there should be cycles with ever increasing amplitude until the host and/or parasitoid goes extinct as seen in Burnett's (1958) experiment. With a host growth rate R of 1.1 and a parasitoid searching efficiency a of 0.1, the nbmod function forecasts the Nicholson-Bailey model and allows a plot of host/parasitoid abundance against time and host-parasitoid numbers in the phase plane (Fig. 16.2)

```
sim = nbmod(R = 1.1, a = 0.1)
time = 1:100
par(mfrow = c(1, 2))
plot(time, sim$H, type = "l", xlab = "Generations",
```

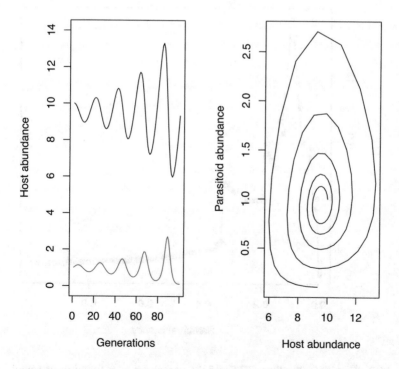

Fig. 16.2: Simulation of the Nicholson-Bailey model with $R = 1.1$ and $a = 0.1$

```
    ylab  =  "Host abundance", ylim = c(0, 14))
points(time, sim$P, type = "l", col = "red")
plot(sim$H, sim$P, type = "l", xlab = "Host abundance",
    ylab = "Parasitoid abundance")
```

A sequence of searching efficiencies between 0 and 1 allows an exploration of how the time to extinction of the host-parasitoid depends on *a*. The functions which and min store the time to extinction. The analysis shows the persistence time is greatest at intermediate search efficiency (Fig. 16.3).

```
aVals = seq(0, 1, by = 0.01)
tte = rep(NA, length(aVals))
for (i in c(1:length(aVals))){
    sim = nbmod(R = 1.1, a = aVals[i], T = 500)
    tte[i] = min(which(sim$P == 0))
    }
plot(aVals, tte, type = "b", ylab = "TTE",
    xlab = "Search efficiency")
```

Burnett (1958) suggested that $R = 2$ and $a = 0.067$ were appropriate values for this system. The previous model fitting ideas of trajectory matching (Sect. 9.3) finds val-

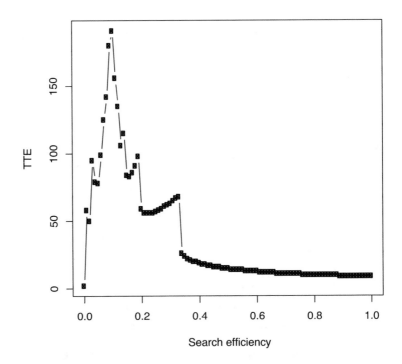

Fig. 16.3: Time to extinction (TTE) of the parasitoid as a function of search efficiency in the Nicholson-Bailey model

ues that minimize the sum-of-squared-errors between observed and predicted abundances to estimate R and a (on a log-scale to make sure they are both strictly positive quantities):

```
ssfn = function(par) {
    R = exp(par[1])
    a = exp(par[2])
    sim = nbmod(R, a, T = 22, H0 = 10.1, P0 = 11.9)
    ss = sum((burnett$NumberofHostsUnparasitized - sim$H)^2 +
        (burnett$NumberofHostsParasitized - sim$P)^2)
    return(ss)
}
par = log(c(2, 0.05))
fit = optim(par, ssfn)
exp(fit$par)

    ## [1] 2.16767130 0.06812596
```

The fit is close to Burnett's numbers. Figure 16.4 shows the model prediction using the MLE best parameters.

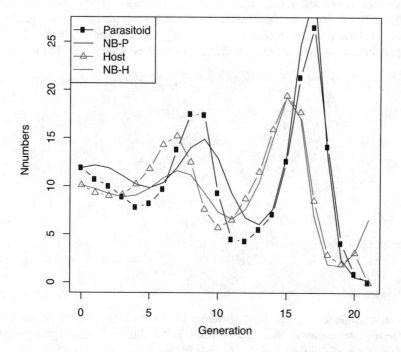

Fig. 16.4: Burnett's data and predictions by the Nicholson-Bailey model with $R = 2.17$ and $a = 0.07$. NB-P and NB-H are the predicted number of parasitoids and hosts from the model

```
sim = nbmod(R = 2.16767, a = 0.06812, T = 22, H0 = 10.1,
    P0 = 11.9)
plot(burnett$Generation,
    burnett$NumberofHostsParasitized, type = "b",
    ylab = "Numbers", xlab = "Generation")
lines(burnett$Generation, sim$P)
lines(burnett$Generation,
    burnett$NumberofHostsUnparasitized, type = "b",
    col = 2, pch = 2)
lines(burnett$Generation, sim$H, col = 2)
legend("topleft", legend = c("Parasitoid", "NB-P",
    "Host", "NB-H"), lty = c(1, 1, 1, 1), pch=c(1, NA, 2, NA),
    col=c(1, 1, 2, 2))
```

16.3 Stability and Resonant Periodicity

Nicholson and Bailey (1935) did a detailed mathematical analysis of their model and showed that the equilibrium is an unstable focus regardless of parameter values. The concepts from Chap. 10 hold all relevant results for this analysis. The equilibrium of the Nicholson-Bailey model is $P^* = log(R)/a$, $H^* = log(R)/(a(R-1))$. The eigenvalues of the Jacobian evaluated at the Burnett experiment equilibrium are:

```
paras = c(R = 2.17, a = 0.068)
eq = with(as.list(paras), c(P = log(R)/a, H = log(R)/(a *
    (R - 1))))
# states
states = c("H", "P")
# equations
elist = c(Heq = quote(R * H * exp(-a * P)), Peq = quote(R *
    H * (1 - exp(-a * P))))
# matrices
JJ = jacobian(states = states, elist = elist, parameters = paras,
    pts = eq)
eigen(JJ, only.values = TRUE)$values

  ## [1] 0.83108+0.8638247i 0.83108-0.8638247i

max(abs(eigen(JJ)$values))

  ## [1] 1.198702
```

It is an unstable focus since the eigenvalues are a pair of complex conjugates whose absolute value is greater than one.[1] Since this is a difference model, the predicted period of the outwards spiral is $2\pi/\tan^{-1}(\frac{Im(\lambda)}{Re(\lambda)})$:

---

[1] Recall that according to local stability theory, stability of discrete-time models requires the absolute value of the largest eigenvalue of the Jacobian evaluated at the equilibrium to be smaller than one. This is as opposed to continuous-time models for which the requirement is that the real part of the dominant eigenvalue must be smaller than zero.

```
2 * pi/atan2(Im(eigen(JJ)$values[1]), Re(eigen(JJ)$values[1]))

   ## [1] 7.807961
```

To revisit on how stability analysis can elucidate how the cycle period depends on key parameters (Sect. 10.2) we can, for example, investigate its dependence on host growth rate (Fig. 16.5):

```
RVals = seq(1.1, 3, by = 0.1)
per = rep(NA, length(RVals))
for(i in 1:length(RVals)){
    paras = c(R = RVals[i], a = 0.068)
    eq = with(as.list(paras), c(P = log(R)/a,
        H= log(R) /(a*(R-1))))
    JJ = jacobian(states = states, elist = elist,
        parameters = paras, pts = eq)
    per[i] = 2 * pi/atan2(Im(eigen(JJ)$values[1]),
        Re(eigen(JJ)$values[1]))
}
plot(RVals, per, type = "b", xlab = "R", ylab = "Period")
```

The higher the host growth rate, the faster the outwards spiral.

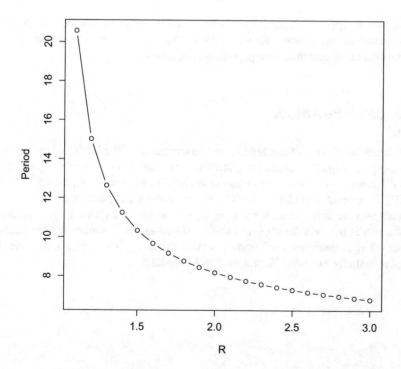

Fig. 16.5: Resonant period of the unstable Nicholson-Bailey model as a function of host growth rate

16.4 Biological Control

Parasitoids have been used for biocontrol of agricultural pest through the ages (Murdoch et al., 1985). Successful biocontrol requires that the natural enemy such as a parasitoid keeps the pest consistently below an economic threshold. The inherent instability predicted by the Nicholson-Bailey model is at odds with successful biocontrol by parasitoids. Many different model modifications have been analyzed to understand when stable regulation can happen. These include: (i) long-lived adult hosts, (ii) density-dependent host growth, (iii) heterogeneity in risk such as aggregated attack rates, spatial heterogeneity, host refugia, and (iv) interference among parasitoids (Murdoch et al., 2003). May (1978) proposed by replacing the Poisson attack assumption with a negative binomial distribution with aggregation parameter k that heterogeneity in risk can stabilize dynamics toward stable successful control. He coined a CV^2 rule which says that if the coefficient of variation in attack rate is greater than 1, the host-parasitoid dynamics stabilizes and control can be achieved. The CV for the negative binomial is $1/\sqrt{k}$. May's (1978) host-parasitoid model is:

$$H_{t+1} \quad = RH_t(1+\tfrac{aP_t}{k})^{-k} \tag{16.3}$$

$$P_{t+1} = RH_t(1-(1+\tfrac{aP_t}{k})^{-k}). \tag{16.4}$$

For a `shinyApp` of this model see below. Finally, (v) as with infectious diseases, host-parasitoid interactions can persist even with local non-persistence through regional consumer–resource metapopulation dynamics...

16.5 Larch Bud Moth

Parasitoids cause violent fluctuations in the dynamics of the larch bud moth across the European Alps. Historical records show recurrent traveling waves of defoliation every 9 years for centuries (Bjørnstad et al., 2002b; Johnson et al., 2010).[2] Turchin (2003) developed a model of the interactions among the larch bud moth, its parasitoids and the host plant. Johnson et al. (2004) showed that a spatial extension of this model predicts the observed waves. However, for the more general purpose of considering spatiotemporal host-parasitoid dynamics it is useful to consider the simpler spatially extended Nicholson-Bailey model.

---

[2] https://tinyurl.com/2v6tusp3 shows an animated GIF of the Larch bud moth defoliation between 1960 and 2000.

16.6 Host-Parasitoid Metapopulation Dynamics

In ecology the type of coupled map lattice models introduced in Chap. 12 was originally introduced in the context of parasitoid-host dynamics (Hassell et al., 1991;
Bjørnstad & Bascompte, 2001; Johnson et al., 2004). Hassell et al. (1991) highlighted the importance of allowing for different mobility of the host and parasitoid.
Define Dh as the proportion of host that disperses to neighboring patches and Dp the
proportion of parasitoid that disperses. Hassell et al. (1991) showed that changing
these can shift the spatial dynamics between spatial chaos, waves or frozen Turing spatial heterogeneity. A Nicholson-Bailey CML along the lines introduced in
Chap. 12 is:

```
# Dh is proportion of hosts that disperses Dp is
# proportion of parasitoids that disperses
Dh = 0.5
Dp = 0.7
# xlen is width of the lattice (E-W) ylen is height
# of the lattice (N-S)
xlen = 30
ylen = 30
```

The hp.dyn function defines the function to update the local abundances of hosts
and parasitoids according to the Nicholson-Bailey model. Previous densities of host,
h, and parasitoids, p, need to be supplied as arguments to the function, in addition
to the host growth rate (R) and parasitoid search efficiency a.

```
hp.dyn = function(h, p, R, a) {
    # hnew is the post-interaction host density
    hnew = R * h * exp(-a * p)
    # pnew is the post-interaction parasitoid
    # density
    pnew = R * h * (1 - exp(-a * p))
    # the two vectors of results are stored in a
    # 'list'
    res = list(h = hnew, p = pnew)
    return(res)
}
```

The spatial coordinates and the distance matrix are:

```
xy = expand.grid(1:xlen, 1:ylen)
dmat = as.matrix(dist(xy))
```

The redistribution matrices are calculated by checking if the distance in dmat is
smaller than two, thus flagging all populations that are first neighbors. Each neigh-
bor is assumed to receive a fraction Dh/8 of the focal host abundance and a fraction
Dp/8 of the parasitoids. The fractions that do not disperse (1-Dh and 1-Dp) are
along the diagonal of the redistribution matrices:

```
kh = ifelse(dmat < 2, Dh/8, 0)
kp = ifelse(dmat < 2, Dp/8, 0)
diag(kh) = 1 - Dh
diag(kp) = 1 - Dp
```

Finally construct matrices to store results and set starting conditions for the simulation. IT is number of generations to be simulated. The initial conditions are zeros everywhere except for an arbitrary population (in this case location 23) which starts with four hosts and one parasitoid:

```
IT = 600
hmat = matrix(NA, nrow = xlen * ylen, ncol = IT)
pmat = matrix(NA, nrow = xlen * ylen, ncol = IT)
hmat[, 1] = 0
pmat[, 1] = 0
hmat[23, 1] = 4
pmat[23, 1] = 1
```

The coupled map lattice formulation assumes, as in Chap. 12, a two-stage process of first local growth (using the hp.dyn function) followed by redistribution according to the host and parasitoid dispersal matrices using matrix multiplication (%*%).

```
for (i in 2:IT) {
    # growth
    tmp = hp.dyn(h = hmat[, i - 1], p = pmat[, i - 1],
        R = 2, a = 1)
    # redistribution
    hmat[, i] = tmp$h %*% kh
    pmat[, i] = tmp$p %*% kp
    cat(i, " of ", IT, "\r")   #progress monitor
}
```

The following is code to make an in-line animation of the last 100 generations for the parasitoid:

```
# plot the last 100 generations for the parasitoid
for (i in 1:100) {
    x = xy[, 1]
    y = xy[, 2]
    z = pmat[, i + 500]
    symbols(x, y, fg = 2, circles = z, inches = 0.1, bg = 2,
        xlab = "", ylab = "")
    Sys.sleep(0.1)   #this is to slow down the plotting
}
```

and the code to write frames to the disk to make a permanent web-optimized movie using ImageMagick is:

```
for (k in 1:50) {
    png(filename = paste("Pplot", k, ".png", sep = ""))
    x = xy[, 1]
    y = xy[, 2]
```

```
    z = pmat[, k + 500]
    symbols(x, y, fg = 2, circles = z, inches = 0.1, bg = 2,
        xlab = "", ylab = "")
    dev.off()
}
system("convert Pplot*.png -delay 500 -coalesce
    -layers OptimizeTransparency cml2.gif")
system("rm Pplot*.png")
```

Low mobility of both host and parasitoid (e.g., Dp = Dh = 0.1) leads to spatially chaotic dynamics and high mobility (e.g., Dh = 0.5, Dp = 0.7) leads to waves (Hassell et al., 1991).[3]

16.7 Parasitoid-Host shinyApps

The epimdr2 package contains a shinyApp to study the negative binomial parasitoid-host model discussed in Sect. 16.4. It can be launched through:

```
require(epimdr2)
runApp(may.app)
```

The nbspat.app shinyApp animates the spatially extended host-parasitoid model discussed in Sect. 16.6. It can be launched through:

```
require(epimdr2)
require(plotly)
runApp(nbspat.app)
```

---

[3] Animated gifs of the two dynamic regimes are on:
https://tinyurl.com/5n7y94v5 and
https://tinyurl.com/mryjr28a.

Chapter 17
Quantifying In-Host Patterns

17.1 Motivation

This chapter is somewhat tangential to the main text but it does loosely loop back to the discussion in Sect. 1.2 on how patterns of in-host persistence are important determinants of population-level dynamics. In-host dynamics results from replication rates of pathogens as molded by the innate and adaptive branches of the host immune system. For example, using the TSIR as a tool for understanding plasmodium replication rates, Metcalf et al. (2011b, see also Sect. 8.9) documented a strong dose-response effect whereby the innate branch seemingly is able to slow the growth from low inocula but not subsequent anemia in the infected mice. Kamiya et al. (2020) provide further discussion of such dose-response effects and consequences for onwards transmission.

Many different immune pathways are regulated through chemical signaling. Graham et al. (2007) reviewed how key signals such as the various cytokines affect in-host pathogen trajectories with an emphasis on chatter during coinfections. It is therefore instructive to study how assemblages of immune markers are triggered to respond to infections. This and Chap. 18 use some haphazardous case studies to introduce some statistical methodology ("beyond multiple t-tests") that may help elucidate the patterns in data. The datasets are chosen because they have been made publicly available and represent the sort of data that are commonly collected in laboratory experiments.

17.2 Two Experiments

The mouse malaria dataset was introduced in Sect. 8.9 and will be further discussed in Sect. 18.4. It represents daily counts of parasitized and non-parasitized red blood cells from several different *Plasmodium chabaudi* strains. This species of rodent

---

This chapter uses the following R packages: ade4 and MASS.

O. N. Bjørnstad, *Epidemics*, Use R!, https://doi.org/10.1007/978-3-031-12056-5_17

malaria has a synchronized life-cycle in which merozoites will infect red blood cells to replicate and burst out at night to invade other red blood cells (Mideo et al., 2013; Greischar et al., 2014). A small fraction of parasites are committed to become sexual gametocytes that can infect mosquitos for onwards transmission (Greischar et al., 2016).

The second dataset is from a coinfection study of Feline Immunodeficiency Virus in domestic cats (Roy et al., 2009). Like HIV, FIV is a retrovirus that targets various white blood cells and uses its generic reverse transcriptase enzyme to transcribe RNA into complementary cDNA that is inserted into the host genome by the integrase enzyme. The experiment was design to study why the feline strain (FIV_f) is so virulent while the cougar (*Puma concolor*) strain (FIV_p) cause no disease. The experiment showed that FIV_f infections in cats is attenuated by prior infection with FIV_p. The data were collected from twenty cats that were experimentally infected with FIV. The background details leading to the data that will be used as illustration of several multivariate statistical methods are that 10 cats were infected with FIV_p on day zero and 10 were sham inoculated. On day 28 five cats from each group were inoculated with FIV_f and the other 10 cats were again sham inoculated. This resulted in four treatment groups: C (control, only sham inoculation), P (FIV_p on day zero and sham on day 28), F (sham on day zero, FIV_f on day 28) and D (dual infection, FIV_p on day zero and FIV_f on day 28). A variety of cytokines and cell counts that were thought to relate to protective immunity were measures approximately every seven days. Details of the experiment can be found in Roy et al. (2009).

17.3 Data

The full datasets from the two experiments can be found in the `epimdr2` package, but for the purpose of illustrating the methods we will consider subsets of the data. For the FIV analysis we focus on the multivariate measures on days 31 and 59 to create two datasets `Day31` and `Day59`, three and 30 days, respectively, after the second treatment (the FIV_f inoculation). In preparation for analyses some columns that are extraneous or were not measured on these days are stripped and lines with missing values are removed (using `na.omit`). Each row is labeled with the animal `Id`.

```
data(fiv)
Day31 = fiv[fiv$Day == 31, ]
dimnames(Day31)[[1]] = Day31$Id
Day31 = na.omit(Day31[, -c(1, 14, 15, 16)])
Day59 = fiv[fiv$Day == 59, ]
dimnames(Day59)[[1]] = Day59$Id
Day59 = na.omit(Day59[, -c(1, 14, 15, 16)])
```

For the malaria analysis we also strip some unnecessary columns that are extraneous so as to focus on the red blood cell count (RBC).

```
data(chabaudi)
chabaudirbc = chabaudi[, -c(1, 3, 4, 7, 8, 10, 11)]
```

In addition to the long format used for the repeated measures analysis (Sect. 18.4), we need "wide" formatted data (denoted ...w) for both the principal component analysis (PCA) and linear discriminant analysis (LDA). The wide formatted data is constructed using reshape. The -seq(4,50,by = 2) strips extraneous columns generated during the reshaping. The names(...)[2] = "Treatment" renames column 2.

```
chabaudirbcw = reshape(chabaudirbc, idvar = "Ind2",
    direction = "wide", timevar = "Day")
chabaudirbcw = chabaudirbcw[, -seq(4, 50, by = 2)]
names(chabaudirbcw)[2] = "Treatment"
```

17.4 PCA of the FIV Data

The FIV data has variables representing counts of various effector cells (lymphocytes, neutrophils and CD4, CD8B, CD25 T cells), virus load (provirus and overall viremia), and measurements on a number of cytokines (IFNγ, IL-4, IL-10, IL-12, TNFα). Cytokines are signaling molecules that helps orchestrate the immune response. The goal of the experiment was to elucidate what immunological conditions best distinguished sever from attenuated infections relative to the base line of control animals.

Principal component analysis is the simplest ways to explore multivariate data. The idea is to think of the data as residing in a hyper volume were each axis (v) corresponds to a variable. The PCA summarizes the dominant variability by projecting the data onto a set of rotated axes that are linear combinations of the original axes ($\dot{v}_1 = c_1v_1 + c_2v_2 + ...$). The first axis is constructed so as to spread out the data points. Each subsequent axis spreads out the remaining variability under the constraint that they have to be orthogonal to previous axes. In the parlance of multivariate statistics, the c's are called the loadings (or sometimes column scores) and the coordinates of each datum in the rotated space are the scores (or row scores). The biplot visualizes the analysis by plotting the loadings as vectors and the scores as points in the space spanned by the first and second PCA axes. Base R contains the princomp function, but the ade4 package has refined statistical and graphical methods for such analyses. According to the French protocol (Dray & Dufour, 2007), as implemented in the ade4 package, biplot-like decompositions are referred to as duality diagrams (because of the vectors and points); thus the naming of dudi.pca for principal component analysis. We use the dudi.pca function to elaborate on the biplot. By providing an explicit fac argument representing each treatment we can add group means as well as group ellipses (which reflect within-group variability) to the biplot using the s.class function.[1] The `add.scatter.eig` function adds a histogram that shows the relative importance of each PCA axis (Fig. 17.1).

```
require(ade4)
pca31 = dudi.pca(Day31[, 1:11], scannf = FALSE, nf = 5)
# select 5 axes
groups = Day31$Treatment
s.arrow(dfxy = pca31$co[, 1:2] * 8, ylim = c(-7, 9), sub = "Day 31",
    possub = "topleft", csub = 2)
s.class(dfxy = pca31$li[, 1:2], fac = groups, cellipse = 2,
    axesell = FALSE, cstar = 0, col = c(2:5), add.plot = TRUE)
add.scatter.eig(pca31$eig, xax = 1, yax = 2, posi = "bottomright")
```

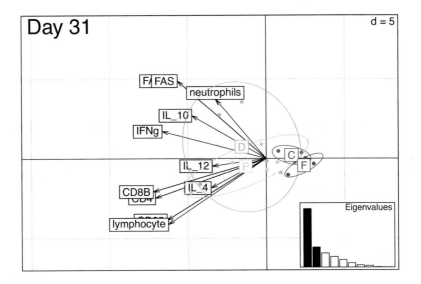

Fig. 17.1: A biplot of the PCA of the in-host measurement in the FIV experiment on day 31 (three days after FIV_p inoculations) with group ellipses and eigenvalues superimposed

On Day 59 patterns are starting to resolve and treatment units are starting to separate with FIV_f infected cats having low white blood cell lymphocyte counts and very high viral loads while the dual infected cats have very attenuated infection (Fig. 17.2). In its natural cougar host FIV_p prevalence is high but the virus appears to be largely avirulent (Biek et al., 2006).[2]

---

[1] Numerically, the PCA decomposition is done through the eigen-decomposition of the correlation matrix of the original data (unless `scale=FALSE` in which case the decomposition is of the variance–covariance matrix) for which each eigenvalue represents the relative importance of each PCA axis and the eigenvectors represents the loadings.

[2] Virgin et al. (2009) provide a review of the many chronic viral infections of humans that all appears to be largely avirulent.

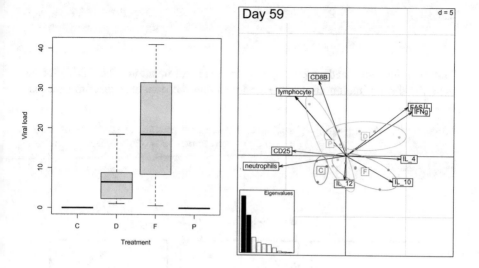

Fig. 17.2: The day 59 analysis. (**a**) Boxplot of viral load by treatment (C = Control, D = Dual infection, F = Fiv$_f$ infection, P = Fiv$_p$ infection). (**b**) The biplot of in-host immune measures with group ellipses and eigenvalues superimposed

```
par(mfrow = c(1, 2))
boxplot(fiv$viremia[fiv$Day == 59]/10000 ~ fiv$Treatment[fiv$Day ==
    59], ylab = "Viral load", xlab = "Treatment")
pca59 = dudi.pca(Day59[, 1:11], scannf = FALSE, nf = 5)
groups = Day59$Treatment
s.arrow(dfxy = pca59$co[, 1:2] * 7, xlim = c(-9, 9), ylim = c(-1,
    5), sub = "Day 59", possub = "topleft", csub = 2)
s.class(dfxy = pca59$li[, 1:2], fac = groups, cellipse = 2,
    axesell = FALSE, cstar = 0, col = c(2:5), add.plot = TRUE)
add.scatter.eig(pca59$eig, xax = 1, yax = 2, posi = "bottomleft")
```

17.5 LDA of the FIV Data

In contrast to the PCA which broadly explores the overall variability in multivariate data, discriminant analysis explicitly considers group membership (such as experimental treatment or other types of grouping) and asks what linear combination of response variables (a kin to the loadings of a PCA) allows for the best discrimination among groups. The MASS package has the lda function to do such analysis. Since the variables are heterogeneous in nature we normalize each prior to the analysis by applying the scale function to each of the first eleven columns of the dataset.

```
require(MASS)
Day31sc = Day31
Day31sc[, 1:11] = apply(Day31[, 1:11], 2, scale)
```

The lda function needs a group~response formulation. The LDA plot depicts the discrimination among the groups along the dominant discriminant axes (Fig. 17.3).

```
lda31 = lda(Treatment ~ CD4 + CD8B + CD25 + FAS + IFNg +
    IL_10 + IL_12 + lymphocyte + neutrophils + TNF_a,
    data = Day31sc)
plot(lda31)
```

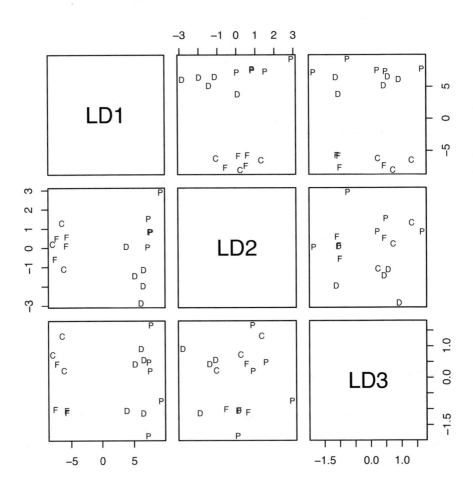

Fig. 17.3: The LDA of in-host measurement in the FIV experiment on day 31

Figure 17.3 shows how discriminant axis 1 clearly discriminates between the Dual (D)/Cougar (P) and the Control (C)/Feline (F) groups. Axis 2 separates the Dual (D) group from the Cougar (P) group. Axis 3 provides imperfect separation between the Control (C) group and the Feline (F) group. We can further check how the predicted LDA group assignments compare to the true treatment groupings:

```
pr = predict(lda31, method = "plug-in")$class
table(pr, Day31sc$Treatment)

   ##
   ## pr  C D F P
   ##   C 2 0 1 0
   ##   D 0 5 0 0
   ##   F 1 0 3 0
   ##   P 0 0 0 5
```

For the most part the discrimination is good, but as Fig. 17.3 suggests there is some difficulty in discriminating between the C and F group on day 31; there is one mis-classification among the groups.

To see how the group-informed LDA ordination differs from the PCA we can represent the LDA analysis as a biplot (Fig. 17.4). The first two lines in the below code calculates the coordinates of each cat along the first two LDA axes to be compatible with the ADE4 package plotting functions. The discrimination is largely along LDA axis one.

```
ld1 = as.matrix(Day31sc[,attr(lda31$terms,
    "term.labels")])%*%matrix(lda31$scaling[, 1], ncol = 1)
ld2 = as.matrix(Day31sc[,attr(lda31$terms,
    "term.labels")])%*%matrix(lda31$scaling[, 2], ncol = 1)
groups = Day31$Treatment

contribs = lda31$svd/sum(lda31$svd)
s.arrow(dfxy = lda31$scaling[,1:2], sub = "Day 31",
    possub = "topleft", csub = 2)
s.class(dfxy = cbind(ld1, ld2) * 2.5, fac = groups,
    cellipse = 2,  axesell = FALSE, cstar = 0,
    col = c(2:5), add.plot = TRUE)
add.scatter.eig(contribs, xax = 1, yax = 2,
    posi = "bottomright")
```

The analysis for the data from day 59 shows that the discrimination among all four groups is very good by this time (Fig. 17.5). The linear discriminant axis 1 separates treatments C from D/F and P and LD 2 separates F from the other treatments.

```
Day59sc = Day59
Day59sc[, 1:11] = apply(Day59[, 1:11], 2, scale)
lda59  =  lda(Treatment ~ CD4 + CD8B + CD25 + FAS +
    IFNg + IL_10 + IL_12 + lymphocyte + neutrophils +
    TNF_a, data = Day59sc)
pr = predict(lda59, method = "plug-in")$class
table(pr, Day59sc$Treatment)
```

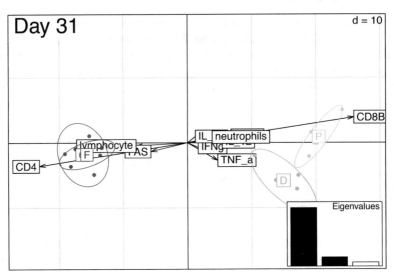

Fig. 17.4: The linear discriminant analysis of the day 31 data represented as a biplot

```
##
## pr  C D F P
##   C 5 0 0 0
##   D 0 5 0 0
##   F 0 0 5 0
##   P 0 0 0 4
ld1 = as.matrix(Day59sc[,attr(lda59$terms,
    "term.labels" )])%*%matrix(lda59$scaling[, 1], ncol = 1)
ld2 = as.matrix(Day59sc[,attr(lda59$terms,
    "term.labels" )])%*%matrix(lda59$scaling[, 2], ncol = 1)
groups = Day59$Treatment

contribs  =  lda59$svd/sum(lda59$svd)
s.arrow(dfxy = lda59$scaling[,1:2], sub = "Day 59",
    possub = "topleft", csub = 2)
s.class(dfxy = cbind(ld1, ld2), fac = groups, cellipse = 2,
    axesell = FALSE, cstar = 0 , col = c(2:5), add.plot = TRUE)
add.scatter.eig(contribs, xax = 1, yax = 2,
    posi = "bottomright")
```

The severe disease (treatment F) is associated with reduction in counts of several
cell types and modulation of the expression of various cytokines with up-regulation
of various interleukins and down-regulation of IFN-γ and TNF-α.

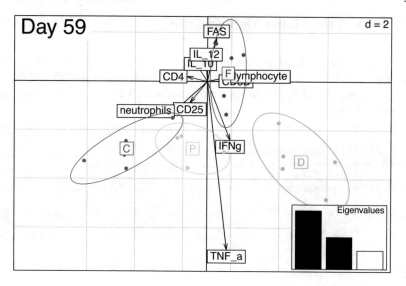

Fig. 17.5: The LDA of Day 59 as a biplot

17.6 MANOVA of the FIV Data

In addition to the exploratory analysis provided by PCA and LDA we may also want to do a formal multivariate test between treatment groups. The most traditional approach is through the use of multivariate analysis of variance (manova). The manova function has many test options. The Hotelling T^2 is the multivariate version of the t-test. According to the R help pages, the Pillai-Bartlett statistic is recommended by Hand and Taylor (1987) and is the default. There are many assumptions involved (including multivariate normality).

```
Y = cbind(Day59sc$CD4, Day59sc$CD8B, Day59sc$CD25,
    Day59sc$FAS, Day59sc$IFNg, Day59sc$IL_10,
    Day59sc$IL_12, Day59sc$lymphocyte,
    Day59sc$neutrophils, Day59sc$TNF_a)
X = Day59$Treatment
mova59 = manova(Y ~ X)
summary(mova59, test = "Pillai")

  ##             Df Pillai approx F num Df den Df  Pr(>F)
  ## X            3 2.1078   1.8901     30     24 0.05676 .
  ## Residuals 15
  ## ---
  ## Signif. codes:  0 '***' 0.001 '**' 0.01 '*' 0.05 '.' 0.1 ' ' 1
```

While this provides a formal significance value, the MANOVA is in some ways less informative than the previous more descriptive analyses.

17.7 PCA of the Mouse Malaria Data

The mouse malaria data were previously analyzed using the in-host TSIR model in
Sect. 8.9. A preliminary PCA of the red blood cell time series reveals that the fate
of the animals completely dominates the patterns since RBCs were scored as 0 after
death (Fig. 17.6).

```
require(ade4)
dead = ifelse(chabaudirbcw[,27] == 0, "dead", "alive")
pcarbc = dudi.pca(chabaudirbcw[, 3:27], scale = FALSE,
    scannf = FALSE, nf = 5)
s.arrow(dfxy = pcarbc$co[, 1:2] * 3, xlim = c(-10, 10),
    ylim = c(-5, 5), sub = "RBC", possub = "topleft", csub = 2)
s.class(dfxy = pcarbc$li[, 1:2]*.3, fac = as.factor(dead),
    cellipse = 2, axesell = FALSE, cstar = 0 ,
    col = c(2:7), add.plot = TRUE)
add.scatter.eig(pcarbc$eig, xax = 1, yax = 2,
    posi = "bottomright")
```

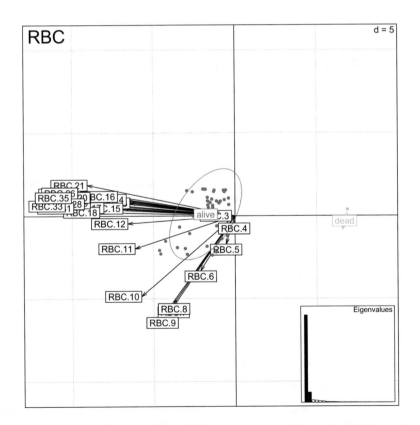

Fig. 17.6: The biplot of the RBC time series of the mouse malaria experiment

The strains are known to have different virulence, with the CB strain causing the most severe disease, so deaths are not random (the dead were seven CB, two AT, one BC, zero AQ and zero control). However, it is instructive to omit the 11 animals that died and redo the analysis to characterize the finer details in the progression of disease.[3] Because the measurements are all of the same nature (all RBC counts),[4] it is most informative to do the analysis based on the variance–covariance matrix as specified by the `scale = FALSE` argument.

```
chabaudirbcw2 = chabaudirbcw[dead == "alive",]
groups = chabaudirbcw2$Treatment
pcarbc2 = dudi.pca(chabaudirbcw2[, 3:27], scale = FALSE, scannf =
    FALSE, nf = 5)
s.arrow(dfxy = pcarbc2$co[, 1:2] * 3, xlim = c(-4,9),
    ylim = c(-5,5), sub = "RBC", possub = "topleft", csub = 2)
s.class(dfxy = pcarbc2$li[,1:2] * 0.3, fac = groups, cellipse = 2,
    axesell = FALSE, cstar = 0 , col = c(2:7), add.plot = TRUE)
add.scatter.eig(pcarbc2$eig, xax = 1, yax = 2,
    posi = "bottomright")
```

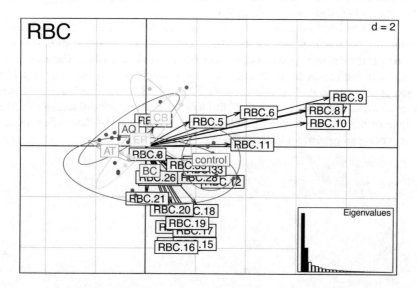

Fig. 17.7: The biplot of the RBC time series of the mouse malaria experiment excluding animals that died

As is often the case when doing eigen-decompositions of covariances all the loadings are of the same sign (arrows are pointing in the same direction) along axis one

---

[3] An approach that uses all available data would be to code dead RBCs as NAs and do a PCA with missing data using nonlinear iterative partial least-squares (`nipals`) as done by Roy et al. (2009).

[4] As opposed to the FIV data that is comprised of cytokine, virus, and cell measures with very different scales so that a PCA analysis based on the correlation matrix is most appropriate.

(Fig. 17.7). This first axis is therefore broadly called the means effect, in this case meaning that individuals with more positive axis one scores tend overall to suffer less severe anemia (with control animals suffering none). Clearly the main driver of the variation in the dataset is between control and treatment animals. There is, however, some further level of separation among the treatment animals along the second axis.

17.8 FDA of the Mouse Malaria Data

It is possible to get some deeper insights into the differences revealed by the PCA by considering how the mouse data is of a functional nature. That is, we can consider each of the time series of RBC counts as sampled along a curve through time. With this perspective one can ask how each curve can be thought of as being generated by adding or subtracting underlying component curves.[5] Generally speaking this multivariate approach is referred to as a functional data analysis (FDA; Ramsay & Silverman, 1997; Bjørnstad et al., 1998).

While specialized packages exist, we can treat the PCA as a simple FDA by considering the loadings along each axis to comprise a component time series—a so called empirical orthogonal function (EOF) (Castro et al., 1986; Bjørnstad et al., 1996)—and the scores for each individual as a weight of how much of that EOF to add or subtract to reconstitute the data. Figure 17.8 depicts the loadings of axis one and two as EOFs and how their addition or subtraction, corresponding to having positive or negative scores, these EOFs modulate the shape of the overall average curve among all experimental animals.

```
par(mfrow = c(1, 2))
# Gets the experimental days
day = unique(chabaudi$Day)
# Calculate the average time series
avg = apply(chabaudirbcw2[, 3:27], 2, mean)
plot(day, avg, type = "b", ylim = range(chabaudirbcw2[,
    3:27]), ylab = "RBC", xlab = "Day")
title("Mean +/- 1 SD eof 1")
lines(day, avg + 1 * pcarbc2$co[, 1], col = 2, type = "b",
    pch = "+")
lines(day, avg - 1 * pcarbc2$co[, 1], col = 2, type = "b",
    pch = "-")
plot(day, avg, type = "b", ylim = range(chabaudirbcw2[,
    3:27]), ylab = "RBC", xlab = "Day")
title("Mean +/- 1 SD eof 2")
lines(day, avg + 1 * pcarbc2$co[, 2], col = 2, type = "b",
    pch = "+")
lines(day, avg - 1 * pcarbc2$co[, 2], col = 2, type = "b",
    pch = "-")
```

---

[5] In some sense analogous to how a time series can be reconstructed as a weighted sum of trigonometric curves as discussed in Sect. 7.11.

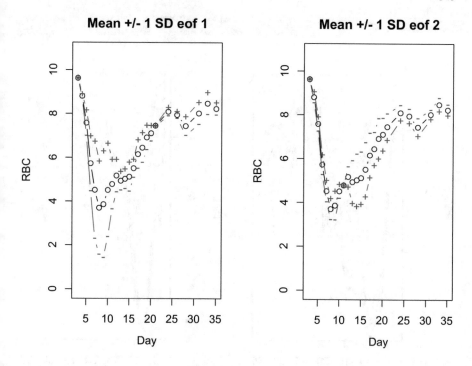

Fig. 17.8: The PCA of the RBC time series represented as a functional data analysis. Open circles are the average trajectories and red "+" and "-" show how the time series are molded by the (**a**) first and (**b**) second EOF

The analysis offers some new insights. As previously suggested, axis one measures the overall anemia. Animals with positive scores experience less anemia. Axis two, in contrast, is more interesting as it reveals that the second most important pattern broadly distinguishes animals that have peak anemia before day 10 (negative scores; broadly comprised of individuals infected with the BC clone) versus the other more slowly progressing infections (positive scores) that have peak anemia around day 15. To confirm the interpretation we can plot the actual time series for the 10 most extreme mice along the first and second EOF axes (Fig. 17.9).

```
par(mfrow = c(1, 2))
so = order(pcarbc2$li[, 1])
plot(day, t(chabaudirbcw2[so[1], 3:27]), type = "l", ylab = "RBC",
    xlab = "Day")
for (i in 1:5) lines(day, t(chabaudirbcw2[so[i], 3:27]))
for (i in 36:41) lines(day, t(chabaudirbcw2[so[i], 3:27]),
    col = 2, lty = 2)
so = order(pcarbc2$li[, 2])
plot(day, t(chabaudirbcw2[so[1], 3:27]), type = "l", ylab = "RBC",
    xlab = "Day")
for (i in 1:5) lines(day, t(chabaudirbcw2[so[i], 3:27]))
for (i in 36:41) lines(day, t(chabaudirbcw2[so[i], 3:27]),
```

col = 2, lty = 2)

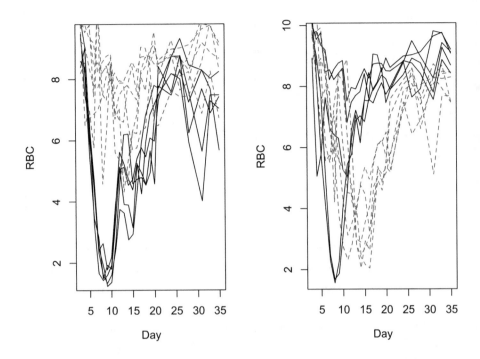

Fig. 17.9: The RBC time series for the five animals with highest (lowest) scores along the (**a**) first and (**b**) second axes. Black lines represent the five mice with the most negative scores and red dashed lines represent the mice with the most positive scores

The dominant feature is thus the depth of anemia and the subdominant feature is whether peak anemia is early or late.

While descriptive multivariate analysis is a vast field of statistics, the above sampling is an attempt to highlight some applications and methodologies that may be useful when considering the type of in-host experimental data commonly collected in the study of infectious diseases.

Chapter 18
Non-Independent Data

18.1 Non-Independence

Many infectious disease experiments result in non-independent data because of spatial autocorrelation across fields (such as discussed in Chap. 13), repeated measures on experimental animals (such as the in-host *Plasmodium* data discussed in Sect. 8.9), or other sources of correlated experimental responses among experimental units (such as the possibility of correlated infection fates among the rabbit littermates discussed in Sect. 5.2). Statistical methods that assume independence of observations are not strictly valid and/or fully effective on such data (e.g., Legendre, 1993; Keitt et al., 2002). Mixed-effects models and generalized linear mix-effects models (GLMMs) have been/are being developed to optimize the analysis of such data (Pinheiro & Bates, 2006; Bolker et al., 2009; Bates et al., 2015).

While this full topic is outside the main scope of this text, it is very pertinent to analyses of disease data, so we will study the three case studies as a sampler of things to consider.

```
require(nlme)
require(ncf)
require(lme4)
require(splines)
```

18.2 Spatial Dependence

The rust example introduced in Sect. 13.2 (Fig. 13.1) can be used to illustrate two approaches to accounting for spatial dependence in disease data: (i) random blocks versus (ii) spatial regression. Recall that this experiment looked at severity of a foliar rust infection on three focal individuals of flat-top goldenrods in each of 120 plots

---

This chapter uses the following R package: nlme, ncf, lme4 and splines.

O. N. Bjørnstad, *Epidemics*, Use R!, https://doi.org/10.1007/978-3-031-12056-5_18

across a field divided into four blocks. The experimental treatments were watering or not and whether surrounding non-focal host plants were conspecifics only, a mixture of conspecifics and an alternative host (the Canadian goldenrod) or the alternative host only.

As in the spatial pattern analysis, `jittered` coordinates allow application of some methods that require unique coordinates for each data point.

```
data(euthamia)
euthamia$jx = jitter(euthamia$xloc)
euthamia$jy = jitter(euthamia$yloc)
```

The randomized block design is the most classic way to deal with spatial dependence.[1] It serves two purposes. First, by randomly allocating treatments it frees experimental effects from underlying spatial structures that could cause spurious conclusions. Second, by stratifying observations into blocks the design enhances the power of the experiment by allowing for variability caused by unknown broader spatial heterogeneities. The `lme` function of the `nlme` package can be used to illustrate two random effect models of increasing nestedness. The first considers individuals in the blocks depicted in Fig. 13.1. The second considers plots nested in blocks.

```
fit = lme(score ~ comp + water, random = ~1 | block,
          data =  euthamia, na.action = na.omit, method="ML")
fit2 = lme(score ~ comp + water, random = ~1 | block / plot,
           data = euthamia, na.action = na.omit, method="ML")
```

A likelihood-ratio test provides a check for the better fit. The likelihood ratio test (provided by the `anova` function) shows that the more nested model provides the most parsimonious fit among the two candidates.

```
anova(fit, fit2)
##          Model df      AIC      BIC   logLik    Test
## fit          1  6 1178.570 1201.887 -583.2850
## fit2         2  7 1072.312 1099.515 -529.1561 1 vs 2
##           L.Ratio p-value
## fit
## fit2 108.2578  <.0001
```

The `intervals` call shows that the between-plot variance is about twice as large as the between-block variance and that watered plots have a significantly higher rust burden.

```
intervals(fit2)
## Approximate 95% confidence intervals
##
##   Fixed effects:
```

---

[1] I have always found it amusing that this most foundational idea in experimental design and statistics was published by R.A. Fisher on the 6th page of a paper in the *Journal of the Ministry of Agriculture* under the heading "A useful method" (Fisher, 1926).

```
##                   lower       est.      upper
## (Intercept)   0.9175659  1.4180556  1.9185452
## compSOL      -0.2457869  0.2083333  0.6624535
## compSYM      -0.1666202  0.2875000  0.7416202
## watermesic    0.2597680  0.6305556  1.0013431
##
##   Random Effects:
##     Level: block
##                       lower       est.      upper
## sd((Intercept))  0.1396334  0.3436512  0.8457586
##     Level: plot
##                       lower       est.      upper
## sd((Intercept))  0.7755296  0.9150862  1.079756
##
##   Within-group standard error:
##       lower       est.      upper
## 0.7315988  0.8001735  0.8751759
```

18.3 Spatial Regression

The above randomized block mixed-effects models is an example of the classic solution to analyzing experiments with spatial structure. An alternative is to formulate a regression model that considers the spatial dependence among observations as a function of separating distance. To investigate how proximate observations on different experimental treatments may be spatially autocorrelated, we can explore the spatial dependence among the residuals from a simple linear analysis of the data using the nonparametric spatial covariance function (as implemented in the spline.correlogram function in the ncf package) discussed in Chap. 13. The simple regression model that ignores space altogether is:

```
fitlm = lm(score ~ comp + water, data = euthamia)
```

The spatial correlation function among the residuals of the fit are (Fig. 18.1):

```
fitc = spline.correlog(euthamia$x, euthamia$y, resid(fitlm))
```

The nonparametric spatial correlation function reveals strong local spatial autocorrelation that decays to zero around 38m (with a CI of 31–43m).

```
plot(fitc, ylim = c(-0.5, 1))
```

The gls function from the nlme package can be used to fit spatial regression models (Pinheiro & Bates, 2006). This function fits mixed models from data that have a single dependence group, i.e., one spatial map, one time series, etc.[2] There are many possible models for spatial dependence as arising, for example, from spatial

---

[2] With multiple groups the lme function provides appropriate fits; see Sect. 18.4.

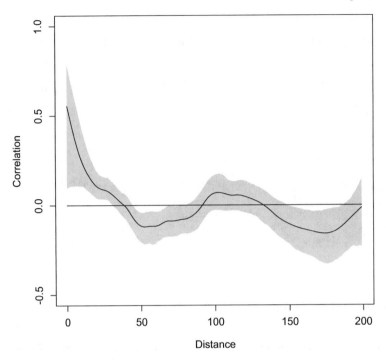

Fig. 18.1: The spline correlogram of the residuals from the regression model of the `euthamia` rust data

processes such as those discussed in Sect. 12.2. As an illustration compare the exponential model (which assumes the correlation to decay with distance proportional to $exp(-d/u)$ where d is distance and u is the scale) and the Gaussian model (proportional to $exp(-(d/u)^2)$. [The `nugget` flag in the below code means that the autocorrelation function is not anchored at one at distance zero.] We can compare these to the non-spatial model (`fitn`) and the best random block model (`fit2`) using the Akaike Information Criterion mentioned in Sect. 9.4.

```
fite = gls(score ~ comp + water, corr = corSpatial(form =
    ~ jx + jy, type = "exponential", nugget = TRUE),
    data = euthamia, na.action = na.omit, method="ML")
fitg = gls(score ~ comp + water, corr = corSpatial(form =
    ~ jx + jy, type = "gaussian", nugget = TRUE),
    data = euthamia, na.action = na.omit, method="ML")
fitn = gls(score ~ comp + water,  data = euthamia,
    na.action = na.omit, method="ML")
ai=matrix(c(extractAIC(fite),
    extractAIC(fitg), extractAIC(fitn),
    extractAIC(fit2)), ncol=2, byrow=TRUE)
dimnames(ai)=list(c("fite", "fitg", "fitn", "fit2"),
    c("edf", "aic"))
```

```
ai
```

```
##         edf      aic
## fite    7 1056.903
## fitg    7 1059.139
## fitn    5 1199.881
## fit2    7 1072.312
```

The AICs show that the exponential model provides the best fit. Moreover, the spatial regression model provides a better fit than the nested random effect model. This is presumably because of the gradual decay in correlation with distance (Fig. 18.1).

```
summary(fite, corr = FALSE)
```

```
## Generalized least squares fit by maximum likelihood
##   Model: score ~ comp + water
##   Data: euthamia
##         AIC       BIC    logLik
##   1056.903 1084.105 -521.4513
##
## Correlation Structure: Exponential spatial
##  correlation
##  Formula: ~jx + jy
##  Parameter estimate(s):
##      range     nugget
## 9.4619981 0.3383328
##
## Coefficients:
##                 Value Std.Error  t-value p-value
## (Intercept) 1.4591343 0.2485970 5.869477  0.0000
## compSOL     0.1911232 0.2016895 0.947611  0.3440
## compSYM     0.2241991 0.1997320 1.122500  0.2624
## watermesic  0.5336263 0.1573116 3.392161  0.0008
##
##  Correlation:
##             (Intr) cmpSOL cmpSYM
## compSOL     -0.412
## compSYM     -0.412  0.552
## watermesic  -0.298  0.033  0.015
##
## Standardized residuals:
##         Min         Q1        Med         Q3
## -1.3689448 -0.7647249 -0.1463925  0.6243239
##         Max
##   3.9923094
##
## Residual standard error: 1.254221
## Degrees of freedom: 360 total; 356 residual
```

The parametrically estimated range of 9.8m is a bit longer (but within the confidence interval) of the e-folding scale (5.5m) estimated via the spline correlogram; 1-nugget = 0.64 is comparable (but a little greater) than the 0.55 y-intercept. We can use the

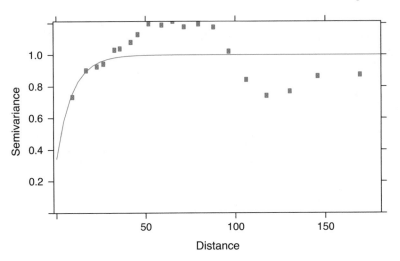

Fig. 18.2: A variogram plot of the fitted and observed spatial dependence for the spatial regression model

Variogram function from the nlme package to see if the spatial model adequately reflects the spatial dependence (Fig. 18.2). It looks like a plausible fit.

```
plot(Variogram(fite))
```

18.4 Repeated Measures

Repeated measurements usually result in non-independent data because of the inherent serial dependence. We can explore this notion using the data on anemia of mice infected of *Plasmodium chabaudi* introduced in Sect. 8.9 and analyzed further in Chap. 17 with lots of measurements taken. Consider the red blood cell counts (RBCs) on days three through 35 of mice infected by one of the five different strains as well as the control group. The sample sizes per treatment were 10 for AQ, BC, CB, and ER, seven for AT and five for control because eleven of the animals died during the course of the experiment. The chabaudi dataset is in long format.[3] As for previous analyses, some columns are extraneous in order to focus on the RBC count:

```
data(chabaudi)
chabaudirbc = chabaudi[, -c(1, 3, 4, 7, 8, 10, 11)]
```

---

[3] With repeated measures data one intermittently move between use both long format with one line for each observation and wide format with one line for each experimental unit.

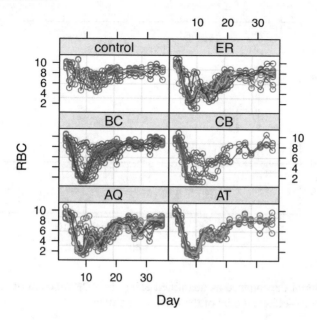

Fig. 18.3: RBC counts of control and *P. chabaudi*-infected mice. Each panel represent a different parasite strain

The repeated measures analyses require a `groupedData` object from the `nmle` package. The below call declares how the RBC counts represent time series for each mouse. Note that mice that died are scored by zero RBC count in the data set and that these zeros end up dominating patterns. It is best to rescore these data as missing (`NA`), and plot the grouped data object to visualize the anemia by treatment (Fig. 18.3).

```
RBC = groupedData(RBC ~ Day | Ind2, data = chabaudirbc)
RBC$RBC[RBC$RBC == 0] = NA
plot(RBC, outer = ~Treatment, key = FALSE)
```

The obvious main difference is between control and treatments, but the maximum and timing of the anemia varies somewhat among strains as previously discussed in Sect. 17.8. To test for significant differences `lme` can build a repeated measures model. In the simplest case, the standard conventions are to model the time series using day as an ordered factor and assume the treatment effect to be additive. The `random= ~ 1 | Ind2` call in the formula assumes there to be individual variation in the intercept (but not the slopes) among individuals. The `ACF` function of the `nlme` package[4] shows evidence of serial dependence in the residuals from the

---

[4] Different from the previously employed `acf` function from R base.

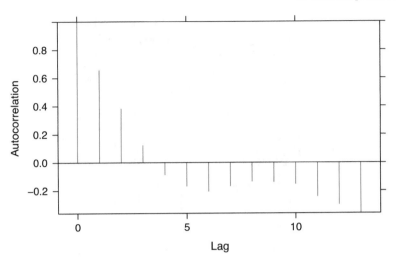

Fig. 18.4: Serial dependence as quantified using the ACF function on the repeated measures mixed-effects model of the chabaudi data

fit. As is apparent from the autocorrelation plot there is temporal autocorrelation in the residuals out to at least 4 days (Fig. 18.4).

```
mle.rbc = lme(RBC ~ Treatment + ordered(Day), random = ~1 |
    Ind2, data = RBC, na.action = na.omit, method = "ML")
plot(ACF(mle.rbc))
```

As with spatial dependence (Sect. 18.3), there are many models for serial dependence. The below use a first order autoregressive AR(1) process. This is specified by the correlation = corAR1(form = ~ Day|Ind2) function call. Note that this is one of a variety of time series models available in the nlme package, the most general of which is the ARMA(p, q) model discussed in Sect. 7.3.

```
mle.rbc2 = lme(RBC ~ Treatment + ordered(Day), random = ~1 |
    Ind2, data = RBC, correlation = corAR1(form = ~Day |
    Ind2), na.action = na.omit, method = "ML")
mle.rbc2

## Linear mixed-effects model
##   Data: RBC
##   Log-likelihood: -1568.255
##   Fixed: RBC ~ Treatment + ordered(Day)
##       (Intercept)        TreatmentAT
##       5.860494309        0.024586193
##       TreatmentBC        TreatmentCB
##       0.947853117       -0.022048465
## Treatmentcontrol        TreatmentER
##       1.560872851        0.325308683
```

```
##     ordered(Day).L    ordered(Day).Q
##       3.339300000       6.015597509
##     ordered(Day).C    ordered(Day)^4
##      -5.057192257       1.498354649
##     ordered(Day)^5    ordered(Day)^6
##       0.067695099      -0.600409959
##     ordered(Day)^7    ordered(Day)^8
##       1.352000127      -1.122142721
##     ordered(Day)^9    ordered(Day)^10
##      -0.394162545       0.312998475
##    ordered(Day)^11    ordered(Day)^12
##      -0.673514349      -0.122937927
##    ordered(Day)^13    ordered(Day)^14
##       0.219014886       0.378460147
##    ordered(Day)^15    ordered(Day)^16
##       0.191963472       0.180627944
##    ordered(Day)^17    ordered(Day)^18
##      -0.024392052       0.032617128
##    ordered(Day)^19    ordered(Day)^20
##      -0.142080994      -0.046539002
##    ordered(Day)^21    ordered(Day)^22
##      -0.054854991      -0.039333282
##    ordered(Day)^23    ordered(Day)^24
##      -0.210031799       0.006591632
##
## Random effects:
##  Formula: ~1 | Ind2
##          (Intercept) Residual
## StdDev: 0.0002332905 1.327223
##
## Correlation Structure: ARMA(1,0)
##  Formula: ~Day | Ind2
##  Parameter estimate(s):
##      Phi1
## 0.7088701
## Number of Observations: 1104
## Number of Groups: 52
```

The Phi1 parameter of 0.7088 represents the estimated day to day correlation, which is substantial. We can plot the predicted and observed correlation. The AR(1) model seems to be a nice fit (Fig. 18.5).

```
tmp = ACF(mle.rbc2)
plot(ACF ~ lag, data = tmp)
lines(0:15, 0.7088^(0:15))
```

Moreover, a formal likelihood-ratio test provided by the anova function reveals that the correlated error model provides a significantly better fit to the data:

```
anova(mle.rbc, mle.rbc2)
```

```
##          Model df      AIC      BIC    logLik
## mle.rbc      1 32 3834.369 3994.583 -1885.184
```

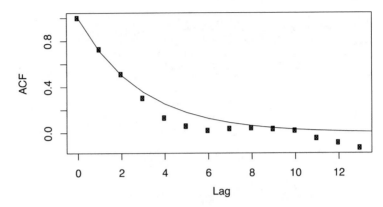

Fig. 18.5: An ACF plot of the fitted and observed serial dependence for the repeated measures regression model

```
## mle.rbc2     2 33 3202.510 3367.731 -1568.255
##                 Test  L.Ratio p-value
## mle.rbc
## mle.rbc2 1 vs 2 633.8586  <.0001
```

Statistically, the time-by-treatment interaction model that assumes that trajectories are treatment specific, rather than the additive model, is better still:

```
mle.rbc3 = lme(RBC ~ Treatment * ordered(Day), random = ~1 |
    Ind2, data = RBC, correlation = corAR1(form = ~Day |
    Ind2), na.action = na.omit, method = "ML")
anova(mle.rbc2, mle.rbc3)
```

```
##              Model df     AIC      BIC    logLik
## mle.rbc2     1  33 3202.510 3367.731 -1568.255
## mle.rbc3     2 153 3163.654 3929.679 -1428.827
##                 Test  L.Ratio p-value
## mle.rbc2
## mle.rbc3 1 vs 2 278.8557  <.0001
```

Finally we can plot the predicted values against time (filtering out predictions for the missing values in the original data) (Fig. 18.6). There is a distinct ordering following from the virulence of the strains:

```
pr = predict(mle.rbc3)
RBC$pr = NA
RBC$pr[!is.na(RBC$RBC)] = pr
plot(RBC$pr ~ RBC$Day, col = as.numeric(RBC$Treatment),
    pch = as.numeric(RBC$Treatment), xlab = "Day",
    ylab = "RBC count")
legend("bottomright",
    legend = c("AQ", "AT", "BC", "CB", "Control", "ER"),
    pch = unique(as.numeric(RBC$Treatment)), col = 1:6)
```

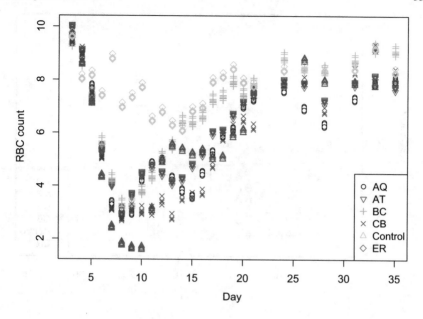

Fig. 18.6: Predicted and observed anemia levels for the best-fitting repeated measures model

Modeling time as an ordered factor is quite parameter wasteful (the full interaction model has 153 parameters). A flexible more economic approach may be to model time using the sort of smoothing splines introduced in Sect. 5.4. The following example uses B-splines with five degrees of freedom (Fig. 18.7). The qualitative features are similar to the more parameter rich model (Fig. 18.6):

```
mle.rbc4 = lme(RBC ~ Treatment * bs(Day, df = 5),
    random = ~1 | Ind2, data = RBC, correlation =
    corAR1(form = ~ Day | Ind2),
      na.action = na.omit, method = "ML")
pr = predict(mle.rbc4)
RBC$pr = NA
RBC$pr[!is.na(RBC$RBC)] = pr
plot(RBC$pr ~ RBC$Day, col = as.numeric(RBC$Treatment),
    pch = as.numeric(RBC$Treatment),  xlab = "Day",
    ylab = "RBC count")
legend("bottomright",
legend = c("AQ", "AT", "BC", "CB", "Control", "ER"),
    pch = unique(as.numeric(RBC$Treatment)), col = 1:6)
```

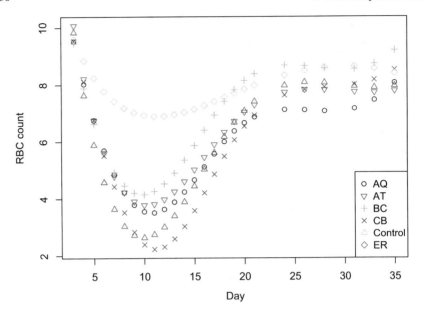

Fig. 18.7: Predicted and observed for the repeated measures RBC data using a spline model in time

18.5 Sibling Correlation

Bordetella bronchiseptica is a respiratory infection of a range of mammals (e.g., Bjørnstad & Harvill, 2005). Its congeners, *B. pertussis* and *B. parapertussis*, cause whooping cough in humans, but *B. bronchiseptica* is usually relatively asymptomatic (though it can cause snuffles in rabbits and kennel cough in dogs). The data comes from a commercial rabbitry which breeds NZW rabbits to study transmission paths in the colony. The data is from the same study as used to study the age-specific force of infection in Sect. 5.2. Nasal swabs of female rabbits and their young were taken at weaning (∼ 4 weeks old). A total of 86 does and 408 kits was included in the study (Long et al., 2010).

```
data(litter)
```

To investigate if (i) offspring of infected mothers have an increased instantaneous risk of becoming infected and (ii) if offspring of the same litter tended to have the same infection fate because of within-litter transmission, we can use a random effect generalized linear mixed (GLMM) logistic regression, with litter as a random effect. Some data formatting prepares for the analysis:

```
tdat = data.frame(lsize = as.vector(table(litter$Litter)),
    Litter = names(table(litter$Litter)),
anysick = sapply(split(litter$sick, litter$Litter), sum))
```

```
ldat = merge(litter, tdat, by = "Litter")
ldat$othersick = ldat$anysick - ldat$sick
ldat$anyothersick = ldat$othersick > 0
ldat$X = 1:408
```

Here, the concern is with whether litter mates share correlated fates. Unlike for spatial or temporal autocorrelation, there are no canned functions to quantify this correlation. However, following the discussion of autocorrelation in Sect. 13.3, it is easy to customize appropriate calculations. In the below, the first double-loop makes a sibling-sibling contact matrix (along the lines of the ideas introduced in Chap. 14), tmp, that flags kittens according to litter membership. After, tmp2 is the scaled binary sick vector that flags whether or not an animal was infected, and tmp3 is the similarity matrix. Finally mean(tmp3*tmp) provides the within-litter autocorrelation in infection status averaged across all litters.

```
tmp = matrix(NA, ncol = length(ldat$Litter),
    nrow = length(ldat$Litter))
    for(i in 1:length(ldat$Litter)) {
        for(j in 1:length(ldat$Litter)) {
            if(ldat$Litter[i] == ldat$Litter[j]) {
                tmp[i, j] = 1
            }
        }
    }
diag(tmp) = NA
tmp2 = scale(ldat$sick)[,1]
tmp3 = outer(tmp2, tmp2, FUN="*")
mean(tmp3 * tmp, na.rm = TRUE)
```

```
## [1] 0.5302508
```

The within-litter correlation of 0.53 represents a substantial interdependence in infection risk among litter mates. Since the response variable is binary (infected versus non-infected) lme does not apply. Instead we can use the lmer function from the lme4 package (Bates et al., 2015) and specify that the response is binomial using the family argument. The AICs compare the fit that incorporates the within-litter correlation (fitL) with the fit that assumes independence (fit0). The appropriate independence fit is generated by declaring that each of the 408 individuals are in their own group (variable X in the data set).

```
fitL = glmer(sick ~ msick + lsize + Facility + anyothersick +
    (1 | Litter), family = binomial(), data = ldat)
fit0 = glmer(sick ~ msick + lsize + Facility + anyothersick +
    (1 | X), family = binomial(), data = ldat)

ai = matrix(c(extractAIC(fitL), extractAIC(fit0)), ncol = 2,
    byrow = TRUE)
dimnames(ai) = list(c("fitL", "fit0"), c("edf", "aic"))
ai
```

```
##       edf      aic
```

```
## fitL   7 291.0263
## fit0   7 316.5853
```

The litter-dependent model is clearly best (no surprise given the strong empirical intra-litter correlation). The summary of the best model reveals that the key predictor of infection fate is whether or not a sibling was infected (anyothersickTRUE). The infection status of the mother is insignificant. The mixed-effect logistic regression thus reveals that the most important route of infection is likely to be sib-to-sib transmission (Long et al., 2010).

```
summary(fitL, corr = FALSE)

## Generalized linear mixed model fit by maximum
##   likelihood (Laplace Approximation)
## Family: binomial   ( logit )
## Formula:
## sick ~ msick + lsize + Facility + anyothersick +
##     (1 | Litter)  Data: ldat
##
##     AIC       BIC    logLik deviance df.resid
##   291.0     319.1    -138.5   277.0      400
##
## Scaled residuals:
##    Min      1Q   Median       3Q      Max
## -1.7277 -0.3199 -0.1333 -0.0386 13.2186
##
## Random effects:
##  Groups Name          Variance Std.Dev.
##  Litter (Intercept) 2.077     1.441
## Number of obs: 407, groups:  Litter, 52
##
## Fixed effects:
##                    Estimate Std. Error z value
## (Intercept)        -3.43236    2.32298  -1.478
## msick               2.74171    1.65447   1.657
## lsize              -0.37908    0.19153  -1.979
## FacilityT3          1.15833    0.80626   1.437
## FacilityT9         -0.01773    0.68553  -0.026
## anyothersickTRUE    2.88387    0.71564   4.030
##                     Pr(>|z|)
## (Intercept)          0.1395
## msick                0.0975 .
## lsize                0.0478 *
## FacilityT3           0.1508
## FacilityT9           0.9794
## anyothersickTRUE 5.58e-05 ***
## ---
## Signif. codes:
## 0 '***' 0.001 '**' 0.01 '*' 0.05 '.' 0.1 ' ' 1
```

18.6 The End

This concludes the text of the 2nd edition of "Epidemics: Models and Data using R". While the 3rd part is somewhat eclectic it was collated in the spirit that some methodology and associated code is very easy to find, but other bits less so. The last three chapters may be seen as providing some additional biological/dynamic perspectives on infectious disease dynamics and otherwise as a repository of more obscure R code.

References

Abbey, H. (1952). An examination of the Reed-Frost theory of epidemics. *Human Biology, 24*(3), 201.

Abbott, K. C., & Dwyer, G. (2008). Using mechanistic models to understand synchrony in forest insect populations: the North American gypsy moth as a case study. *The American Naturalist, 172*(5), 613–624.

Aitkin, M. A., Francis, B., & Hinde, J. (2005). *Statistical modelling in GLIM 4*. Oxford University Press.

Althouse, B. M., & Scarpino, S. V. (2015). Asymptomatic transmission and the resurgence of *Bordetella pertussis*. *BMC Medicine, 13*(1), 146.

Altizer, S., Dobson, A., Hosseini, P., Hudson, P., Pascual, M., & Rohani, P. (2006). Seasonality and the dynamics of infectious diseases. *Ecology Letters, 9*(4), 467–484.

Anagnostakis, S. L. (1987). Chestnut blight: the classical problem of an introduced pathogen. *Mycologia, 79*(1), 23–37.

Anderson, R. M., Jackson, H. C., May, R. M., & Smith, A. M. (1981). Population dynamics of fox rabies in Europe. *Nature, 289*(5800), 765–771.

Anderson, R. M., & May, R. M. (1982). Directly transmitted infectious diseases: Control by vaccination. *Science, 215*, 1053–1060.

Anderson, R. M., & May, R. M. (1991). *Infectious diseases of humans: Dynamics and control*. Oxford University Press, Oxford.

Anselin, L. (1995). Local indicators of spatial association—LISA. *Geographical Analysis, 27*(2), 93–115.

Antonovics, J. (2004). Long-term study of a plant-pathogen metapopulation. In Hanski, I., & Gaggiotti, O., (Eds.), *Ecology, genetics, and evolution of metapopulations* (pp. 471–488). Amsterdam: Elsevier.

Arias, E., Rostron, B. L., & Tejada-Vera, B. (2010). National vital statistics reports. *National Vital Statistics Reports, 58*(10).

Aron, J. L., & May, R. M. (1982). The population dynamics of malaria. In *The population dynamics of infectious diseases: Theory and applications* (pp. 139–179). Springer.

Aron, J. L., & Schwartz, I. B. (1984). Seasonality and period-doubling bifurcations in an epidemic model. *Journal of Theoretical Biology, 110*(4), 665–679.

Axelsen, J. B., Yaari, R., Grenfell, B. T., & Stone, L. (2014). Multiannual forecasting of seasonal influenza dynamics reveals climatic and evolutionary drivers. *Proceedings of the National Academy of Sciences, 111*(26), 9538–9542.

Bailey, B. A., Ellner, S., & Nychka, D. W. (1997). Chaos with confidence: Asymptotics and applications of local lyapunov exponents. *Nonlinear dynamics and time series: building a bridge between the natural and statistical sciences. American Mathematical Society, Providence, Rhode Island, USA* (pp. 115–133).

Bailey, N. T. J. (1956). On estimating the latent and infectious periods of Measles: I. Families with two susceptibles only. *Biometrika, 43*(1/2), 15–22.

Bailey, N. T. J. (1957). *The mathematical theory of epidemics*. London: Griffin.

Bailey, N. T. J., & Alff-Steinberger, C. (1970). Improvements in the estimation of the latent and infectious periods of a contagious disease. *Biometrika, 57*(1), 141–153.

Baker-Austin, C., Trinanes, J. A., Taylor, N. G., Hartnell, R., Siitonen, A., & Martinez-Urtaza, J. (2013). Emerging vibrio risk at high latitudes in response to ocean warming. *Nature Climate Change, 3*(1), 73–77.

Bansal, S., Grenfell, B. T., & Meyers, L. A. (2007). When individual behaviour matters: Homogeneous and network models in epidemiology. *Journal of the Royal Society Interface, 4*(16), 879–891.

Barabási, A.-L., & Albert, R. (1999). Emergence of scaling in random networks. *Science, 286*(5439), 509–512.

Barbour, A., & Mollison, D. (1990). Epidemics and random graphs. In *Stochastic processes in epidemic theory* (pp. 86–89). Springer.

Bartlett, M. S. (1956). Deterministic and stochastic models for recurrent epidemics. In Neyman, J., (Ed.), *Proceedings of the third Berkeley symposium on mathematical statistics and probability* (pp. 81–109). University of California Press.

Bartlett, M. S. (1960a). *Stochastic population models in ecology and epidemiology*. Wiley.

Bartlett, M. S. (1960b). The critical community size for measles in the U.S. *Journal of Royal Statistical Society A, 123*, 37–44.

Bascompte, J., & Solé, R. V. (1995). Rethinking complexity: Modelling spatiotemporal dynamics in ecology. *Trends in Ecology and Evolution, 10*(9), 361–366.

Bates, D., Mächler, M., Bolker, B. M., & Walker, S. C. (2015). Fitting linear mixed-effects models using lme4. *Journal of Statistical Software, 67*(1), 1–48.

Bauch, C. T., & Earn, D. J. D. (2003). Interepidemic intervals in forced and unforced SEIR models. *Dynamical Systems and their Applications in Biology, 36*, 33–44.

Becker, A. D., & Grenfell, B. T. (2017). tsiR: An R package for time-series Susceptible-Infected-Recovered models of epidemics. *PloS One, 12*(9), e0185528.

Becker, A. D., Wesolowski, A., Bjørnstad, O. N., & Grenfell, B. T. (2019). Long-term dynamics of measles in london: Titrating the impact of wars, the 1918 pandemic, and vaccination. *PLoS Computational Biology, 15*(9), e1007305.

Bhattacharyya, S., Gesteland, P. H., Korgenski, K., Bjørnstad, O. N., & Adler, F. R. (2015). Cross-immunity between strains explains the dynamical pattern of paramyxoviruses. *Proceedings of the National Academy of Sciences, 112*(43), 13396–13400.

Biek, R., Drummond, A. J., & Poss, M. (2006). A virus reveals population structure and recent demographic history of its carnivore host. *Science, 311*(5760), 538–541.

Bjørnstad, O. N. (2000). Cycles and synchrony: Two historical 'experiments' and one experience. *Journal of Animal Ecology*, 869–873.

Bjørnstad, O. N., & Bascompte, J. (2001). Synchrony and second-order spatial correlation in host-parasitoid systems. *Journal of Animal Ecology, 70*(6), 924–933.

Bjørnstad, O. N., & Bolker, B. (2000). Canonical functions for dispersal-induced synchrony. *Proceedings of the Royal Society of London B, 267*(1454), 1787–1794.

Bjørnstad, O. N., Champely, S., Stenseth, N. C., & Saitoh, T. (1996). Cyclicity and stability of grey-sided voles, *Clethrionomys rufocanus*, of Hokkaido: Spectral and principal components analyses. *Philosophical Transactions of the Royal Society of London. Series B: Biological Sciences, 351*(1342), 867–875.

Bjørnstad, O. N., & Falck, W. (2001). Nonparametric spatial covariance functions: Estimation and testing. *Environmental and Ecological Statistics, 8*(1), 53–70.

Bjørnstad, O. N., Finkenstadt, B. F., & Grenfell, B. T. (2002a). Dynamics of measles epidemics: Estimating scaling of transmission rates using a time series sir model. *Ecological Monographs, 72*(2), 169–184.

Bjørnstad, O. N., & Grenfell, B. T. (2001). Noisy clockwork: time series analysis of population fluctuations in animals. *Science, 293*(5530), 638–643.

Bjørnstad, O. N., & Harvill, E. T. (2005). Evolution and emergence of *Bordetella* in humans. *Trends in Microbiology, 13*(8), 355–359.

Bjørnstad, O. N., Ims, R. A., & Lambin, X. (1999b). Spatial population dynamics: Analyzing patterns and processes of population synchrony. *Trends in Ecology and Evolution, 14*(11), 427–432.

Bjørnstad, O. N., Nelson, W. A., & Tobin, P. C. (2016). Developmental synchrony in multivoltine insects: Generation separation versus smearing. *Population Ecology, 58*(4), 479–491.

Bjørnstad, O. N., Nisbet, R. M., & Fromentin, J.-M. (2004). Trends and cohort resonant effects in age-structured populations. *Journal of Animal Ecology, 73*(6), 1157–1167.

Bjørnstad, O. N., Peltonen, M., Liebhold, A. M., & Baltensweiler, W. (2002b). Waves of larch budmoth outbreaks in the European Alps. *Science, 298*(5595), 1020–1023.

Bjørnstad, O. N., Robinet, C., & Liebhold, A. M. (2010). Geographic variation in North American gypsy moth cycles: Subharmonics, generalist predators, and spatial coupling. *Ecology, 91*(1), 106–118.

Bjørnstad, O. N., Sait, S. M., Stenseth, N. C., Thompson, D. J., & Begon, M. (2001). The impact of specialized enemies on the dimensionality of host dynamics. *Nature, 409*(6823), 1001.

Bjørnstad, O. N., Shea, K., Krzywinski, M., & Altman, N. (2020a). Modeling infectious epidemics. *Nature Methods, 17*(5), 455–456.

Bjørnstad, O. N., Shea, K., Krzywinski, M., & Altman, N. (2020b). The SEIRS model for infectious disease dynamics. *Nature Methods, 17*(6), 557–559.

Bjørnstad, O. N., Stenseth, N. C., & Saitoh, T. (1999a). Synchrony and scaling in dynamics of voles and mice in northern Japan. *Ecology, 80*(2), 622–637.

Bjørnstad, O. N., Stenseth, N. C., Saitoh, T., & Lingjærde, O. C. (1998). Mapping the regional transition to cyclicity in *Clethrionomys rufocanus*: Spectral densities and functional data analysis. *Population Ecology, 40*(1), 77–84.

Bjørnstad, O. N., & Viboud, C. (2016). Timing and periodicity of influenza epidemics. *Proceedings of the National Academy of Sciences*, 201616052.

Black, F. L. (1959). Measles antibodies in the population of New Haven, Connecticut. *Journal of Immunology, 83*, 74–83.

Blehert, D. S., Hicks, A. C., Behr, M., Meteyer, C. U., Berlowski-Zier, B. M., Buckles, E. L., Coleman, J. T., Darling, S. R., Gargas, A., Niver, R., et al. (2009). Bat white-nose syndrome: an emerging fungal pathogen? *Science, 323*(5911), 227–227.

Blumberg, S., & Lloyd-Smith, J. O. (2013a). Comparing methods for estimating R^0 from the size distribution of subcritical transmission chains. *Epidemics, 5*(3), 131–145.

Blumberg, S., & Lloyd-Smith, J. O. (2013b). Inference of R^0 and transmission heterogeneity from the size distribution of stuttering chains. *PLoS Computational Biology, 9*(5), e1002993.

Blythe, S. P., Nisbet, R. M., & Gurney, W. S. C. (1984). The dynamics of population models with distributed maturation periods. *Theoretical Population Biology, 25*(3), 289–311.

Bobashev, G. V., Ellner, S. P., Nychka, D. W., & Grenfell, B. T. (2000). Reconstructing susceptible and recruitment dynamics from measles epidemic data. *Mathematical Population Studies, 8*(1), 1–29.

Bolker, B. M. (2008). *Ecological models and data in R.* Princeton: Princeton University Press.

Bolker, B. M., Brooks, M. E., Clark, C. J., Geange, S. W., Poulsen, J. R., Stevens, M. H. H., & White, J.-S. S. (2009). Generalized linear mixed models: A practical guide for ecology and evolution. *Trends in Ecology and Evolution, 24*(3), 127–135.

Bolker, B. M., & Grenfell, B. T. (1993). Chaos and biological complexity in measles dynamics. *Proceedings of the Royal Society of London B, 251*(1330), 75–81.

Breda, D., Diekmann, O., De Graaf, W. F., Pugliese, A., & Vermiglio, R. (2012). On the formulation of epidemic models (an appraisal of Kermack and McKendrick). *Journal of Biological Dynamics, 6*(sup2), 103–117.

Broadbent, S., & Kendall, D. G. (1953). The random walk of *Trichostrongylus retortaeformis*. *Biometrics, 9*(4), 460–466.

Brooks, J. (1996). The sad and tragic life of Typhoid Mary. *Canadian Medical Association Journal, 154*(6), 915.

Bruno, J. F., Ellner, S. P., Vu, I., Kim, K., & Harvell, C. D. (2011). Impacts of aspergillosis on sea fan coral demography: Modeling a moving target. *Ecological Monographs, 81*(1), 123–139.

Bukreyev, A., Yang, L., Fricke, J., Cheng, L., Ward, J. M., Murphy, B. R., & Collins, P. L. (2008). The secreted form of respiratory syncytial virus G glycoprotein helps the virus evade antibody-mediated restriction of replication by acting as an antigen decoy and through effects on Fc receptor-bearing leukocytes. *Journal of Virology, 82*(24), 12191–12204.

Burnett, T. (1958). A model of host-parasite interaction. In *Proceedings of the 10th International Congress of Entomology* (vol. 2, pp. 679–686).

Burnham, K. P., & Anderson, D. R. (2003). *Model selection and multimodel inference: A practical information-theoretic approach.* Springer.

Canini, L., & Carrat, F. (2011). Population modeling of influenza A/H1N1 virus kinetics and symptom dynamics. *Journal of Virology, 85*(6), 2764–2770.

Carrat, F., Vergu, E., Ferguson, N. M., Lemaitre, M., Cauchemez, S., Leach, S., & Valleron, A. J. (2008). Time lines of infection and disease in human influenza: A review of volunteer challenge studies. *American Journal of Epidemiology, 167*(7), 775–785.

Castro, P. E., Lawton, W. H., & Sylvestre, E. (1986). Principal modes of variation for processes with continuous sample curves. *Technometrics, 28*(4), 329–337.

Caswell, H. (2001). *Matrix population models: Construction, analysis, and interpretation (2nd edn).* Sinauer Associates.

Chambers, J. M. (1998). *Programming with data: A guide to the S language.* Springer.

Cheng, B., & Tong, H. (1992). On consistent nonparametric order determination and chaos. *Journal of the Royal Statistical Society B*, 427–449.

Childs, J. E., Curns, A. T., Dey, M. E., Real, L. A., Feinstein, L., Bjørnstad, O. N., & Krebs, J. W. (2000). Predicting the local dynamics of epizootic rabies among raccoons in the united states. *Proceedings of the National Academy of Sciences, 97*(25), 13666–13671.

Choi, K., & Thacker, S. B. (1981). An evaluation of influenza mortality surveillance, 1962–1979: I. Time series forecasts of expected pneumonia and influenza deaths. *American Journal of Epidemiology, 113*(3), 215–226.

Chowell, G., Echevarría-Zuno, S., Viboud, C., Simonsen, L., Tamerius, J., Miller, M. A., & Borja-Aburto, V. H. (2011). Characterizing the epidemiology of the 2009 influenza A/H1N1 pandemic in Mexico. *PLoS Medicine, 8*(5).

Clark, D. A., & Clark, D. B. (1984). Spacing dynamics of a tropical rain forest tree: Evaluation of the Janzen-Connell model. *The American Naturalist, 124*(6), 769–788.

Clark, J. S. (1998). Why trees migrate so fast: Confronting theory with dispersal biology and the paleorecord. *The American Naturalist, 152*(2), 204–224.

Clark, J. S., & Bjørnstad, O. N. (2004). Population time series: Process variability, observation errors, missing values, lags, and hidden states. *Ecology, 85*(11), 3140–3150.

Codeço, C. T. (2001). Endemic and epidemic dynamics of cholera: The role of the aquatic reservoir. *BMC Infectious Diseases* 1.

Connell, J. H. (1971). On the role of natural enemies in preventing competitive exclusion in some marine animals and in rain forest trees. In Boer, P. J. D., & Gradwell, G., editors, *Dynamics of populations* (pp. 298–312). Wageningen: Centre for Agricultural Publishing and Documentation.

Cowling, B. J., Fang, V. J., Riley, S., Peiris, J. S. M., & Leung, G. M. (2009). Estimation of the serial interval of influenza. *Epidemiology, 20*(3), 344–347.

Coyne, M. J., Smith, G., & McAllister, F. E. (1989). Mathematic model for the population biology of rabies in raccoons in the mid-Atlantic states. *American Journal of Veterinary Research, 50*(12), 2148–2154.

Cummings, D. A. T., Irizarry, R. A., Huang, N. E., Endy, T. P., Nisalak, A., Ungchusak, K., & Burke, D. S. (2004). Travelling waves in the occurrence of dengue haemorrhagic fever in Thailand. *Nature, 427*(6972), 344–347.

Cushing, J. M., Dennis, B., Desharnais, R. A., & Costantino, R. F. (1998). Moving toward an unstable equilibrium: Saddle nodes in population systems. *Journal of Animal Ecology*, 298–306.

Dalziel, B. D., Bjørnstad, O. N., van Panhuis, W. G., Burke, D. S., Metcalf, C. J. E., & Grenfell, B. T. (2016). Persistent chaos of measles epidemics in the prevaccination United States caused by a small change in seasonal transmission Patterns. *PLoS Computationmal Biology, 12*(2), e1004655.

Dalziel, B. D., Kissler, S., Gog, J. R., Viboud, C., Bjørnstad, O. N., Metcalf, C. J. E., & Grenfell, B. T. (2018). Urbanization and humidity shape the intensity of influenza epidemics in US cities. *Science, 362*(6410), 75–79.

De, P., Singh, A. E., Wong, T., Yacoub, W., & Jolly, A. (2004). Sexual network analysis of a gonorrhoea outbreak. *Sexually Transmitted Infections, 80*(4), 280–285.

De Castro, F., & Bolker, B. (2005). Mechanisms of disease-induced extinction. *Ecology Letters, 8*(1), 117–126.

de Jong, M., Diekmann, O., & Heesterbeek, H. (1995). How does transmission of infection depend on population size? In Mollison, D., (Ed.), *Epidemic models: Their structure and relation to data* (pp. 84–94). Cambridge University Press.

Delatte, H., Gimonneau, G., Triboire, A., & Fontenille, D. (2009). Influence of temperature on immature development, survival, longevity, fecundity, and gonotrophic cycles of *Aedes albopictus*, vector of chikungunya and dengue in the Indian Ocean. *Journal of Medical Entomology, 46*(1), 33–41.

Dennis, B., Desharnais, R. A., Cushing, J., Henson, S. M., & Costantino, R. (2003). Can noise induce chaos? *Oikos, 102*(2), 329–339.

Diekmann, O., Heesterbeek, J. A. P., & Metz, J. A. J. (1990). On the definition and the computation of the basic reproduction ratio R^0 in models for infectious diseases in Heterogeneous Populations. *Journal of Mathematical Biology, 28*(4), 365–382.

Dietz, K. (1993). The estimation of the basic reproduction number for infectious diseases. *Statistical Methods in Medical Research, 2*, 23–41.

Dietz, K., & Heesterbeek, J. (2002). Daniel Bernoulli's epidemiological model revisited. *Mathematical Biosciences, 180*(1), 1–21.

Dietz, K., & Schenzle, D. (1985). Proportionate mixing models for age-dependent infection transmission. *Journal of Mathematical Biology, 22*(1), 117–120.

Dixon, M. G., Ferrari, M., Antoni, S., Li, X., Portnoy, A., Lambert, B., Hauryski, S., Hatcher, C., Nedelec, Y., Patel, M., et al. (2021). Progress toward regional measles elimination worldwide, 2000–2020. *Morbidity and Mortality Weekly Report, 70*(45), 1563.

Donoghue, H. D., Marcsik, A., Matheson, C., Vernon, K., Nuorala, E., Molto, J. E., Greenblatt, C. L., & Spigelman, M. (2005). Co-infection of *Mycobacterium tuberculosis* and *Mycobacterium leprae* in human archaeological samples: A possible explanation for the historical decline of leprosy. *Proceedings of the Royal Society B, 272*(1561), 389–394.

Dowdle, W. R. (1999). Influenza A virus recycling revisited. *Bulletin of the World Health Organization, 77*(10), 820.

Dray, S., & Dufour, A.-B. (2007). The ade4 package: Implementing the duality diagram for ecologists. *Journal of Statistical Software, 22*(4), 1–20.

Duarte, J. H. (2016). Functional switching. *Nature Immunology, 17*(1), S12–S12.

Dushoff, J., Plotkin, J. B., Levin, S. A., & Earn, D. J. (2004). Dynamical resonance can account for seasonality of influenza epidemics. *Proceedings of the National Academy of Sciences, 101*(48), 16915–16916.

Dwyer, G., Dushoff, J., Elkinton, J. S., & Levin, S. A. (2000). Pathogen-driven outbreaks in forest defoliators revisited: Building models from experimental data. *The American Naturalist, 156*(2), 105–120.

Dwyer, G., Dushoff, J., & Yee, S. H. (2004). The combined effects of pathogens and predators on insect outbreaks. *Nature, 430*(6997), 341–345.

Dye, C. (2015). *The population biology of tuberculosis* (vol. 54). Princeton University Press.

Eames, K. T. D., Tilston, N. L., & Edmunds, W. J. (2011). The impact of school holidays on the social mixing patterns of school children. *Epidemics, 3*(2), 103–108.

Earn, D. J. D., Levin, S. A., & Rohani, P. (2000a). Coherence and conservation. *Science, 290*(5495), 1360–1364.

Earn, D. J. D., Rohani, P., Bolker, B. M., & Grenfell, B. T. (2000b). A simple model for complex dynamical transitions in epidemics. *Science, 287*(5453), 667–670.

Eckmann, J.-P., & Ruelle, D. (1985). Ergodic theory of chaos and strange attractors. *Reviews of Modern Physics, 57*(3), 617.

Elkinton, J. S., & Liebhold, A. M. (1990). Population dynamics of gypsy moth in North America. *Annual review of Entomology, 35*(1), 571–596.

Ellner, S. P., Bailey, B. A., Bobashev, G. V., Gallant, A. R., Grenfell, B. T., & Nychka, D. W. (1998). Noise and nonlinearity in measles epidemics: Combining mechanistic and statistical approaches to population modeling. *The American Naturalist, 151*(5), 425–440.

Ellner, S. P., Seifu, Y., & Smith, R. H. (2002). Fitting population dynamic models to time-series data by gradient matching. *Ecology, 83*(8), 2256–2270.

Ellner, S. P., & Turchin, P. (2005). When can noise induce chaos and why does it matter: A critique. *Oikos, 111*(3), 620–631.

Engen, S., Tian, H., Yang, R., Bjørnstad, O. N., Whittington, J. D., & Stenseth, N. C. (2021). The ecological dynamics of the coronavirus epidemics during transmission from outside sources when R^0 is successfully managed below one. *Royal Society Open Science, 8*(6), 202234.

Erdős, P. & Rényi, A. (1959). On random graphs i. *Publicationes Mathematicae, 6*, 290–297.

Erlander, S., & Stewart, N. F. (1990). *The gravity model in transportation analysis: Theory and extensions* (vol. 3). VSP.

Fan, J., Yao, Q., & Tong, H. (1996). Estimation of conditional densities and sensitivity measures in nonlinear dynamical systems. *Biometrika, 83*(1), 189–206.

Farrington, C. P., & Grant, A. D. (1999). The distribution of time to extinction in subcritical branching processes: Applications to outbreaks of infectious disease. *Journal of Applied Probability, 36*(3), 771–779.

Farrington, C. P., Kanaan, M. N., & Gay, N. J. (2003). Branching process models for surveillance of infectious diseases controlled by mass vaccination. *Biostatistics, 4*(2), 279–295.

Ferguson, N. M., Anderson, R. M., & Garnett, G. P. (1996). Mass vaccination to control chickenpox: The influence of zoster. *Proceedings of the National Academy of Sciences, 93*(14), 7231–7235.

Ferguson, N. M., Keeling, M. J., Edmunds, W. J., Gani, R., Grenfell, B. T., Anderson, R. M., & Leach, S. (2003). Planning for smallpox outbreaks. *Nature, 425*(6959), 681–685.

Ferrari, M. J., Bansal, S., Meyers, L. A., & Bjørnstad, O. N. (2006a). Network frailty and the geometry of herd immunity. *Proceedings of the Royal Society of London B, 273*(1602), 2743–2748.

Ferrari, M. J., Bjørnstad, O. N., & Dobson, A. P. (2005). Estimation and inference of R^0 of an infectious pathogen by a removal method. *Mathematical Biosciences, 198*(1), 14–26.

Ferrari, M. J., Bjørnstad, O. N., Partain, J. L., & Antonovics, J. (2006b). A gravity model for the spread of a pollinator-borne plant pathogen. *The American Naturalist, 168*(3), 294–303.

Ferrari, M. J., Djibo, A., Grais, R. F., Grenfell, B. T., & Bjørnstad, O. N. (2010). Episodic outbreaks bias estimates of age-specific force of infection: A corrected method using measles as an example. *Epidemiology and Infection, 138*(1), 108–116.

Ferrari, M. J., Grais, R. F., Bharti, N., Conlan, A. J., Bjørnstad, O. N., Wolfson, L. J., Guerin, P. J., Djibo, A., & Grenfell, B. T. (2008). The dynamics of measles in sub-Saharan Africa. *Nature, 451*(7179), 679–684.

Ferrari, M. J., Perkins, S. E., Pomeroy, L. W., & Bjørnstad, O. N. (2011). Pathogens, social networks, and the paradox of transmission scaling. *Interdisciplinary Perspectives on Infectious Diseases, 2011*.

Fine, P. E. M., & Clarkson, J. A. (1982). Measles in England and Wales. I. An analysis of factors underlying seasonal patterns. *International Journal of Epidemiology, 11*, 5–15.

Finkenstädt, B. F., Bjørnstad, O. N., & Grenfell, B. T. (2002). A stochastic model for extinction and recurrence of epidemics: Estimation and inference for measles outbreaks. *Biostatistics, 3*(4), 493–510.

Finkenstädt, B. F., & Grenfell, B. T. (2000). Time series modelling of childhood diseases: A dynamical systems approach. *Journal of the Royal Statistical Society C, 49*(2), 187–205.

Fisher, R. A. (1926). The arrangement of field experiments. *Journal of the Ministry of Agriculture, 33*, 503–515.

Fonnesbeck, C. J., Shea, K., Carran, S., Cassio de Moraes, J., Gregory, C., Goodson, J. L., & Ferrari, M. J. (2018). Measles outbreak response decision-making under uncertainty: A retrospective analysis. *Journal of The Royal Society Interface, 15*(140), 20170575.

Fotheringham, A. S. (1984). Spatial flows and spatial patterns. *Environment and Planning A, 16*(4), 529–543.

Freuling, C. M., Hampson, K., Selhorst, T., Schröder, R., Meslin, F. X., Mettenleiter, T. C., & Müller, T. (2013). The elimination of fox rabies from Europe: Determinants of success and lessons for the future. *Philosophical Transactions of the Royal Society B, 368*(1623), 20120142.

Fu, F., Rosenbloom, D. I., Wang, L., & Nowak, M. A. (2011). Imitation dynamics of vaccination behaviour on social networks. *Proceedings of the Royal Society B, 278*(1702), 42–49.

Funk, S., Salathé, M., & Jansen, V. A. (2010). Modelling the influence of human behaviour on the spread of infectious diseases: A review. *Journal of the Royal Society Interface*, rsif20100142.

Gammaitoni, L., Hänggi, P., Jung, P., & Marchesoni, F. (1998). Stochastic resonance. *Reviews of Modern Physics, 70*(1), 223.

Gillespie, D. T. (1977). Exact stochastic simulation of coupled chemical reactions. *The Journal of Physical Chemistry, 81*(25), 2340–2361.

Gillespie, D. T. (2001). Approximate accelerated stochastic simulation of chemically reacting systems. *The Journal of Chemical Physics, 115*(4), 1716–1733.

Glass, G. E., Cheek, J. E., Patz, J. A., Shields, T. M., Doyle, T. J., Thoroughman, D. A., Hunt, D. K., Enscore, R. E., Gage, K. L., Irland, C., et al. (2000). Using remotely sensed data to identify areas at risk for hantavirus pulmonary syndrome. *Emerging Infectious Diseases, 6*(3), 238.

Glass, K., Xia, Y., & Grenfell, B. T. (2003). Interpreting time-series analyses for continuous-time biological models—measles as a case study. *Journal of Theoretical Biology, 223*(1), 19–25.

Gog, J. R., Ballesteros, S., Viboud, C., Simonsen, L., Bjornstad, O. N., Shaman, J., Chao, D. L., Khan, F., & Grenfell, B. T. (2014). Spatial transmission of 2009 pandemic influenza in the US. *PLoS Computational Biology, 10*(6), e1003635.

Goldstein, J., Park, J., Haran, M., Liebhold, A., & Bjørnstad, O. N. (2019). Quantifying spatio-temporal variation of invasion spread. *Proceedings of the Royal Society B, 286*(1894), 20182294.

Graham, A. L., Cattadori, I. M., Lloyd-Smith, J. O., Ferrari, M. J., & Bjørnstad, O. N. (2007). Transmission consequences of coinfection: Cytokines writ large? *Trends in Parasitology, 23*(6), 284–291.

Graham, M., Winter, A. K., Ferrari, M., Grenfell, B., Moss, W. J., Azman, A. S., Metcalf, C. J. E., & Lessler, J. (2019). Measles and the canonical path to elimination. *Science, 364*(6440), 584–587.

Grais, R. F., Conlan, A. J. K., Ferrari, M. J., Djibo, A., Le Menach, A., Bjørnstad, O. N., & Grenfell, B. T. (2008). Time is of the essence: Exploring a measles outbreak response vaccination in Niamey, Niger. *Journal of the Royal Society Interface, 5*(18), 67–74.

Grais, R. F., Dubray, C., Gerstl, S., Guthmann, J. P., Djibo, A., Nargaye, K. D., Coker, J., Alberti, K. P., Cochet, A., Ihekweazu, C., et al. (2007). Unacceptably high mortality related to measles epidemics in Niger, Nigeria, and Chad. *PLoS Medicine, 4*(1), e16.

Greischar, M. A., Mideo, N., Read, A. F., & Bjørnstad, O. N. (2016). Predicting optimal transmission investment in malaria parasites. *Evolution, 70*(7), 1542–1558.

Greischar, M. A., Read, A. F., & Bjørnstad, O. N. (2014). Synchrony in malaria infections: How intensifying within-host competition can be adaptive. *The American Naturalist, 183*(2), E36–E49.

Grenfell, B., & Harwood, J. (1997). (meta)population dynamics of infectious diseases. *Trends in Ecology and Evolution, 12*(10), 395–399.

Grenfell, B. T., & Anderson, R. M. (1985). The estimation of age-related rates of infection from case notifications and serological data. *Journal of Hygene, 95*, 419–436.

Grenfell, B. T., & Anderson, R. M. (1989). Pertussis in England and Wales: An investigation of transmission dynamics and control by mass vaccination. *Proceedings of the Royal Society B, 236*(1284), 213–252.

Grenfell, B. T., Bjørnstad, O. N., & Finkenstadt, B. F. (2002). Dynamics of measles epidemics: Scaling noise, determinism, and predictability with the TSIR model. *Ecological Monographs, 72*(2), 185–202.

Grenfell, B. T., Bjørnstad, O. N., & Kappey, J. (2001). Travelling waves and spatial hierarchies in measles epidemics. *Nature, 414*(6865), 716–723.

Grenfell, B. T., Williams, C. S., Bjørnstad, O. N., & Banavar, J. R. (2006). Simplifying biological complexity. *Nature Physics, 2*(4), 212–214.

Gupta, S., Ferguson, N., & Anderson, R. (1998). Chaos, persistence, and evolution of strain structure in antigenically diverse infectious agents. *Science, 280*(5365), 912–915.

Hajek, A. E., & St. Leger, R. J. (1994). Interactions between fungal pathogens and insect hosts. *Annual Review of Entomology, 39*(1), 293–322.

Hall, A. J., Jepson, P. D., Goodman, S. J., & Härkönen, T. (2006). Phocine distemper virus in the North and European seas—Data and models, nature and nurture. *Biological Conservation, 131*(2), 221–229.

Hall, P., & Patil, P. (1994). Properties of nonparametric estimators of autocovariance for stationary random fields. *Probability Theory and Related Fields, 99*(3), 399–424.

Hammill, M. O., Stenson, G. B., Mosnier, A., & Doniol-Valcroz, T. (2021). *Trends in Abundance of Harp Seals,* Pagophilus Groenlandicus, *in the Northwest Atlantic, 1952–2019.* Canadian Science Advisory Secretariat.

Hand, D. J., & Taylor, C. C. (1987). *Multivariate analysis of variance and repeated measures: A practical approach for behavioural scientists* (vol. 5). CRC Press.

Handcock, M. S., Hunter, D. R., Butts, C. T., Goodreau, S. M., & Morris, M. (2008). statnet: Software tools for the representation, visualization, analysis and simulation of network data. *Journal of Statistical Software, 24*(1), 1548.

Hanski, I. (1994). A practical model of metapopulation dynamics. *Journal of Animal Ecology, 63*(1), 151–162.

Hanski, I. (1998). Metapopulation dynamics. *Nature, 396*(6706), 41–49.

Hanski, I. A., & Gaggiotti, O. E. (2004). *Ecology, genetics and evolution of metapopulations.* Academic Press.

Hardin, G. (1960). The competitive exclusion principle. *Science, 131*(3409), 1292–1297.

Harding, K. C., Härkönen, T., & Caswell, H. (2002). The 2002 European seal plague: Epidemiology and population consequences. *Ecology Letters, 5*(6), 727–732.

Härdle, W. (1990). *Applied nonparametric regression.* Cambridge university press.

Harty, J. T., & Badovinac, V. P. (2008). Shaping and reshaping CD8+ T-cell memory. *Nature Reviews Immunology, 8*(2), 107–119.

Hassell, M. P., Comins, H. N., & May, R. M. (1991). Spatial structure and chaos in insect population dynamics. *Nature, 353*(6341), 255–258.

Hastie, T. J., & Tibshirani, R. J. (1990). *Generalized additive models.* CRC press.

Heesterbeek, J. A. P., & Dietz, K. (1996). The concept of R^0 in epidemic theory. *Statistica Neerlandica, 50*(1), 89–110.

Heisey, D. M., Joly, D. O., & Messier, F. (2006). The fitting of general force-of-infection models to wildlife disease prevalence data. *Ecology, 87*(9), 2356–2365.

Hemelaar, J. (2012). The origin and diversity of the HIV-1 pandemic. *Trends in Molecular Medicine, 18*(3), 182–192.

Henderson, D. A., & Klepac, P. (2013). Lessons from the eradication of smallpox: An interview with DA Henderson. *Philosophical Transactions of the Royal Society B, 368*(1623), 20130113.

Hens, N., Aerts, M., Faes, C., Shkedy, Z., Lejeune, O., Van Damme, P., & Beutels, P. (2010). Seventy-five years of estimating the force of infection from current status data. *Epidemiology and Infection, 138*(6), 802–812.

Herzog, C. M., De Glanville, W. A., Willett, B. J., Kibona, T. J., Cattadori, I. M., Kapur, V., Hudson, P. J., Buza, J., Cleaveland, S., & Bjørnstad, O. N. (2019). Pastoral production is associated with increased peste des petits ruminants seroprevalence in northern Tanzania across sheep, goats and cattle. *Epidemiology and Infection, 147*, e242.

Holme, P., & Litvak, N. (2017). Cost-efficient vaccination protocols for network epidemiology. *PLoS Computational Biology, 13*(9), e1005696.

Hope-Simpson, R. E. (1952). Infectiousness of communicable diseases in the household. *The Lancet, 2*, 549–554.

Hope-Simpson, R. E. (1981). The role of season in the epidemiology of influenza. *Journal of Hygiene, 86*(01), 35–47.

House, T., & Keeling, M. J. (2011). Epidemic prediction and control in clustered populations. *Journal of Theoretical Biology, 272*(1), 1–7.

House, T., Ross, J. V., & Sirl, D. (2013). How big is an outbreak likely to be? methods for epidemic final-size calculation. *Proceedings of the Royal Society A, 469*(2150), 20120436.

Hoyt, J. R., Kilpatrick, A. M., & Langwig, K. E. (2021). Ecology and impacts of white-nose syndrome on bats. *Nature Reviews Microbiology, 19*(3), 196–210.

Iacono, G. L., Cunningham, A. A., Fichet-Calvet, E., Garry, R. F., Grant, D. S., Khan, S. H., Leach, M., Moses, L. M., Schieffelin, J. S., Shaffer, J. G., et al. (2015). Using modelling to disentangle the relative contributions of zoonotic and anthroponotic transmission: The case of Lassa fever. *PLoS Negl ectedTropical Diseases, 9*(1), e3398.

Inglesby, T. V. (2020). Public health measures and the reproduction number of SARS-CoV-2. *Journal of the American Medical Association, 323*(21), 2186–2187.

Janzen, D. H. (1970). Herbivores and the number of tree species in tropical forests. *The American Naturalist, 104*(940), 501–528.

Johnson, D. M., Bjørnstad, O. N., & Liebhold, A. M. (2004). Landscape geometry and travelling waves in the larch budmoth. *Ecology Letters, 7*(10), 967–974.

Johnson, D. M., Büntgen, U., Frank, D. C., Kausrud, K., Haynes, K. J., Liebhold, A. M., Esper, J., & Stenseth, N. C. (2010). Climatic warming disrupts recurrent Alpine insect outbreaks. *Proceedings of the National Academy of Sciences, 107*(47), 20576–20581.

Jones, C. G., Ostfeld, R. S., Richard, M. P., Schauber, E. M., & Wolff, J. O. (1998). Chain reactions linking acorns to gypsy moth outbreaks and lyme disease risk. *Science, 279*(5353), 1023–1026.

Kamiya, T., Greischar, M. A., Schneider, D. S., & Mideo, N. (2020). Uncovering drivers of dose-dependence and individual variation in malaria infection outcomes. *PLoS Computational Biology, 16*(10), e1008211.

Kaneko, K. (1993). *Theory and applications of coupled map lattices.* John Wiley and Son.

Keeling, M. J., Bjørnstad, O. N., & Grenfell, B. T. (2004). Metapopulation dynamics of infectious diseases. In Hanski, I., & Gaggiotti, O., (Eds.), *Ecology, Genetics, and Evolution of Metapopulations* (pp. 415–445). Elsevier.

Keeling, M. J., & Eames, K. T. D. (2005). Networks and epidemic models. *Journal of the Royal Society Interface, 2*(4), 295–307.

Keeling, M. J., & Grenfell, B. T. (1997). Disease extinction and community size: Modeling the persistence of measles. *Science, 275*(5296), 65–67.

Keeling, M. J., & Rohani, P. (2002). Estimating spatial coupling in epidemiological systems: A mechanistic approach. *Ecology Letters, 5*(1), 20–29.

Keeling, M. J., & Rohani, P. (2008). *Modeling infectious diseases in humans and animals.* Princeton University Press.

Keeling, M. J., Rohani, P., & Grenfell, B. T. (2001). Seasonally forced disease dynamics explored as switching between attractors. *Physica D: Nonlinear Phenomena, 148*(3), 317–335.

Keeling, M. J., Wilson, H., & Pacala, S. W. (2002). Deterministic limits to stochastic spatial models of natural enemies. *The American Naturalist, 159*(1), 57–80.

Keitt, T. H., Bjørnstad, O. N., Dixon, P. M., & Citron-Pousty, S. (2002). Accounting for spatial pattern when modeling organism-environment interactions. *Ecography, 25*(5), 616–625.

Kendall, B. E., Bjørnstad, O. N., Bascompte, J., Keitt, T. H., & Fagan, W. F. (2000). Dispersal, environmental correlation, and spatial synchrony in population dynamics. *The American Naturalist, 155*(5), 628–636.

Kendall, B. E., Briggs, C. J., Murdoch, W. W., Turchin, P., Ellner, S. P., McCauley, E., Nisbet, R. M., & Wood, S. N. (1999). Why do populations cycle? a synthesis of statistical and mechanistic modeling approaches. *Ecology, 80*(6), 1789–1805.

Kendall, D. G. (1949). Stochastic processes and population growth. *Journal of the Royal Statistical Society B, 11*(2), 230–282.

Kennedy, D. A., & Read, A. F. (2017). Why does drug resistance readily evolve but vaccine resistance does not? *Proceedings of the Royal Society of London B, 284*(1851), 20162562.

Kermack, W. O., & McKendrick, A. G. (1927). A contribution to the mathematical theory of epidemics. *Proceedings of the Royal Society of London A, 115*(772), 700–721.

Keyfitz, N., & Littman, G. (1979). Mortality in a heterogeneous population. *Population Studies, 33*(2), 333–342.

King, A. A., de Celles, M. D., Magpantay, F. M. G., & Rohani, P. (2015a). Avoidable errors in the modelling of outbreaks of emerging pathogens, with special reference to Ebola. *Proceedings of the Royal Society B, 282*(1806).

King, A. A., Ionides, E. L., Pascual, M., & Bouma, M. J. (2008). Inapparent infections and cholera dynamics. *Nature, 454*(7206), 877–880.

King, A. A., Nguyen, D., & Ionides, E. L. (2015b). Statistical inference for partially observed Markov processes via the R package pomp. Preprint. arXiv:1509.00503.

Kirimanjeswara, G. S., Agosto, L. M., Kennett, M. J., Bjornstad, O. N., & Harvill, E. T. (2005). Pertussis toxin inhibits neutrophil recruitment to delay antibody-mediated clearance of *Bordetella pertussis*. *The Journal of Clinical Investigation, 115*(12), 3594–3601.

Klepac, P., Metcalf, C. J. E., McLean, A. R., & Hampson, K. (2013). Towards the endgame and beyond: Complexities and challenges for the elimination of infectious diseases. *Philosophical transactions of the Royal Society B*.

Klepac, P., Pomeroy, L. W., Bjørnstad, O. N., Kuiken, T., Osterhaus, A. D., & Rijks, J. M. (2009). Stage-structured transmission of phocine distemper virus in the Dutch 2002 outbreak. *Proceedings of the Royal Society B, 276*(1666), 2469–2476.

Klovdahl, A. S., Potterat, J. J., Woodhouse, D. E., Muth, J. B., Muth, S. Q., & Darrow, W. W. (1994). Social networks and infectious disease: The Colorado Springs study. *Social Science and Medicine, 38*(1), 79–88.

Knox, E. G. (1980). Strategy for rubella vaccination. *International Journal of Epidemiology, 9*(1), 13–23.

Koelle, K., Cobey, S., Grenfell, B., & Pascual, M. (2006). Epochal evolution shapes the phylodynamics of interpandemic influenza A (H3N2) in humans. *Science, 314*(5807), 1898–1903.

Koenig, W. D. (1999). Spatial autocorrelation of ecological phenomena. *Trends in Ecology and Evolution, 14*(1), 22–26.

Kooperberg, C., Stone, C. J., & Truong, Y. K. (1995). Logspline estimation of a possibly mixed spectral distribution. *Journal of Time Series Analysis, 16*(4), 359–388.

Kot, M., Lewis, M. A., & van den Driessche, P. (1996). Dispersal data and the spread of invading organisms. *Ecology, 77*(7), 2027–2042.

Kröger, M., Turkyilmazoglu, M., & Schlickeiser, R. (2021). Explicit formulae for the peak time of an epidemic from the SIR model. Which approximant to use? *Physica D, 425*, 132981.

Kucharski, A. J., Conlan, A. J. K., & Eames, K. T. D. (2015). School's out: Seasonal variation in the movement patterns of school children. *PloS One, 10*(6), e0128070.

Kundrick, A., Huang, Z., Carran, S., Kagoli, M., Grais, R. F., Hurtado, N., & Ferrari, M. (2018). Sub-national variation in measles vaccine coverage and outbreak risk: a case study from a 2010 outbreak in Malawi. *BMC Public Health, 18*(1), 1–10.

Kurosaki, T., Kometani, K., & Ise, W. (2015). Memory B cells. *Nature Reviews Immunology, 15*(3), 149–159.

Lau, M. S. Y., Becker, A. D., Korevaar, H. M., Caudron, Q., Shaw, D. J., Metcalf, C. J. E., Bjørnstad, O. N., & Grenfell, B. T. (2020). A competing-risks model explains hierarchical spatial coupling of measles epidemics en route to national elimination. *Nature Ecology and Evolution, 4*, 934–939.

Lau, M. S. Y., Dalziel, B. D., Funk, S., McClelland, A., Tiffany, A., Riley, S., Metcalf, C. J. E., & Grenfell, B. T. (2017). Spatial and temporal dynamics of superspreading events in the 2014–2015 West Africa Ebola epidemic. *Proceedings of the National Academy of Sciences, 114*(9), 2337–2342.

Lavine, J. S., Bjornstad, O. N., & Antia, R. (2021). Immunological characteristics govern the transition of COVID-19 to endemicity. *Science, 371*(6530), 741–745.

Lavine, J. S., King, A. A., Andreasen, V., & Bjørnstad, O. N. (2013). Immune boosting explains regime-shifts in prevaccine-era pertussis dynamics. *PLoS One, 8*(8), e72086.

Lavine, J. S., King, A. A., & Bjørnstad, O. N. (2011). Natural immune boosting in pertussis dynamics and the potential for long-term vaccine failure. *Proceedings of the National Academy of Sciences, 108*(17), 7259–7264.

Legendre, L., Frechette, M., & Legendre, P. (1981). The contingency periodogram: A method of identifying rhythms in series of nonmetric ecological data. *The Journal of Ecology, 69*, 965–979.

Legendre, P. (1993). Spatial autocorrelation: Trouble or new paradigm? *Ecology, 74*(6), 1659–1673.

Legendre, P., & Fortin, M. J. (1989). Spatial pattern and ecological analysis. *Vegetatio, 80*(2), 107–138.

Legrand, J., Grais, R. F., Boelle, P. Y., Valleron, A. J., & Flahault, A. (2007). Understanding the dynamics of Ebola epidemics. *Epidemiology and Infection, 135*(4), 610–621.

Leslie, P. H. (1945). On the use of matrices in certain population mathematics. *Biometrika, 33*(3), 183–212.

Leynaert, B., Downs, A. M., de Vincenzi, I., & European Study Group on Heterosexual Transmission of HIV (1998). Heterosexual transmission of human immunodeficiency virus: Variability of infectivity throughout the course of infection. *American Journal of Epidemiology, 148*(1), 88–96.

Li, R., Bjørnstad, O. N., & Stenseth, N. C. (2021a). Switching vaccination among target groups to achieve improved long-lasting benefits. *Royal Society Open Science, 8*(6), 210292.

Li, R., Metcalf, C. J. E., Stenseth, N. C., & Bjørnstad, O. N. (2021b). A general model for the demographic signatures of the transition from pandemic emergence to endemicity. *Science Advances, 7*(33), eabf9040.

Li, S.-L., Bjørnstad, O. N., Ferrari, M. J., Mummah, R., Runge, M. C., Fonnesbeck, C. J., Tildesley, M. J., Probert, W. J., & Shea, K. (2017). Essential information: Uncertainty and optimal control of Ebola outbreaks. *Proceedings of the National Academy of Sciences, 114*(22), 5659–5664.

Li, T.-Y., & Yorke, J. A. (2004). Period three implies chaos. In Hunt, B. R., Li, T.-Y., Kennedy, J. A., & Nusse, H. E., (Eds.), *The theory of chaotic attractors* (pp. 77–84). Springer.

Lietman, T., Porco, T., & Blower, S. (1997). Leprosy and tuberculosis: The epidemiological consequences of cross-immunity. *American Journal of Public Health, 87*(12), 1923–1927.

Linthicum, K. J., Anyamba, A., Tucker, C. J., Kelley, P. W., Myers, M. F., & Peters, C. J. (1999). Climate and satellite indicators to forecast Rift Valley fever epidemics in Kenya. *Science, 285*(5426), 397–400.

Lipsitch, M., Cohen, T., Cooper, B., Robins, J. M., Ma, S., James, L., Gopalakrishna, G., Chew, S. K., Tan, C. C., Samore, M. H., et al. (2003). Transmission dynamics and control of severe acute respiratory syndrome. *Science, 300*(5627), 1966–1970.

Liu, W.-M., Levin, S. A., & Iwasa, Y. (1986). Influence of nonlinear incidence rates upon the behavior of SIRS epidemiological models. *Journal of Mathematical Biology, 23*(2), 187–204.

Lloyd, A. L. (2001). Destabilization of epidemic models with the inclusion of realistic distributions of infectious periods. *Proceedings of the Royal Society of London B, 268*(1470), 985–993.

Lloyd-Smith, J. O., George, D., Pepin, K. M., Pitzer, V. E., Pulliam, J. R. C., Dobson, A. P., Hudson, P. J., & Grenfell, B. T. (2009). Epidemic dynamics at the human-animal interface. *Science, 326*(5958), 1362–1367.

Lloyd-Smith, J. O., Schreiber, S. J., Kopp, P. E., & Getz, W. M. (2005). Superspreading and the effect of individual variation on disease emergence. *Nature, 438*(7066), 355–359.

Loader, C. (2006). *Local regression and likelihood.* Springer.

Lomb, N. R. (1976). Least-squares frequency analysis of unequally spaced data. *Astrophysics and Space Science, 39*(2), 447–462.

London, W. P., & Yorke, J. A. (1973). Recurrent outbreaks of measles, chickenpox and mumps: I. Seasonal variation in contact rates. *American Journal of Epidemiology, 98*(6), 453–468.

Long, G. H., Sinha, D., Read, A. F., Pritt, S., Kline, B., Harvill, E. T., Hudson, P. J., & Bjornstad, O. N. (2010). Identifying the ge cohort responsible for transmission in a natural outbreak of *Bordetella bronchiseptica*. *Plos Pathogens, 6*(12).

Lowen, A. C., Mubareka, S., Steel, J., & Palese, P. (2007). Influenza virus transmission is dependent on relative humidity and temperature. *PLoS Pathogens, 3*(10), e151.

Luis, A. D., Douglass, R. J., Mills, J. N., & Bjørnstad, O. N. (2015). Environmental fluctuations lead to predictability in Sin Nombre hantavirus outbreaks. *Ecology, 96*(6), 1691–1701.

Mahmud, A. S. (2017). *A map for all seasons: Tracking transmission dynamics and mortality of childhood infections through the year.* phdthesis, Princeton University.

Mahmud, A. S., Metcalf, C. J. E., & Grenfell, B. T. (2017). Comparative dynamics, seasonality in transmission, and predictability of childhood infections in Mexico. *Epidemiology and Infection, 145*(3), 607–625.

Mari, L., Bertuzzo, E., Righetto, L., Casagrandi, R., Gatto, M., Rodriguez-Iturbe, I., & Rinaldo, A. (2012). Modelling cholera epidemics: The role of waterways, human mobility and sanitation. *Journal of the Royal Society Interface, 9*(67), 376–388.

Martinez-Bakker, M., Bakker, K. M., King, A. A., & Rohani, P. (2014). Human birth seasonality: Latitudinal gradient and interplay with childhood disease dynamics. *Proceedings of the Royal Society of London B, 281*(1783), 20132438.

May, R. M. (1978). Host-parasitoid systems in patchy environments: a phenomenological model. *The Journal of Animal Ecology*, 833–844.

McCaffrey, D. F., Ellner, S., Gallant, A. R., & Nychka, D. W. (1992). Estimating the lyapunov exponent of a chaotic system with nonparametric regression. *Journal of the American Statistical Association, 87*(419), 682–695.

McCullagh, P., & Nelder, J. A. (1989). *Generalized Linear models* (2nd edn.). Chapman and Hall.

Metcalf, C. J. E., & Barrett, A. (2016). Invasion Dynamics of Teratogenic Infections in Light of rubella Control: Implications for Zika Virus. *PLoS Currents*, 8.

Metcalf, C. J. E., Bjørnstad, O. N., Ferrari, M. J., Klepac, P., Bharti, N., Lopez-Gatell, H., & Grenfell, B. T. (2011a). The epidemiology of rubella in Mexico: seasonality, stochasticity and regional variation. *Epidemiology and Infection, 139*(7), 1029–1038.

Metcalf, C. J. E., Bjørnstad, O. N., Grenfell, B. T., & Andreasen, V. (2009). Seasonality and comparative dynamics of six childhood infections in pre-vaccination Copenhagen. *Proceedings of the Royal Society of London B, 276*(1676), 4111–4118.

Metcalf, C. J. E., Graham, A. L., Huijben, S., Barclay, V. C., Long, G. H., Grenfell, B. T., Read, A. F., & Bjørnstad, O. N. (2011b). Partitioning regulatory mechanisms of within-host malaria dynamics using the effective propagation number. *Science, 333*(6045), 984–988.

Metcalf, C. J. E., Hampson, K., Tatem, A. J., Grenfell, B. T., & Bjørnstad, O. N. (2013). Persistence in epidemic metapopulations: quantifying the rescue effects for measles, mumps, rubella and whooping cough. *PloS One, 8*(9), e74696.

Metcalf, C. J. E., Long, G. H., Mideo, N., Forester, J. D., Bjørnstad, O. N., & Graham, A. L. (2012). Revealing mechanisms underlying variation in malaria virulence: Effective propagation and host control of uninfected red blood cell supply. *Journal of The Royal Society Interface, 9*, 2804–2813.

Metcalf, C. J. E., Munayco, C. V., Chowell, G., Grenfell, B. T., & Bjornstad, O. N. (2011c). Rubella metapopulation dynamics and importance of spatial coupling to the risk of congenital rubella syndrome in Peru. *Journal of the Royal Society Interface, 8*(56), 369–376.

Metz, J. A. J., & Diekmann, O. (1991). Exact finite dimensional representations of models for physiologically structured populations. I: The abstract foundations of linear chain trickery. *Differential Equations with Applications in Biology, Physics and Engineering. Lecture Notes in Pure and Applied mathematics, 133*, 269–289.

Mideo, N., Reece, S. E., Smith, A. L., & Metcalf, C. J. E. (2013). The cinderella syndrome: Why do malaria-infected cells burst at midnight? *Trends in Parasitology, 29*(1), 10–16.

Miller, C. L., & Fletcher, W. (1976). Severity of notified whooping cough. *British Medical Journal, 1*(6002), 117–119.

Mollison, D. (1991). Dependence of epidemic and population velocities on basic parameters. *Mathematical Biosciences, 107*(2), 255–287.

Morens, D. M., & Fauci, A. S. (2007). The 1918 influenza pandemic: Insights for the 21st century. *The Journal of Infectious Diseases, 195*(7), 1018–1028.

Morris, S. E., Yates, A. J., de Swart, R. L., de Vries, R. D., Mina, M. J., Nelson, A. N., Lin, W.-H. W., Kouyos, R. D., Griffin, D. E., & Grenfell, B. T. (2018). Modeling the measles paradox reveals the importance of cellular immunity in regulating viral clearance. *PLoS Pathogens, 14*(12), e1007493.

Mossong, J., Hens, N., Jit, M., Beutels, P., Auranen, K., Mikolajczyk, R., Massari, M., Salmaso, S., Tomba, G. S., Wallinga, J., et al. (2008). Social contacts and mixing patterns relevant to the spread of infectious diseases. *PLoS Medicine, 5*(3), e74.

Muench, H. (1959). *Catalytic models in epidemiology.* Harvard University Press.

Murdoch, W. W., Briggs, C. J., & Nisbet, R. M. (2003). *Consumer-resource dynamics* (vol. 36). Princeton University Press.

Murdoch, W. W., Chesson, J., & Chesson, P. L. (1985). Biological control in theory and practice. *The American Naturalist, 125*(3), 344–366.

Murray, J. D., Stanley, E. A., & Brown, D. L. (1986). On the spatial spread of rabies among foxes. *Proceedings of the Royal Society of London. Series B*, 111–150.

Newman, M. E. J. (2002). Spread of epidemic disease on networks. *Physical Review E, 66*(1), 016128.

Newman, M. E. J. (2006). Modularity and community structure in networks. *Proceedings of the National Academy of Sciences, 103*(23), 8577–8582.

Nicholson, A. J., & Bailey, V. A. (1935). The balance of animal populations. Part I. *Proceedings of the Zoological Society of London, 105*(3), 551–598.

Niewiesk, S. (2014). Maternal antibodies: Clinical significance, mechanism of interference with immune responses, and possible vaccination strategies. *Frontiers in Immunology, 5*, 446.

Nisbet, R. M., & Gurney, W. (1982). *Modelling fluctuating populations*. John Wiley and Sons Limited.

Panagiotopoulos, T., Berger, A., Valassi-Adam, E., et al. (1999). Increase in congenital rubella occurrence after immunisation in Greece: Retrospective survey and systematic review. *British Medical Journal, 319*(7223), 1462–1467.

Peel, A. J., Pulliam, J., Luis, A., Plowright, R., O'Shea, T., Hayman, D., Wood, J., Webb, C., & Restif, O. (2014). The effect of seasonal birth pulses on pathogen persistence in wild mammal populations. *Proceedings of the Royal Society of London B, 281*(1786), 20132962.

Petermann, J. S., Fergus, A. J., Turnbull, L. A., & Schmid, B. (2008). Janzen-Connell effects are widespread and strong enough to maintain diversity in grasslands. *Ecology, 89*(9), 2399–2406.

Pinheiro, J., & Bates, D. (2006). *Mixed-effects models in S and S-plus*. Springer.

Pitzer, V. E., Patel, M. M., Lopman, B. A., Viboud, C., Parashar, U. D., & Grenfell, B. T. (2011). Modeling rotavirus strain dynamics in developed countries to understand the potential impact of vaccination on genotype distributions. *Proceedings of the National Academy of Sciences, 108*(48), 19353–19358.

Pitzer, V. E., Viboud, C., Alonso, W. J., Wilcox, T., Metcalf, C. J., Steiner, C. A., Haynes, A. K., & Grenfell, B. T. (2015). Environmental drivers of the spatiotemporal dynamics of respiratory syncytial virus in the United States. *PLoS Pathogens, 11*(1), e1004591.

Plotkin, S. A. (2011). *History of vaccine development*. Springer Science & Business Media.

Pomeroy, L. W., Bjørnstad, O. N., Kim, H., Jumbo, S. D., Abdoulkadiri, S., & Garabed, R. (2015). Serotype-specific transmission and waning immunity of endemic foot-and-mouth disease virus in Cameroon. *PLoS One, 10*(9), e0136642.

Priestley, M. B. (1981). *Spectral analysis and time series*. Academic press.

Ramsay, J. O., & Silverman, B. W. (1997). *Functional data analysis*. Springer.

Rand, D. A., & Wilson, H. B. (1991). Chaotic stochasticity: A ubiquitous source of unpredictability in epidemics. *Proceedings of the Royal Society of London B, 246*(1316), 179–184.

Reluga, T. C., Medlock, J., & Galvani, A. P. (2006). A model of spatial epidemic spread when individuals move within overlapping home ranges. *Bulletin of Mathematical Biology, 68*(2), 401–416.

Relyveld, E. H. (2011). A history of toxoids. In *History of vaccine development* (pp. 57–64). Springer.

Riley, S., Fraser, C., Donnelly, C. A., Ghani, A. C., Abu-Raddad, L. J., Hedley, A. J., Leung, G. M., Ho, L.-M., Lam, T.-H., Thach, T. Q., et al. (2003). Transmission dynamics of the etiological agent of SARS in Hong Kong: Impact of public health interventions. *Science, 300*(5627), 1961–1966.

Rimoin, A. W., Mulembakani, P. M., Johnston, S. C., Smith, J. O. L., Kisalu, N. K., Kinkela, T. L., Blumberg, S., Thomassen, H. A., Pike, B. L., Fair, J. N., et al. (2010). Major increase in human monkeypox incidence 30 years after smallpox vaccination campaigns cease in the Democratic Republic of Congo. *Proceedings of the National Academy of Sciences, 107*(37), 16262–16267.

Roberts, M., & Heesterbeek, H. (1993). Bluff your way in epidemic models. *Trends in Microbiology, 1*(9), 343–348.

Rohani, P., Earn, D. J., & Grenfell, B. T. (1999). Opposite patterns of synchrony in sympatric disease metapopulations. *Science, 286*(5441), 968–971.

Rohani, P., Keeling, M. J., & Grenfell, B. T. (2002). The interplay between determinism and stochasticity in childhood diseases. *The American Naturalist, 159*(5), 469–481.

Rohani, P., & King, A. A. (2010). Never mind the length, feel the quality: The impact of long-term epidemiological data sets on theory, application and policy. *Trends in Ecology and Evolution, 25*(10), 611–618.

Rosatte, R., Sobey, K., Donovan, D., Allan, M., Bruce, L., Buchanan, T., & Davies, C. (2007). Raccoon density and movements after population reduction to control rabies. *Journal of Wildlife Management, 71*(7), 2373.

Rousseeuw, P. J., & Molenberghs, G. (1994). The shape of correlation matrices. *The American Statistician, 48*(4), 276–279.

Roy, S., Lavine, J., Chiaromonte, F., Terwee, J., VandeWoude, S., Bjornstad, O., & Poss, M. (2009). Multivariate statistical analyses demonstrate unique host immune responses to single and dual lentiviral infection. *PloS One, 4*(10), e7359.

Ruelle, D. (1993). *Chance and chaos.* Princeton University Press.

Ruiz-Moreno, D., Pascual, M., Bouma, M., Dobson, A., & Cash, B. (2007). Cholera seasonality in Madras (1901–1940): Dual role for rainfall in endemic and epidemic regions. *EcoHealth, 4*(1), 52–62.

Ruxton, G. D. (1994). Low levels of immigration between chaotic populations can reduce system extinctions by inducing asynchronous regular cycles. *Proceedings of the Royal Society of London B, 256*(1346), 189–193.

Schaffer, W. M. (1985). Can nonlinear dynamics elucidate mechanisms in ecology and epidemiology? *IMA Journal of Mathematics Applied in Medicine and Biology, 2*(4), 221–252.

Schenzle, D. (1984). An age-structured model of pre-and post-vaccination measles transmission. *Mathematical Medicine and Biology A, 1*(2), 169–191.

Scherer, A., & McLean, A. (2002). Mathematical models of vaccination. *British Medical Bulletin, 62*(1), 187–199.

Schwartz, I. B. (1985). Multiple stable recurrent outbreaks and predictability in seasonally forced nonlinear epidemic models. *Journal of Mathematical Biology, 21*(3), 347–361.

Seabloom, E. W., Bjørnstad, O. N., Bolker, B. M., & Reichman, O. J. (2005). Spatial signature of environmental heterogeneity, dispersal, and competition in successional grasslands. *Ecological Monographs, 75*(2), 199–214.

Shaman, J., & Kohn, M. (2009). Absolute humidity modulates influenza survival, transmission, and seasonality. *Proceedings of the National Academy of Sciences, 106*(9), 3243–3248.

Shea, K., Bjørnstad, O. N., Krzywinski, M., & Altman, N. (2020). Uncertainty and the management of epidemics. *Nature Methods, 17*(9), 867–869.

Shea, K., Tildesley, M. J., Runge, M. C., Fonnesbeck, C. J., & Ferrari, M. J. (2014). Adaptive management and the value of information: Learning via intervention in epidemiology. *PLoS Biology, 12*(10), e1001970.

Shrestha, S., Bjørnstad, O. N., & King, A. A. (2014). Evolution of acuteness in pathogen metapopulations: Conflicts between "classical" and invasion-persistence trade-offs. *Theoretical Ecology, 7*(3), 299–311.

Simonsen, L., Clarke, M. J., Schonberger, L. B., Arden, N. H., Cox, N. J., & Fukuda, K. (1998). Pandemic versus epidemic influenza mortality: A pattern of changing age distribution. *Journal of Infectious Diseases, 178*(1), 53–60.

Smith, D. L., Battle, K. E., Hay, S. I., Barker, C. M., Scott, T. W., & McKenzie, F. E. (2012). Ross, Macdonald, and a theory for the dynamics and control of mosquito-transmitted pathogens. *PLoS Pathogens, 8*(4), e1002588.

Smith, D. L., Ericson, L., & Burdon, J. J. (2003). Epidemiological patterns at multiple spatial scales: an 11-year study of a *Triphragmium ulmariae–Filipendula ulmaria* metapopulation. *Journal of Ecology, 91*(5), 890–903.

Smith, D. L., Lucey, B., Waller, L. A., Childs, J. E., & Real, L. A. (2002a). Predicting the spatial dynamics of rabies epidemics on heterogeneous landscapes. *Proceedings of the National Academy of Sciences, 99*(6), 3668–3672.

Smith, G. J., Vijaykrishna, D., Bahl, J., Lycett, S. J., Worobey, M., Pybus, O. G., Ma, S. K., Cheung, C. L., Raghwani, J., Bhatt, S., et al. (2009a). Origins and evolutionary genomics of the 2009 swine-origin H1N1 influenza A epidemic. *Nature, 459*(7250), 1122–1125.

Smith, M. J., Telfer, S., Kallio, E. R., Burthe, S., Cook, A. R., Lambin, X., & Begon, M. (2009b). Host-pathogen time series data in wildlife support a transmission function between density and frequency dependence. *Proceedings of the National Academy of Sciences, 106*(19), 7905–7909.

Smith, T. G., Walliker, D., & Ranford-Cartwright, L. C. (2002b). Sexual differentiation and sex determination in the apicomplexa. *Trends in Parasitology, 18*(7), 315–323.

Special Commitee on Seals. (2002). Scientific advice on matters related to the management of seal populations. Technical report, Sea Mammal Research Unit, St Adrews University.

Stern, A., Nickel, P., Meyer, T. F., & So, M. (1984). Opacity determinants of *Neisseria gonorrhoeae*: Gene expression and chromosomal linkage to the gonococcal pilus gene. *Cell, 37*(2), 447–456.

Sugihara, G., Grenfell, B., & May, R. M. (1990). Distinguishing error from chaos in ecological time series. *Philosophical Transactions of the Royal Society of London B, 330*, 235–250.

Swinton, J. (1998). Extinction times and phase transitions for spatially structured closed epidemics. *Bulletin of Mathematical Biology, 60*(2), 215–230.

Swinton, J., Harwood, J., Grenfell, B. T., & Gilligan, C. A. (1998). Persistence thresholds for phocine distemper virus infection in harbour seal *Phoca vitulina* metapopulations. *Journal of Animal Ecology, 67*, 54–68.

Taber, S. W., & Pease, C. M. (1990). Paramyxovirus phylogeny: Tissue tropism evolves slower than host specificity. *Evolution, 44*(2), 435–438.

Takahashi, S., Liao, Q., Van Boeckel, T. P., Xing, W., Sun, J., Hsiao, V. Y., Metcalf, C. J. E., Chang, Z., Liu, F., Zhang, J., et al. (2016). Hand, foot, and mouth disease in China: Modeling epidemic dynamics of enterovirus serotypes and implications for vaccination. *PLoS Medicine, 13*(2), e1001958.

Takahashi, S., Metcalf, C. J. E., Ferrari, M. J., Moss, W. J., Truelove, S. A., Tatem, A. J., Grenfell, B. T., & Lessler, J. (2015). Reduced vaccination and the risk of measles and other childhood infections post-Ebola. *Science, 347*(6227), 1240–1242.

Tettelin, H., Saunders, N. J., Heidelberg, J., Jeffries, A. C., Nelson, K. E., Eisen, J. A., Ketchum, K. A., Hood, D. W., Peden, J. F., Dodson, R. J., et al. (2000). Complete genome sequence of Neisseria meningitidis serogroup B strain MC58. *Science, 287*(5459), 1809–1815.

Tian, H., Liu, Y., Li, Y., Wu, C.-H., Chen, B., Kraemer, M. U., Li, B., Cai, J., Xu, B., Yang, Q., et al. (2020). An investigation of transmission control measures during the first 50 days of the COVID-19 epidemic in China. *Science, 368*(6491), 638–642.

Tilman, D. (1976). Ecological competition between algae: Experimental confirmation of resource-based competition theory. *Science, 192*, 463–465.

Tong, H. (1995). A personal overview of nonlinear time-series analysis from a chaos perspective. *Scandinavian Journal of Statistics, 22*(4), 399–421.

Torrence, C., & Compo, G. P. (1998). A practical guide to wavelet analysis. *Bulletin of the American Meteorological Society, 79*(1), 61–78.

Truscott, J., & Ferguson, N. M. (2012). Evaluating the adequacy of gravity models as a description of human mobility for epidemic modelling. *PLoS Computational Biology, 8*(10), e1002699.

Turchin, P. (2003). *Complex population dynamics: A theoretical/empirical synthesis* (vol. 35). Princeton University Press.

Turing, A. M. (1990). The chemical basis of morphogenesis. *Bulletin of Mathematical Biology, 52*(1), 153–197.

Van Bressem, M.-F., Duignan, P. J., Banyard, A., Barbieri, M., Colegrove, K. M., De Guise, S., Di Guardo, G., Dobson, A., Domingo, M., Fauquier, D., et al. (2014). Cetacean morbillivirus: Current knowledge and future directions. *Viruses, 6*(12), 5145–5181.

van den Bosch, F., Metz, J. A. J., & Diekmann, O. (1990). The velocity of spatial population expansion. *Journal of Mathematical Biology, 28*(5), 529–565.

Vaupel, J. W., Manton, K. G., & Stallard, E. (1979). The impact of heterogeneity in individual frailty on the dynamics of mortality. *Demography, 16*(3), 439–454.

Vaupel, J. W., & Yashin, A. I. (1985). Heterogeneity's ruses: Some surprising effects of selection on population dynamics. *The American Statistician, 39*(3), 176–185.

Venables, W., & Ripley, B. D. (2013). *S programming*. Springer.

Verity, R., Okell, L. C., Dorigatti, I., Winskill, P., Whittaker, C., Imai, N., Cuomo-Dannenburg, G., Thompson, H., Walker, P. G., Fu, H., et al. (2020). Estimates of the severity of coronavirus disease 2019: A model-based analysis. *The Lancet Infectious Diseases, 20*(6), 669–677.

Viboud, C., Bjørnstad, O. N., Smith, D. L., Simonsen, L., Miller, M. A., & Grenfell, B. T. (2006). Synchrony, waves, and spatial hierarchies in the spread of influenza. *Science, 312*(5772), 447–451.

Vijgen, L., Keyaerts, E., Moës, E., Thoelen, I., Wollants, E., Lemey, P., Vandamme, A.-M., & Van Ranst, M. (2005). Complete genomic sequence of human coronavirus OC43: Molecular clock analysis suggests a relatively recent zoonotic coronavirus transmission event. *Journal of Virology, 79*(3), 1595–1604.

Vink, M. A., Bootsma, M. C. J., & Wallinga, J. (2014). Serial intervals of respiratory infectious diseases: A systematic review and analysis. *American Journal of Epidemiology, 180*(9), 865–875.

Virgin, H. W., Wherry, E. J., & Ahmed, R. (2009). Redefining chronic viral infection. *Cell, 138*(1), 30–50.

Waller, L. A., & Gotway, C. A. (2004). Linking spatial sxposure data to health events. In *Applied spatial statistics for public health data* (pp. 325–443). John Wiley and Sons.

Walsh, P. D., Biek, R., & Real, L. A. (2005). Wave-like spread of Ebola Zaire. *PLoS Biology, 3*(11), e371.

Warfel, J. M., Zimmerman, L. I., & Merkel, T. J. (2014). Acellular pertussis vaccines protect against disease but fail to prevent infection and transmission in a nonhuman primate model. *Proceedings of the National Academy of Sciences, 111*(2), 787–792.

Watts, D. J., & Strogatz, S. H. (1998). Collective dynamics of 'small-world' networks. *Nature, 393*(6684), 440–442.

White, L. F., & Pagano, M. (2008). A likelihood-based method for real-time estimation of the serial interval and reproductive number of an epidemic. *Statistics in Medicine, 27*(16), 2999–3016.

WHO (2011). Rubella vaccines: WHO position paper. *Weekly Epidemiological Record, 86*(29), 301–316.

WHO Ebola Response Team (2014). Ebola virus disease in West Africa—the first 9 months of the epidemic and forward projections. *New England Journal of Medicine, 2014*(371), 1481–1495.

Wiesenfeld, K., & Moss, F. (1995). Stochastic resonance and the benefits of noise: From ice ages to crayfish and squids. *Nature, 373*(6509), 33–36.

Wood, S. N. (2003). Thin plate regression splines. *Journal of the Royal Statistical Society B, 65*(1), 95–114.

Wood, S. N. (2010). Statistical inference for noisy nonlinear ecological dynamic systems. *Nature, 466*(7310), 1102–1104.

Woodhouse, D. E., Rothenberg, R. B., Potterat, J. J., Darrow, W. W., Muth, S. Q., Klovdahl, A. S., Zimmerman, H. P., Rogers, H. L., Maldonado, T. S., Muth, J. B., et al. (1994). Mapping a social network of heterosexuals at high risk for HIV infection. *Aids, 8*(9), 1331–1336.

Woolhouse, M. E., Dye, C., Etard, J.-F., Smith, T., Charlwood, J., Garnett, G., Hagan, P., Hii, J., Ndhlovu, P., Quinnell, R., et al. (1997). Heterogeneities in the transmission of infectious agents: Implications for the design of control programs. *Proceedings of the National Academy of Sciences, 94*(1), 338–342.

Xia, Y., Bjørnstad, O. N., & Grenfell, B. T. (2004). Measles metapopulation dynamics: A gravity model for epidemiological coupling and dynamics. *The American Naturalist, 164*(2), 267–281.

Yao, Q., & Tong, H. (1994). On prediction and chaos in stochastic systems. *Philosophical Transactions of the Royal Society of London A, 348*(1688), 357–369.

Yao, Q., & Tong, H. (1998). A bootstrap detection for operational determinism. *Physica D, 115*(1-2), 49–55.

Yao, Q., & Tong, H. (2000). Nonparametric estimation of ratios of noise to signal in stochastic regression. *Statistica Sinica*, 751–770.

Ye, H., Beamish, R. J., Glaser, S. M., Grant, S. C., Hsieh, C.-h., Richards, L. J., Schnute, J. T., & Sugihara, G. (2015). Equation-free mechanistic ecosystem forecasting using empirical dynamic modeling. *Proceedings of the National Academy of Sciences, 112*(13), E1569–E1576.

Yoshikawa, Y., Ochikubo, F., Matsubara, Y., Tsuruoka, H., Ishii, M., Shirota, K., Nomura, Y., Sugiyama, M., & Yamanouchi, K. (1989). Natural infection with canine distemper virus in a Japanese monkey (*Macaca fuscata*). *Veterinary Microbiology, 20*(3), 193–205.

Index

A

Age
  age-incidence, 1, 50, 74, 75, 77, 98
  catalytic model, 1, 88, 89
  WAIFW, 70, 72, 74
Animation, 140, 259, 328
Autocorrelation, 121, 122, 252, 261, 263–267,
    345, 347, 348, 352, 357
Autocorrelation function, 121–123, 354
Autoregressive moving-average model, 123,
    125, 205

C

Catalytic model, 1, 88, 89
Chain-binomial model, 25, 37, 43, 44, 143,
    144, 168, 246, 285
Chaos, 113, 233, 251
Chickenpox, 221, 224–227, 231, 233, 234
Correlogram, 265, 266, 268, 269, 348
Coupled-map lattice model, 250, 251, 279,
    327
Critical community size, 4, 296, 299, 300, 308
Critical host density, 33, 68, 197, 198, 305
Cycles, 2, 13, 21, 24, 105, 109, 112, 113, 126,
    132, 136, 137, 160, 172, 195, 201, 223,
    228, 230, 233, 248, 314, 315, 319, 321

D

Dampening period, 22, 24, 117, 128
Differential equations, 14, 22, 111, 143, 162
Dynamics
  chaos, 113, 233, 251
  cycles, 2, 13, 21, 24, 105, 109, 112, 113,
    126, 132, 136, 137, 160, 172, 195, 201,
    223, 228, 230, 233, 248, 314, 315, 319,
    321

dampening period, 22, 24, 117, 128
eigenvalues, 22–24, 84, 111, 186, 187, 192,
    196, 197, 202, 324, 334, 335
invasion orbits, 226, 227
isoclines, 20–22, 163
Jacobian matrix, 22–24, 52, 112, 118, 119,
    187, 190, 195, 196, 199, 200, 210, 212,
    213, 222, 324
Lyapunov exponent, 210, 212–216
phase plane, 20–22, 108, 109, 114, 115,
    119, 146, 163, 195, 196, 211, 213, 214,
    225–227, 321
resonant frequency, 192, 195, 201
stability analysis, 186, 325

E

Ebola, 13, 34, 35, 44, 46, 47, 50, 54, 55, 67,
    168, 261, 296
Eigenvalues, 22–24, 84, 111, 186, 187, 192,
    196, 197, 202, 324, 334, 335
Epidemics
  recurrent, 5, 37, 115, 300
  simple, 37, 143, 170, 172, 185
  virgin, 76, 77, 79

F

Feline immunodeficiency virus, 332–336, 339,
    341
Force of infection, 38, 54, 67, 68, 73, 74,
    87–89, 91–103, 155, 219, 234, 242, 243,
    247, 248, 255, 310, 356
Functional data analysis, 342

G

Gonorrhea, 5, 6, 51, 52, 279, 290, 291
Gravity model, 254–257, 308, 309